A Vital Issue

John S. Sinacore / Angela C. Sinacore

introductory health

A Vital Issue

Macmillan Publishing Co., Inc.
NEW YORK
Collier Macmillan Publishers
LONDON

Printed in the United States of America

Macmillan Publishing Co., Inc.
866 Third Avenue, New York, New York 10022

Collier-Macmillan Canada, Ltd.

Library of Congress Cataloging in Publication Data

Sinacore, John S
Introductory health.

Includes bibliographical references and index.
1. Hygiene. I. Sinacore, Angela C., joint author. II. Title. [DNLM: 1. Hygiene. 2. Public health. WA4 S615i]
RA776.S615 613 74-3803
ISBN 0-02-410690-9

Printing: 2 3 4 5 6 7 8 Year: 6 7 8 9 0

Preface

One of the basic purposes of this text is to put to eternal rest the false notion that a person's health or lack of it is a happening over which the individual or society has little or no control. As stated in the text, "Health used to be regarded as a gift from the gods. It is still an entity that is not well understood, one that people alternately drink to, pray for, take for granted, abuse, or become sick about." The recent advances in the health sciences have provided enormous amounts of health knowledge that need to become a part of our decisions concerning health. There is the growing realization that the kind of life-style a person leads may promote health or predispose him to disease and death. The decisions a person makes as to how he will live can be more important than any actions a doctor may try to take in restoring health sometimes beyond repair.

The text also reveals how the solutions to our environmental health problems of air and water pollution, of pesticide and radiation control need the informed concerted actions of citizen groups and health professionals. There is also a straightforward discussion of such critical and controversial health issues as drug use and abuse, food faddism, and fraudulent consumer practices.

The text is presented in ten chapters. Chapter 1, "That Quality Called Health," seeks to define the term *health* and presents some of the basic purposes and issues of the book.

Chapter 2, "Maintaining Personal Health," discusses such issues as physical fitness, the health food–organic food movement, overweight problems, food additives, and the areas of vision, hearing, and foot care.

Chapter 3, "Disease Prevention and Control," presents the advances in, and some of the present problems of, communicable disease control. It also discusses ways in which the individual and society can prevent and exert greater control over such problems as heart disease, cancer, and genetic disorders, as well as other chronic and degenerative diseases. A discussion of mental retardation lends understanding to the causes and prevention of this problem. It also presents the changing attitudes toward the retarded.

Chapter 4, "Mental Health," is concerned with the various influences on man's mental health. These include the complex patterns of living presented by "civilization," the individual's basic needs, as well as man's psychological and physiological influences. The chapter also discusses mental health problems and varied ways that the individual and society strive to cope with them and to correct them.

Chapter 5, "Human Relationships and Family Life," presents the varying concepts of masculinity and femininity, the feminist movement and its implications, and some of the wholesome and unwholesome reasons for sexual and marital involvement. The section "On Having Children" presents the many points of view on whether couples should or should not have children. Genetic counseling and the issues related to abortion are also discussed.

Chapter 6 is concerned with the consumer of health products and services. It deals with such issues as outright quackery as well as misleading advertisements and practices of industry under question. The activities of consumer protection agencies and their relative effectiveness are also discussed. Criteria for the evaluation of health products and services are offered along with a discussion of the issues related to a changing health-care delivery system.

Chapter 7, "Our Drug-Oriented Society," discusses drug use and abuse in a social-health context rather than a legal-moral one. It presents the benefits drugs can effect as well as the devastation they can wreak when abused. Discussed also are the appropriate and inappropriate reactions of society to its drug abuse problems. Discussions of alcohol use and abuse are presented in this chapter. Alcohol is discussed as a drug and how it has become a part of the social fiber of societies. The cigarette and its mass contributions to emphysema, cancer, and heart disease are also presented.

Chapter 8, "Man and His Environment," is concerned with the issues related to air, water, and land pollution as well as the issues of pesticide and radiation control. It seeks to help the student evaluate society's reaction to these problems and discusses what the responsibilities of the individual are in this context.

Chapter 9, "Living Safely," discusses one of the neglected epidemics of our times—the accident. The issue of the automobile as an accident factor is presented. The implications of the expanded use of the motorbike and snowmobile are also presented. Home, electrical, and industrial safety are also issues of concern.

Chapter 10, "Community Health," discusses and helps the students to evaluate our current community organization for health at the local, state, national, and international levels. It also discusses the relationship that the student can have to these organizations.

In the appendix, "Emergency First Aid," is found a detailed presentation for the preparation of the student in the area of first aid.

J. S. S.
A. C. S.

Contents

Our Drug-Oriented Society 253

Man and His Environment 298

Living Safely 329

Community Health 353

1. That Quality Called Health

IT IS PERHAPS one of the great ironies of our times that our society should view in such negative terms what it has expressed as its most precious possession—namely its health. It attempts to measure its levels of health by the use of charts showing death rates from different diseases. Because the death rate goes down in a given community, does it mean that people are healthier? It could mean they are living longer but unhealthier lives. Our concerns should go beyond how long a person lives, to how *well* he lives; in other words, his quality of life.

There are various means of measuring one's quality of health that do not fall into the all-or-none categories of life or death, disease or lack of disease. To cite several examples, a person's visual acuity could serve as such a measurement. Vision may vary considerably from person to person without illness being a part of the consideration. Nutritional status would also qualify as a standard which could include the iron level in the red blood cells. This could serve as an indication of the amount of iron taken in the diet and reflected in the person's ability to function. Other criteria could include one's physical fitness, levels of resistance to disease, fat levels in the blood, sensitivity to allergens, the degree of emotional stability, and body weight, among others.

Our society trains and pays its physicians to treat disease, not to keep people healthy in the first place. We are overly concerned with treatment and not concerned enough with prevention. Many years ago the Chinese introduced a positive approach to maintaining health. They devised a system whereby the individual paid his physician while he was healthy. When he became ill, the payments stopped until he was once more returned to a state of health.

Ideally, everyone in the population should undergo a periodic medical examination to determine his health status. The current shortage of physicians makes such a procedure impossible. There just are not enough physicians to perform such a broad-scale task. Some experimentation has been done in which the mechanics of the examination (vision testing, blood testing, blood pressure measurement, and many others) are performed by technicians or nurses with the test results then subject to review by the doctor. This procedure saves the physician time and permits him to review the test results of many more people.

A recent contribution along these lines has been made by Dr. Ernest L. Wynder. This physician was the first to produce evidence that cigarette smoking is a major cause of lung cancer, and now he is working on another first. Dr. Wynder has automated the medical examination at the Health Maintenance Center he directs. The person to be examined is initially asked to complete a 378-item questionnaire on his own and his family's medical history. With the aid of technicians, the person goes through a medical assembly line with blood and urine samples tested, and with electrocardiograms taken. The results are checked through a computer with any suspected abnormalities double checked. The entire procedure is completed in one hour. The physician reviews the report of the examination and makes any necessary recommendations. If the examinee has a smoking, an overweight, or a physical fitness problem, he may be assigned to one or more of the center's intervention clinics. Here he may be placed on a diet or on an exercise regimen, or asked to attend a smoking withdrawal clinic. The objective is to correct any patterns of living that will ultimately prove destructive to the individual. The question raised is that it may be necessary to reexamine medical care procedures and their organization if the mere measurement of personal health is to become a reality.

ENVIRONMENTAL INFLUENCES

Generally, in the past, the level of health a person achieved was considered to be pretty much a personal matter. The attitude implied that it was up to the individual to decide how healthy he wanted to be. While this was never completely true in the past, it is even less so now. Increasingly a person's level of health is becoming more dependent on other facilities, conditions, and people. The individual is less a master of his fate than he ever was, and the trend can be expected to continue.

While man is still privileged to bring on his own lung cancer through cigarette smoking, he has little control over the pollutants in the air he breathes if he lives in an urban area. He relies on the health department to safequard the water he drinks and the food he eats. He must to some extent rely on the "other driver" for his safety while on the highway. How well-made and therefore how safe are his car and tires may determine his life expectancy. Yet, how much control can he exert over private industry to guarantee his safety? Man therefore can no longer go it alone, so far as his health is concerned. Where broadly based environmental factors or problems arise, man's only control of them can be through interested, well-informed citizen groups and those organizations in the community that have health responsibilities. In the absence of these alternatives, he must eat the food, drink the water, breathe the air, and drive the cars provided him.

The National Health Survey (a continuous study conducted by the United States Public Health Service to determine the health status of the nation) has shown that there is a "positive" relationship between poor health and low income. It has also indicated that the low-income groups receive less medical care in spite of greater need. It is, of course, not always possible to ascertain if the low income caused the poor health or vice versa. It can, however, be

Figure 1–1

There is a relationship between poor health and low income.

(Susan Johns)

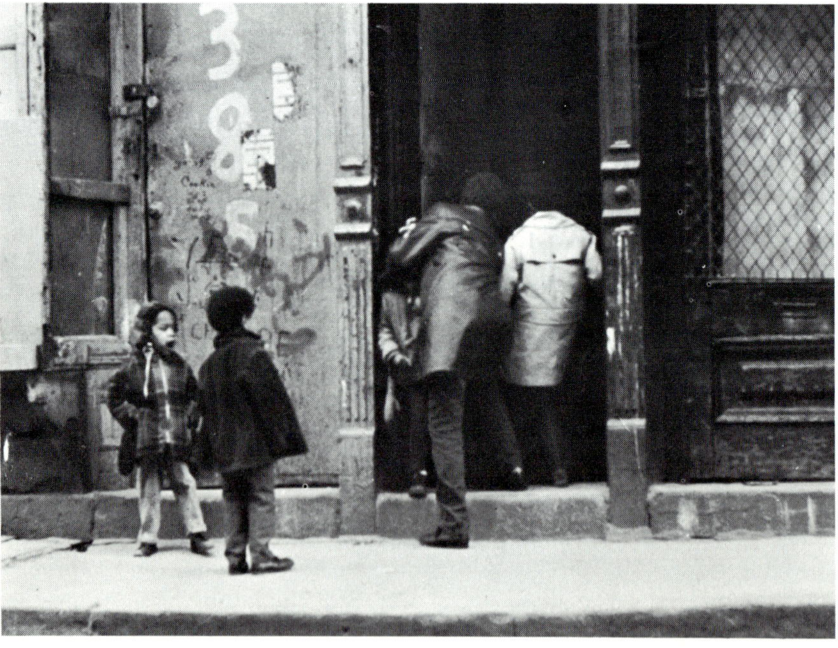

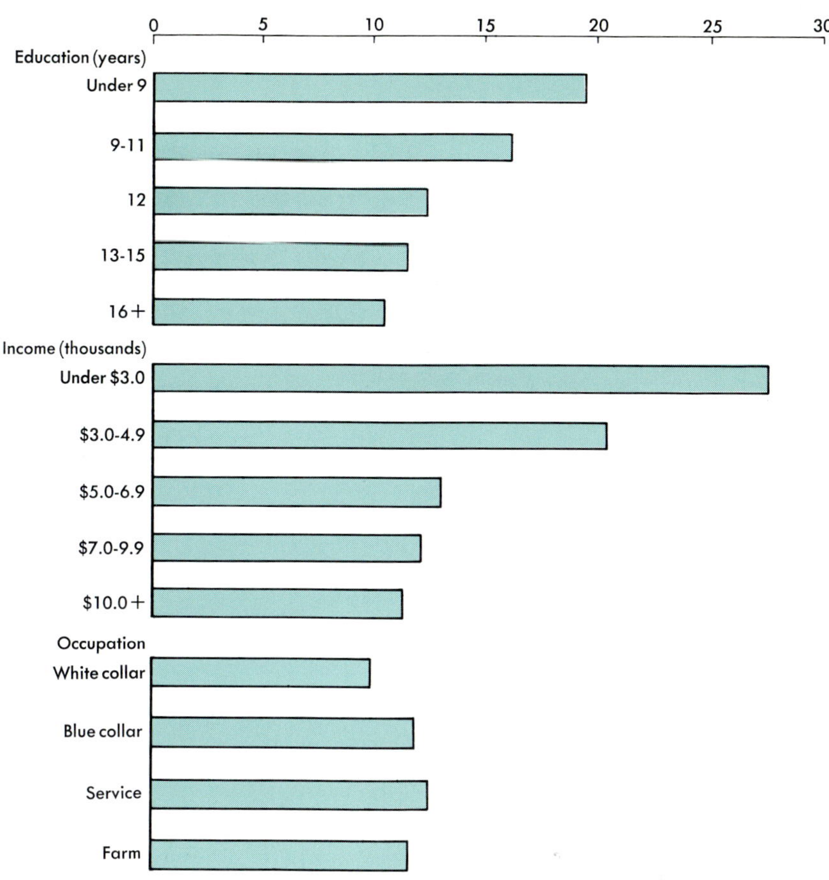

Disability by Socioeconomic Level

United States Noninstitutionalized Civilian Population, 1969, ages 17-64

Days of restricted activity per person

Figure 1–2

Total impact of illness is measured by the number of days on which people missed work or school or otherwise had to reduce their usual activities. The graph shows that lower-income people have more "restricted-activity days."

(Adapted from unpublished data from the National Center for Health Statistics)

concluded that the ability to secure medical care is related to the person's earning power and therefore the ability to maintain health. The availability of health services is rarely viewed as an environmental factor. Yet it is an essential element for the maintenance of health and a segment of man's surroundings that must be considered important. The dental health of a

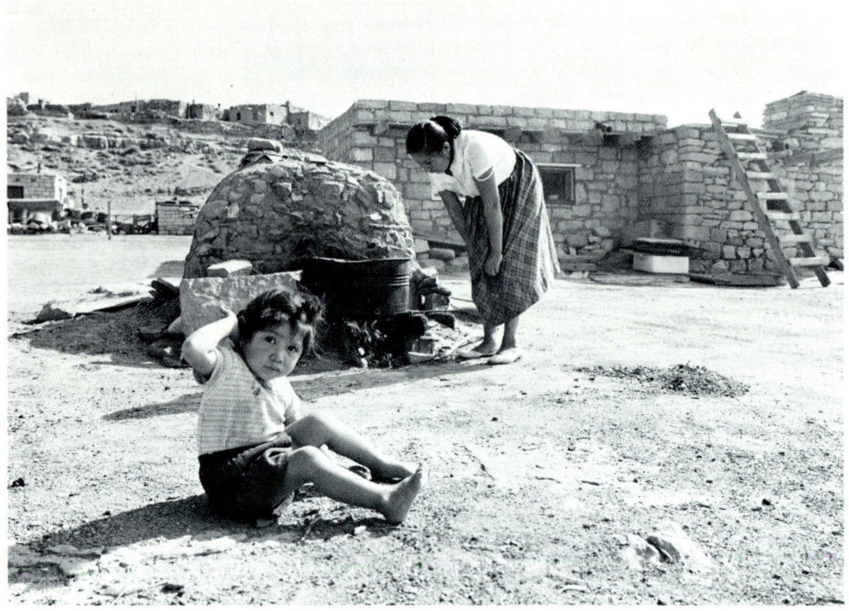

Figure 1–3

Within our population we have groups who do not have access to adequate medical care.

(HEW: Indian Health Service)

community without a dentist cannot be expected to compare with that of one well supplied with dental services. Likewise, the community without medical services would find its health status considerably lowered. Its people would lack the protection of vaccines for smallpox, polio, diphtheria, and whooping cough, to mention a few. Routine cases of appendicitis could mean death. We could easily regress to the level of primitive societies where life is a struggle for existence. In a more sophisticated society such as our own, the question is not one of having or not having dental and medical services. Rather it is a question of their extensiveness, their quality, and their accessibility to all in the community. A person who suffers a heart attack has a better chance of survival if it occurs in a community that has prompt, well-equipped ambulance service and whose hospitals are well prepared to deal with these emergencies. As important, though less dramatic, is the community's preparedness to function in the area of medical rehabilitation. Having the personnel and facilities to return a person suffering an infirmity to useful living could prove as important as saving his life.

THE INDIVIDUAL'S HEALTH RESPONSIBILITIES

While we are to a greater extent looking outward to the community for means of attaining and maintaining health status, we have by no means outgrown our need for personal health responsibilities. Advances in the health sciences make it important for the individual to keep informed of these developments so that he may modify his behavior in accordance with their findings. As a nation we have always enthusiastically supported research. The results of research have been met with equal enthusiasm if they take the form of a vaccine that will prevent disease or a drug that will cure it. If research results indicate that cancer can be prevented by not smoking or some accidents by not speeding, the enthusiasm somehow wanes. Part of the explanation of this is our built-in resistance to change. An additional factor involved is that when we are asked to give up something we enjoy doing, we then have to make a value judgment as to whether the possible results justify the change. Certainly, in some instances we will continue a pattern of behavior even though it contradicts what is considered the healthy thing to do. A fireman who charges into a flaming house to save the life of another is not doing the healthy thing—he has other motivations.

Research results that produce health information are also ignored because people view "the magic pill" or the "miracle drugs" as the only kind of contribution to be made by health research. This attitude probably prevails because concerted efforts have not been made to inform the populace of health research informational findings and of their significance to the individual. The attitude has also persisted that new health information is for the physician or other health professionals but not for the lay public. The result has been that the American public does not enjoy a high level of health information. This conclusion was borne out by the National Health Test conducted by CBS.

It is somewhat ironic to note that the broadcasting system whose fine efforts went into the development and administration of this examination is also part of a pattern of mass media that have contributed to the low scores registered on this health test. The mass media in the United States have long been known as sources of misleading or outright false information in the health area. This was substantiated by a study conducted by medical students at Wayne State University School of Medicine who

> found that during a typical 130-hour week on one commercial television channel health-related content was used 7.2 per cent of the time, including both actual programs and commercials, and that only 30 per cent of the

> information was "useful." The study cited as examples of misleading health information in commercials the claim that a cough medicine was as strong as codeine, and a commercial implying that a medicated foam might cure psoriasis, which has no cure.[1]

In Europe, if a health measure is to be put into effect, health officials make an announcement of it and proceed to implement the program. In the United States, before action can be taken on a recommended health measure it must in one form or another have the approval of the people. Vital public health decisions are thus being asked of a public that is not nearly as informed as it should be for this responsibility. One need only view a public forum on the fluoridation of drinking water to see an unfortunate result of these circumstances. The meeting often becomes mired in distortions, untruths, and inappropriate flag-waving reflecting a resounding lack of good old American know-how.

In addition, the individual is called upon daily to make a number of personal health decisions that will affect his well-being. He must decide if and when to seek medical help, whether or not to use self-prescribed drugs, and the nature of his diet, to mention just a few. It has, for instance, been estimated that half of all blindness and a great deal of impaired vision are due to the failure of people to perform some comparatively simple functions. Glaucoma, a leading cause of blindness in this country, can be controlled in most cases by early detection and treatment. Strabismus (cross-eyed condition), a cause of one-eyed blindness, is usually permitted to advance to have its deleterious effects on children because parents waited for them to "outgrow" the condition. Similarly, a great deal of hearing loss that now occurs is either preventable or results from improper treatment. The lack of sophistication with regard to the basic care and preservation of vital senses seems to be a rather extraordinary complacency of our society.

Fraudulent consumer health practices are also as prevalent today as they ever have been. The sale of cancer and arthritis cures, the half a billion dollar business of food faddists and weight-reducing quackery are but a few examples of practices that are monetarily wasteful and many times dangerous to health. In addition, a real lack of sophistication exists with regard to the utilization of medical care services and facilities. The distinction between medical, paramedical, and other practitioners is not clear to many people.

Statements by various health authorities indicate health knowledge deficiencies related to a number of health problems. Dr. Leona Baumgartner, former Health Commissioner of New York City, stated at a three day conference sponsored by the National Health Council:

> There is widespread evidence that the health professions are not communicating what they know about control and prevention of certain diseases

[1] "Bad Health Information on TV," *Today's Health* (June 1972), p. 7.

to the public. We can cure an estimated one-half of all cases of cancer today by finding them soon enough, and doing for them what we already know how to do.[2]

A national study by the Food and Drug Administration on health practices and opinions revealed the following:

- □ A sample representing 50 million adults, would not be convinced by almost unanimous expert opinion that a hypothetical "cancer cure" was worthless. Only 45% thought such a medicine should be banned by law.
- □ Three-fourths of the public believe that extra vitamins provide more pep and energy, the most common of the mis-conceptions investigated in the survey.
- □ Although their condition had never been diagnosed by a physician, a sample representing about 16 million adults, reported they had arthritis or rheumatism, asthma, allergies, hemorrhoids, heart trouble, high blood pressure, or diabetes.
- □ Twelve percent of the sample also indicated they would self-medicate without seeing a doctor, for longer than two weeks for ailments such as sore throats, coughs, sleeplessness or upset stomach.
- □ Twenty-six percent, representing about 35 million adults, had used nutritional supplements expecting specific observable benefits.[3]

LIFE-STYLE AND ONE'S HEALTH

Health is a topic that has not been well understood. It is something that people will alternately drink to, pray for, take for granted, abuse or become sick about. We still appear to be suffering from the "medicine man complex" regarding health as a gift from the gods rather than something we can do something about. We react with shock when someone suffers a heart attack even though the life-style the person was following made such an occurrance a distinct possibility. We react with sorrow when someone loses his eyesight, yet half of all blindness that occurs in this country is preventable.

It is becoming increasingly evident that how one lives will strongly affect one's quality of health and life expectancy. For example, at the present time the leading cause of death and disability in the United States is heart disease—a disease of "civilization." What are the major risk factors associated with the condition? Cigarette smoking, lack of exercise and overweight, or other factors

[2] Leona Baumgartner, M.D., former Health Commissioner of New York City, in a speech to the National Health Forum as quoted by *The New York Times.*

[3] *HEW News,* "Study of Health Practices and Opinions," news release: October 9, 1972.

"Nutrition supplements benefit few people, but the power of suggestion appears to be a big factor."
VITAMIN
VITAMIN
"About three percent of the total sample had tried to reduce by sweating, an erroneous concept that confuses a very temporary water loss with a reduction in fat . . . . . Most admitted they later gained back the weight."
JANUARY
"The concept that body wastes are so toxic that clock-like regularity must be induced survives from early 19th century medicine."

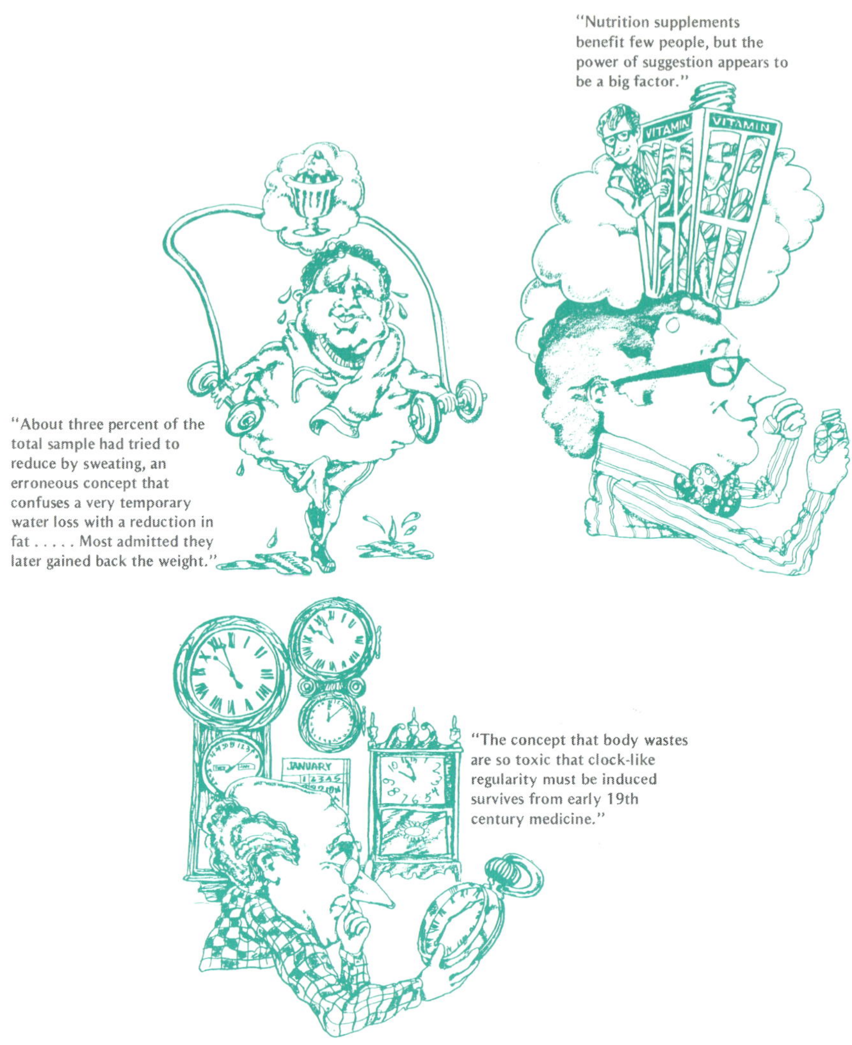

Figure 1–4

("A Study of Health Practices and Opinions." Conducted for Food and Drug Administration, HEW. *FDA Consumer,* October 1972)

related to poor nutrition. In essence a great deal of heart disease could be prevented if people were to change their life-styles and eat properly, exercise adequately, and avoid cigarette smoking. If the person survives his first heart attack, then he begins hopefully to reorder his way of living—literally under the threat of death.

In the epidemic incidence of alcoholism, drug addiction, emphysema, and lung cancer, we find other examples of how the manner in which one lives affects his health status. The overuse or inappropriate use of alcohol, drugs, and cigarettes serve as the vehicle for serious societal health problems. When the individual lives in an environment that encourages the misuse of these substances, it becomes clear that his decisions on these matters are not made in a vacuum.

A factor further complicating these problems is that our medical care system is disease-oriented. It sits back waiting for people to become ill, then goes into action attempting to correct the problem. The difficulty is that with many modern-day health problems (i.e., heart disease, alcoholism, drug abuse, emphysema, or lung cancer) the person is either already seriously damaged by the time he is seen by the physician or the physician has no effective "cure" for the problem. We have in essence painted ourselves into a corner developing life-styles that often include substance use and other factors that predispose us to serious health problems that our medical care system cannot effectively handle.

> For our cigarette users we build heart, cancer and respiratory disease institutes. For our alcoholics, addicts and venereal disease sufferers, we build diagnostic and rehabilitation centers, with mental hospitals and correctional institutes held in reserve. All of these with so little thought or research given to support the thesis that if our youth were given relevant information systematically and professionally, at a time in their lives when it could be of some value, they might very well solve the majority of these problems themselves with that selfsame common sense that we do not give them credit for having. I propose to you, that if a solution to these medical problems does not come by the positive decisions of an enlightened youth, the solution is not likely to come at all.[4]

It would seem that no health problem is under control until it can be prevented. This principle even applies to the problem of venereal diseases where effective treatment is available, but where the epidemic of VD still rages out of control. Since life-styles are learned—not born—it becomes necessary to inform people at early ages of the advantages and consequences of various life-styles. Obviously this kind of education should not belatedly occur in the intensive care unit of a hospital.

While the health professions are reorienting themselves from a disease and therapeutic orientation to one embracing the concepts of health and prevention, each individual needs to assess his own health values. He must do this, recognizing that if he makes mistakes there may be no one available who is capable of correcting them.

[4] Ronald G. Vincent, M.D., "The Physician's Role in the Health Program," *New York State Journal of Health, Physical Education and Recreation,* Vol. 22, No. 3, p. 28.

HEREDITY AND HEALTH

One cannot overlook the hereditary factor in any discussion of health. As every physician knows, a family history is as important as the individual's medical history. We are, after all, the products of our parents and to some extent our grandparents and great-grandparents. Their genes in varying combinations become our genes—both the desirable ones and the undesirable ones. Physicians are often on the alert for the appearance of disorders in an individual simply because the disorder appeared with such frequency in the family. We know for instance that there is a genetic factor associated with diabetes. If this disorder has been present in the family (particularly on both sides of the family), the physician knows that there is a greater possibility for this disease to appear in this patient. Because the tendency for diabetes is passed on by a recessive gene, a minority in the family will be thus affected. It will be in this case a larger minority than normally found in a family group.

The advances made in the medical sciences has increased the survival rate as well as the degree of comfort of those who have disorders that are genetically influenced. The life expectancy of the diabetic has been extended. Epilepsy is largely controlled now by drug therapy, and so it goes for a number of other such disorders. The once hopeless reaction to genetic-borne diseases has changed rather radically. There are some, however, who have viewed this progress with jaundiced eye. They point out that the increased survival rate of people with these disorders results in their reproducing increased numbers of individuals to whom these deficiencies would be transmitted. The claim is made that advances in the medical sciences will effect some short-term gains in dealing with these genetic conditions, but in the long run will result in disadvantages to man. Others feel that the continued advances in medical science will result in man's complete control of these deficiencies and render them to be unimportant.

Under the focus of the health sciences it has now been assessed that health is measurable, qualitatively and quantitatively. The varied hereditary and environmental health factors singly, in combinations, or in interaction with each other are being studied with regard to their positive and negative health contributions. Maintaining and raising levels of man's health can now be planned and educated for and the results measured and evaluated. This is not to imply that the sciences concerned with the study of health have attained an ultimate in their field. But they have begun.

REVIEW QUESTIONS

1 What are the bases of your concern for your health?

2 How have the advances in the health sciences changed the traditional criteria for measuring the quality of health?

3 How have some environmental factors complicated man's quest for a long and healthful life?

4 Discuss those elements of man's environment that contribute to his health status.

5 Research that produces new health information is often not applied as enthusiastically as a new drug or vaccine. Explain.

6 The level of health knowledge of the American public leaves much to be desired. Cite evidence to support this statement.

7 Heredity is related to health. Explain.

8 Having effective treatment for a disease condition does not guarantee control of it. Explain.

9 Explain why the health professions need to shift their emphasis from treatment to one of promoting health and preventing health problems.

10 How can altering one's life-style affect one's health status?

2. Maintaining Personal Health

IN A MODERN technological society, we have sophisticated hearing aids for those who do not hear well. There are well-made eyeglasses with safety lenses and almost invisible contact lenses for those whose vision needs correction. However, there are some things that have not changed. We must still get our nutrition by eating foods that contain the needed nutrients. A well-conditioned body capable of carrying us through our life's activities still requires routine physical exercise if its strength is to be maintained. While man is reaching for the stars he cannot ignore those basic needs that stem from his earliest days.

PHYSICAL FITNESS

The human body was made to be used and therefore thrives on being active. We know from training athletes that if we gradually increase the work load, the body adapts to meet the increased demands and ultimately works more efficiently. For example, in the trained runner, the heart beats more slowly and with greater force, thereby providing more blood to the body than the heart of the person who is inactive. Thus we see improvement in blood vessel and heart fitness. The football player who lifts weights for the improvement of muscular strength to overpower his opponent sees as a result of his training the toughening and strengthening of muscular tissue.

Because our society has become so mechanized, work is often *not* a source of activity. The many appliances used in the home have decreased the amount of physical activity for the housewife. The man at work is often reduced to watching the dials on a machine doing the work that he used to do by hand. Some industries have gone so far as to give their employees exercise breaks to encourage activity. In West Germany, industrial concerns have made some efforts to develop broad-scale physical reconditioning programs for thousands of their workers who have jobs that do not require physical labor. A great deal of evidence points to inactivity as at least one factor related to heart disease. The fat American is no doubt one whose caloric intake exceeds caloric output. Overweight is invariably accompanied by a greater susceptibility to a number of diseases and a shortened life-span. In recent years, the increases in the number of people who die from heart disease among relatively young men have caused particular concern. Lack of exercise in combination with emotional stress, cigarette smoking, and overweight often proves to be lethal. The need to reverse this trend relates not only to the desirability of increasing longevity of life but to a higher quality of living as well. When young women lack proper muscle tone and strength for such natural functions as childbirth, we begin to realize how basic fitness can be. The vigorous, successful, professional often needs the physical mechanism as well as the mental abilities to carry on a strenuous schedule of professional activity.

> Suffice it to conclude here that the development of obesity (and of heart disease as well as a number of other pathologic conditions) is to a large extent the result of the lack or foresight of a civilization which spends tens of billions annually on cars, but is unwilling to include a swimming pool and tennis courts in the plans of every high school.[1]

It is an accepted conclusion that the activity once demanded by people's work must now be provided as part of their leisure time activity. There are those who would compound the error by following a leisure time program of being among the thousands in the stands or among the millions of home viewers watching the athletes perform. The person who would become a chronic watcher of an activity rather than a participant has developed a disease of civilization known as "spectatoritis."[2] The man who worked in order to support his family and the woman who worked to maintain a home were understandably strongly motivated to do so. Is it possible to have motivations of equal strength related to leisure time activities? The question no doubt

[1] Jean Mayer, *Overweight—Causes, Cost, and Control.* A special publication of Consumers Union (Englewood Cliffs, N.J.: Prentice-Hall, 1968), p. 83.

[2] A term coined by Dr. Jay B. Nash.

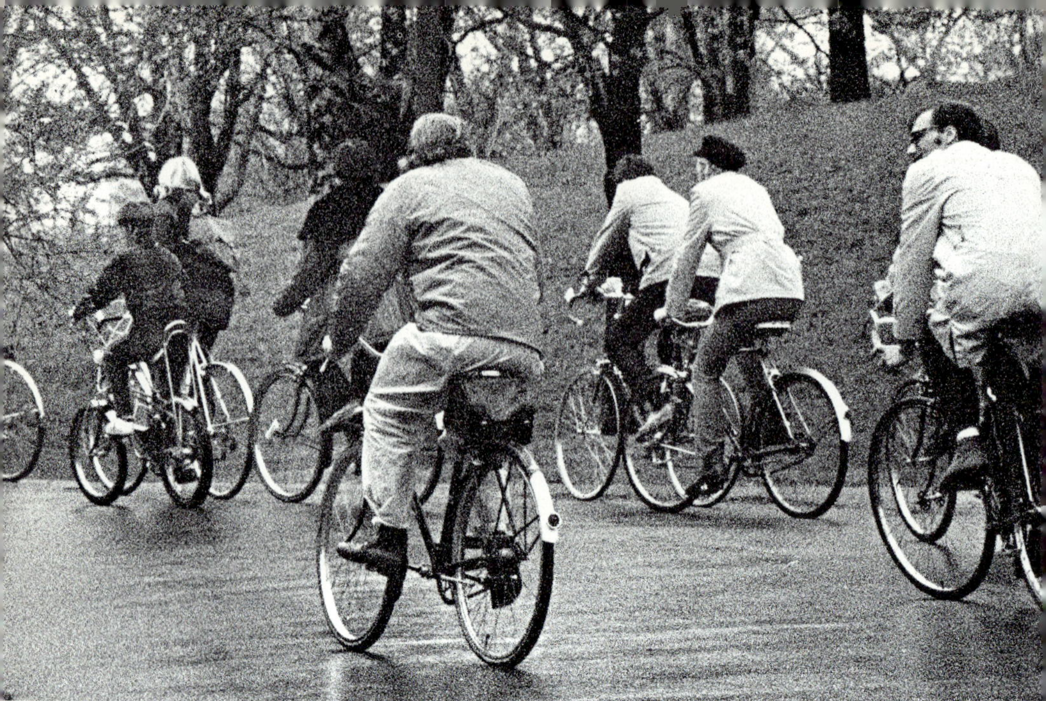

Figure 2–1

Bicycle riding is rapidly becoming an activity for people of all ages.

(Capital Newspapers, Albany, N.Y.)

presents a challenge to the professionals in the areas of physical education and recreation. The answer appears to lie in those activities that one has developed enough skill and interest in to enjoy. The person who becomes a golf bug hardly needs to be motivated to get out to the golf course. If anything, the problem may be one of getting him home! We are witnessing for example, the largest wave of bicycle popularity in its 154-year history. Greater numbers of people are riding bikes for physical fitness reasons, or in other cases the bike is being used by environmentalists as a partial solution to our pollution and energy problems. It makes little difference whether the motivations come from wanting to strengthen one's internal environment or to cleanse our external environment—the results are praiseworthy.

Those, on the other hand, who participate in activities because "it's good for me" are placing exercise in the category of a pill. In this group are those who exercise on the living room floor to the count of a shoulder-padded television personality. The interest in this "game" does not usually last long. There are also those who visit "health" clubs for a dosage of fitness. Fitness cannot be prescribed. It is often best attained as the side effect of one's intense interest in one or preferably several kinds of physical activity. Many of our present-day gropings for exercise and fitness appear to be inappropriate, with "commercialized exercise" being packaged and sold. The result is the loss of those satisfactions that should be derived from physical accomplishment. Lost also are the exhilarations of the baseball well hit, the bowling ball well delivered, the swimming stroke executed with power and grace. The skill of the fencer, the persistence of the runner, the tenaciousness of the mountain climber, and the freedom of the camper are lost to those who would buy fitness by the dollar.

In schools, physical education programs aimed at developing those skills that can be used after the age of 30 can make a major contribution to the present and future fitness of its participants. While big-muscle sports, like basketball, baseball, and football, are fine they do not represent lifelong kinds of activity. We are all too familiar with the college varsity athlete who graduates and suddenly finds himself divorced from the source of intense activity that once occupied major portions of his time. If his job requires that he work from behind a desk, his life could become a very sedentary one with the usual weight gain and deconditioning of muscles.

Physical education and recreation programs should include activities such as swimming, tennis, badminton, volleyball, handball, as well as other activities that can be used for most if not all of one's life. The success of such programs may be measured not only by proficiency of performance in a formal class but the degree to which the individual uses these activities as part of his pattern of living.

NUTRITION ISSUES OF CONCERN

In the past, man suffered from a number of vitamin deficiency diseases such as scurvy, beri-beri, and rickets. To correct these conditions people were made aware of foods that contained needed vitamins. In addition, vitamins were added to certain foods as part of a vitamin enrichment program. As if this was not enough, vitamin pills then became available at food and drug stores. As people began to douse themselves with vitamins, a new vitamin disorder began to appear, *hypervitaminosis*—overdoses of vitamins producing vitamin poisoning.

While lack of food is still a problem for a number of Americans, the prevailing problem in the country is overweight from overeating. We have apparently been dealing with some nutrition problems by overcorrecting for them.

In our efforts to make food more plentiful, thousands of chemicals are used in the form of food additives and pesticides. Checking the safety of food additives and what constitutes safe amounts of pesticide residue on fruits and vegetables has already become a routine public health procedure. The nutritional status of the American people has improved, as indicated by the relative absence of nutritional or related diseases and a taller, presumably healthier generation of youth, but a plentiful food supply does not insure adequate nutrition for all. While significant progress has been made in nutrition, it would be worthwhile to consider the shifting personal and public health concerns in this area and their implications.

POVERTY, HUNGER, AND MALNUTRITION

In the last several years, the problems of hunger and malnutrition associated with poverty have come to the forefront of the nation's social and political conscience. In 1967 and 1968, several reports documented the existence of hunger and malnutrition among poor people in the United States. The age groups most vulnerable to malnutrition seemed to be children through the age of 16 and the elderly, especially black and Spanish-speaking individuals over 60 years of age. In all areas surveyed, income showed a positive correlation with overall nutritional status, with the poorest of the poor having the least adequate diets and the greatest vulnerability to malnutrition. Impaired growth of children, low hemoglobin levels (reflecting low iron intakes), low plasma vitamin A levels especially in children, and poor dental health were major problems.

Some programs specifically aimed at improving the nutrition of children have developed. Government subsidized nutrition programs include a National School Lunch Program, School Breakfast Program, Special Food Service Program, and a Special Milk Program. The purpose of the National School Lunch Program is to provide nutritionally adequate lunches and to educate children about good food practices during their formative years. Schools must serve lunches that provide at least one-third of the Recommended Dietary Allowances for a child. Since 1968 schools must make lunches available free or at reduced prices to children unable to pay the full price. The system for determining which children get free or reduced prices is determined by the local school board, but must be a matter of public record and must not discriminate in any way against children receiving free or reduced-price lunches.

The purpose of the School Breakfast Program is similar to that of the lunch program, that is to serve nutritious breakfasts to children from needy homes and/or those children traveling long distances to school.

In addition to the Child Nutrition Programs, several other governmental programs have been developed to combat hunger and malnutrition among the poor. One of these government Family Feeding Programs is the Donated Commodities Program. This program was initially established to help the needy and provide a market for agricultural commodities in surplus. About 3.8 million people now participate in the commodity program. The government provides food bought on the open market, not necessarily in surplus, including staples such as flour, cornmeal, and dry milk, but also including canned meat, canned chicken and turkey, canned vegetables, and fruit juice. Though the variety of foods has been improved, a trend toward the utilization of food stamps seems to be taking place.

The Food Stamp program was the result of food stamp legislation initially introduced in 1961 by President Kennedy. The Food Stamp Act went into effect in 1967. A family pays for food stamps depending on income and the number of people in the family. These food stamps are worth much more than the actual price paid and may be spent in any supermarket or grocery store that accepts them. More than 10 million people are currently participating in the Food Stamp Program.

These governmental programs have recently been subject to review with the republican administration seeking to delimit or curtail them. On the other hand democratic Senators Humphrey and McGovern have sought to pass legislation that would maintain or expand them.

WEIGHT CONTROL

In spite of the fact that some individuals do not get enough to eat, a far larger number have the problem of obesity resulting from an excess of food intake and/or a lack of exercise. Obesity is by far the most common nutritional problem in the United States today.

Problems of weight control are often considered to be solely related to overeating and gluttony. Increasingly, evidence is being gathered to indicate that this is not necessarily so. There are studies which show that some overweight people eat less than individuals of normal weight. Current information indicates that how fat is formed in the bodies of some obese people may differ from that found in people of normal weight. If this is so, a purely dietary approach to the correction of this kind of obesity would prove inadequate. It is becoming increasingly apparent that there are a number of factors involved in weight control.

One of these factors is that of exercise. Weight control is based on achieving a balance between caloric intake and caloric output. To concentrate solely on diet (caloric intake) is to focus on only one-half of the problem. It has many times been found that weight control can be adequately achieved by increasing the level of exercise alone. Studies have shown that overweight people are, in many instances, not as active as they might be. Observations of overweight children in physical education classes have indicated that these children are frequently much less active than individuals of normal weight.

Increasingly, the relationship between heredity and obesity is being explored. One study[3] has demonstrated that only 10 percent of the children whose parents were of normal weight are obese, and that the proportion will rise to 40 per

[3] Jean Mayer, *Overweight—Causes, Cost, and Control.*

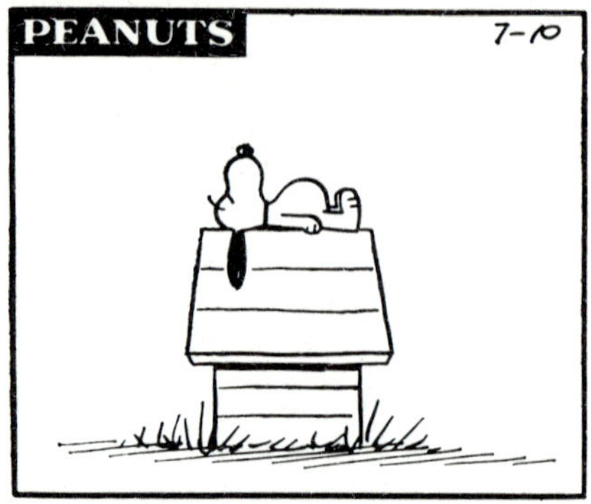

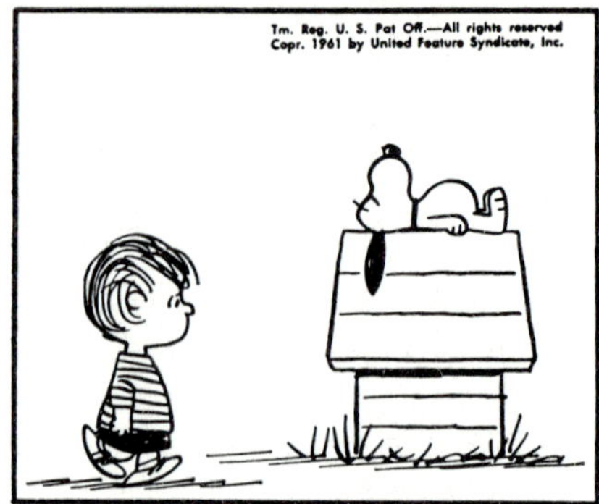

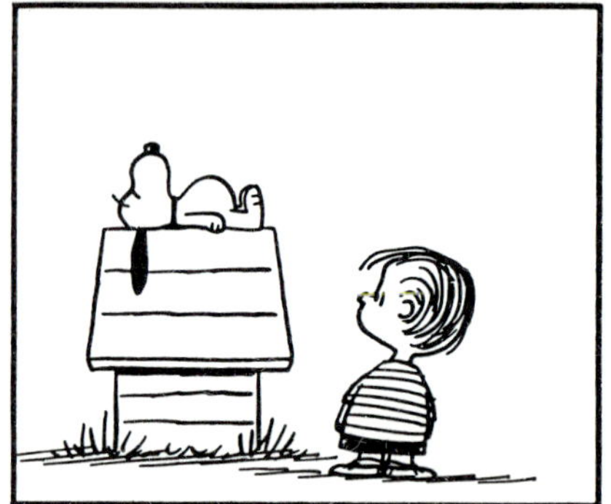

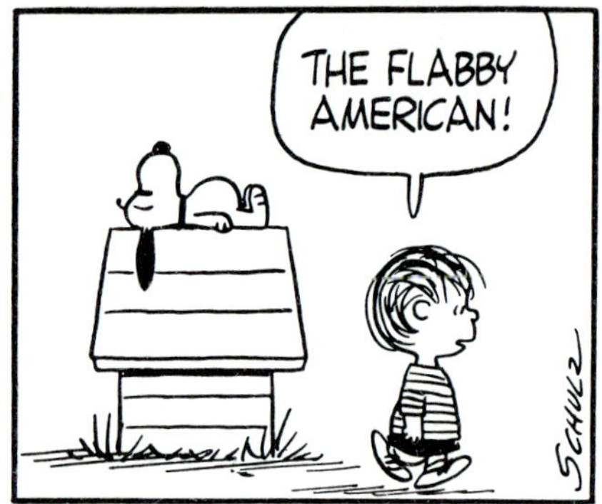

Figure 2–2

Peanuts cartoon by Charles M. Schulz.

(© 7/10/61 by United Feature Syndicate, Inc.)

cent if one parent is obese. Where both parents are obese, the percentage of overweight children in the family rises to 80 per cent. Additional studies in this area indicate that where obesity runs in families, genetic as well as environmental factors may be involved. "Comparative lifetime studies of identical and fraternal twins have strongly pointed toward possible hereditary factors in their obesity. Food habits are not the only or even the main factor in their obesity."[4] Obesity, like any other health concern, deserves early attention. Pediatricians become increasingly concerned where this kind of problem is ignored in childhood, when corrective measures can best be undertaken.

Emotional and psychological factors also have a role to play here. Such factors as grief, lack of affection, success, or popularity are involved as motivators of abnormal eating patterns. Many people will eat out of just plain nervousness. Tensions before an examination or any situation contributing to

[4] *Obesity and Health* (Washington, D.C.: U.S. Dept. of Health, Education and Welfare, U.S. Public Health Service Publication No. 1485), p. 42.

stress might precipitate an evening-long session of "nervous eating." It has been found in those cases where emotional or psychological factors are involved that restriction of food is not necessarily the best solution to the problem. We may be sometimes superimposing an additional difficulty for the individual. If the person can be induced to increase his energy output by some kind of activity, the problem is more easily resolved.

Lack of information with regard to basic nutrition is an additional factor that might complicate the management of obesity. People are too often unaware of which foods are of high calorie value and which ones are not. Basic information in this area alone could prevent much obesity.

It is an established fact that the overweight do not live as long as those of normal weight. Cardiovascular disease, high blood pressure, diabetes, arthritis, cerebral hemorrhage, and nephritis are some of the conditions that occur more often in the overweight. In a study reported by the Metropolitan Life Insurance Company, it was found that excess mortality rose rapidly with an increased degree of overweight. Since several of these disease conditions may be related to diet, nutrition is one means of attacking the problem. A lower fat intake, including less saturated fat (primarily that from animal sources such as in butter, whole milk, meat, and lard), and a lower intake of refined sugar might be beneficial in lowering the rate of heart disease in the population. In addition, the most important nutritional prevention that can be taken by the individual is the attaining and maintaining of normal weight early in life.

DIETING

In considering diets, the first concern should be with nutritional adequacy and balance. Often people establish a diet pattern that is unbalanced with regard to one or more nutrients. The result is the addition of a deficiency problem to the overweight problem they already have. Dieting patterns are also found

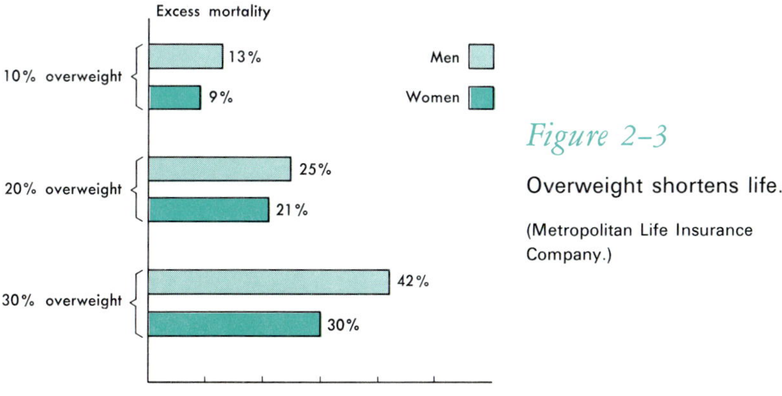

Figure 2–3

Overweight shortens life.

(Metropolitan Life Insurance Company.)

too often to be temporary and emotional in nature. Individuals will attempt to modify their diet for one or two weeks when what is really needed is a change of eating patterns that will last for that individual's lifetime. The emotional nature with which some people approach dieting is exemplified by the woman who felt that she needed to have a banana split smothered with whipped cream and nuts in order to "reinforce" herself before undertaking the "ordeal" of dieting for the next two weeks. This approach immediately condemns the attempt at weight control to obvious failure. Diets that also exclude exercise as indicated earlier are narrow and shortsighted in scope; it must be remembered that some individuals who do not exercise extensively, in order to maintain their weight, go through life feeling constantly hungry.

Dieting to lose weight is usually more successful when done in groups with some professional help. "In the New York City antiobesity program, a survey of almost 2600 obesity clinic patients has shown . . . that group methods supervised by the physician and nutritionist were more successful than individual instruction."[5] Restricting food intake is not always easy. Having the social pressure of a group of people who have similar concerns can serve to reinforce the dietary goals. The professional can help to keep the dieting balanced in terms of needed nutrients and to discount the many faddish and quackish diets that are constantly being offered.

QUACKERY AND SPECIAL DIETS

Quackery in the area of nutrition, and particularly with regard to weight control, is literally running rampant in the United States. Wherever we run across a problem that is difficult to control, invariably people of questionable ethics will move in to sell quick cures. The market at the present time is flooded with publications that give what appear to be easy solutions to the problem. These books come under varying titles intimating that you can eat all you want and lose weight, provided you include some magic ingredient. These ingredients include vegetable oils, special dietary supplements, and homespun but unscientific regimens. We have seen the increased sale of vibrating couches, belts, and other gadgets of this type. The federal government, after extensive testing, has indicated that there is no evidence to support the thesis that these vibrating gadgets will be helpful in weight reduction. For some, the most that can be said for them is that they can be relaxing; however, for others, the possibility for harm is present. The Relax-A-cizer, which promises to reduce girth by electrically stimulating muscles, is one such device.

> In April 1970 a permanent injunction against the distribution of the *Relax-A-cizer* was issued by a U.S. district court. After a trial which heard

[5] Corinne H. Robinson, *Normal and Therapeutic Nutrition,* 14th ed. (New York: Macmillan, Inc., 1972), p. 421.

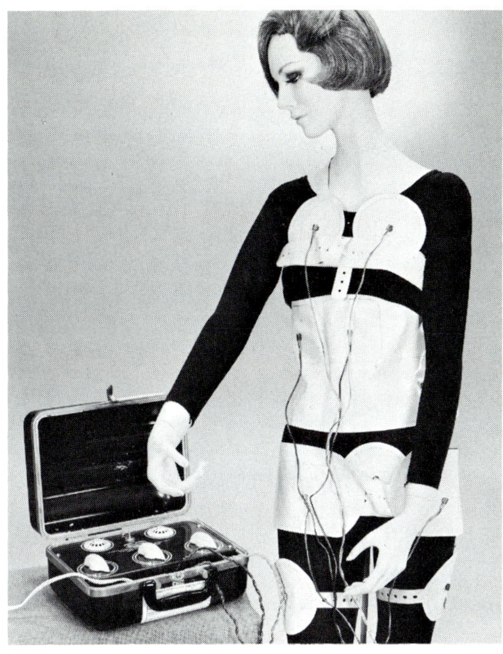

Figure 2–4

The Relaxacizor is an electrical device that has been sold for several years for exercising and reducing specific parts of the body. It provides electrical shocks to the body through contact pads and has proved to be dangerous.

(U.S. Food and Drug Administration.)

> the testimony of thirty-one medical authorities, the device was declared to be dangerous to health, having the potential effect of damaging the heart and other vital organs, and disseminating preexisting cancer cells throughout the body.[6]

Before-meal candies are often sold as a means of suppressing appetite. The person is supposed to eat two candies with the idea of raising the blood sugar level, which in turn is supposed to kill the appetite. The difficulty with this approach is that the caloric content of the candy is much too low to have any effect on the blood sugar level.

Some people are misled into believing that steam baths are a means of losing weight. The unhappy fact is that temporary loss in body fluids is regained with the first intakes of water and other fluid material, but the dollars and time invested are not.

NUTRITIONAL MISINFORMATION

One problem area in nutrition against which little progress has been made is food faddism. The only thing that has changed here is the scene of the crime. The old food faddist sold his wares from the back of a covered wagon.

[6] *The Medicine Show* (Mount Vernon, N.Y.: Consumers Union, 1971), p. 114.

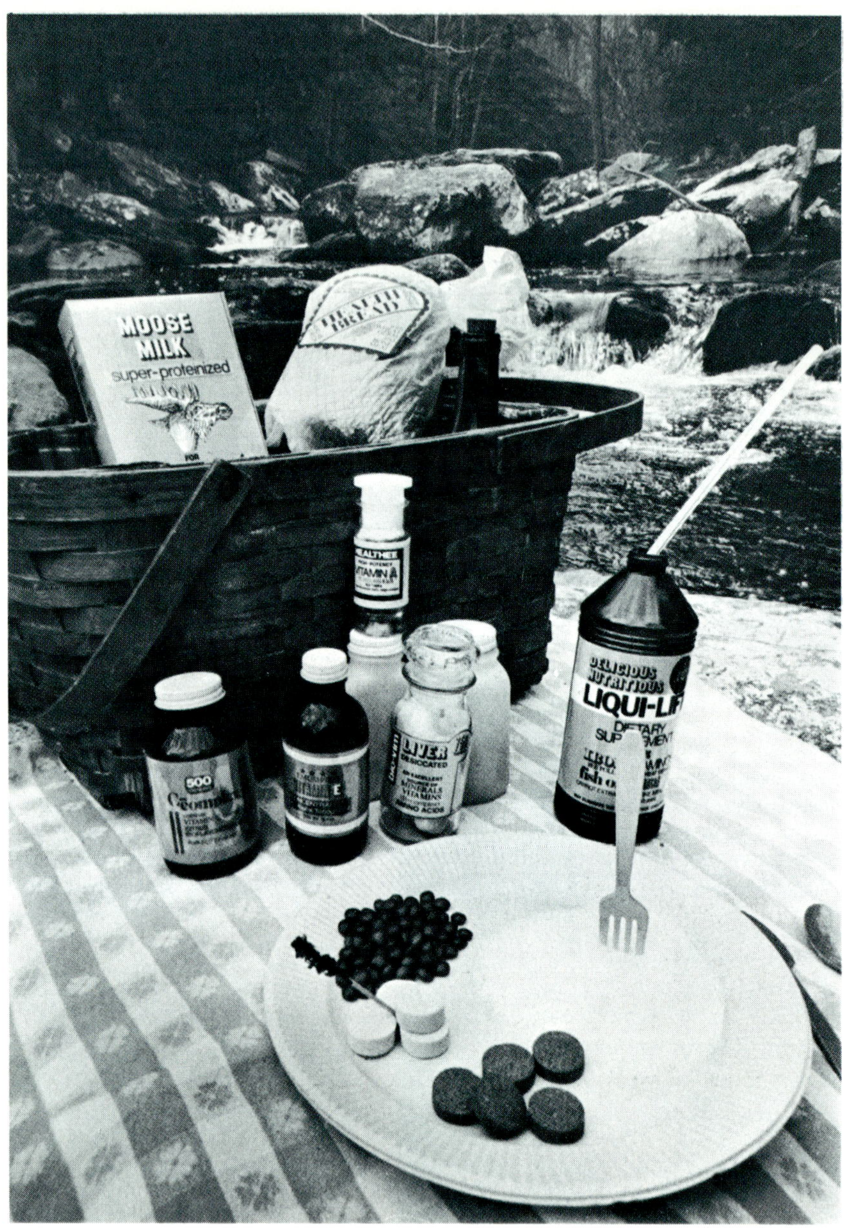

Figure 2–5

So-called health foods take a variety of forms including superproteinized Moose Milk. The major difference between "health foods" and foods found in normal diets is the price.

(*FDA Consumer,* December 1973–January 1974)

Now he has the facilities of television and book publishers who have national distribution. Charlatans using twentieth-century methods are deluding the American public who have in very many cases nineteenth-century nutritional information. It is estimated that almost one billion dollars a year is spent in the United States in the area of food quackery. The range of activity here is a broad one, including the sale of food supplements, books, health foods, weight control plans, and "cures" for a wide range of ailments that even medical science cannot completely control.

Some books persist on best-seller lists in spite of condemnation by the American Medical Association and leading nutritionists. In 1962 the best-selling book in the nation was *Calories Don't Count,* by Herman Taller, M.D., with an estimated sales of 2 million copies. The author was later convicted of conspiracy and violation of federal drug laws because of a commercial tie-in of the book with safflower oil capsules. His license to practice medicine was revoked for three years in addition to being fined.

In 1973 a diet book called *Dr. Atkins' Diet Revolution,* by Robert C. Atkins, M.D., suddenly became a best seller. It told its readers what they apparently wanted to hear—that they could eat large amounts of food and still lose weight. What the author advocated was a high protein and fat diet and one low in carbohydrates. Nutritionists immediately labeled it as another rehashing of the "DuPont diet," the "Drinking Man's Diet," "The Mayo Diet" (not related in any way to the renowned Mayo Clinic) *Calories Don't Count,* and "The Air Force Diet." Nothing is new—at least not in this context.

The AMA Council on Foods and Nutrition reviewed not only the Atkins' publication, but the history of similar diets that have been presented to the public. The Council described the diet as unscientific and potentially dangerous for the following reasons:

1. A high-fat diet would pose greater risk for the development of heart disease, particularly in susceptible individuals.
2. A feeling of fatigue was a common complaint of individuals on this diet. The fatigue promptly disappeared following addition of carbohydrates to the diet.
3. The Atkins' diet would increase the blood uric acid level aggravating gout conditions or inducing a gout condition.
4. The Council felt it was unfortunate that no reliable mechanism exists to help the public evaluate and put into proper perspective the great volume of nutritional information and misinformation with which it is constantly being bombarded. Bizarre concepts of nutrition and dieting should not be promoted to the public as if they were established scientific principles.
5. Further, physicians were warned to counsel their patients as to the potentially harmful results that might occur because of adherence to the "ketogenic diet," and to report adverse effects from this diet in the medical literature just as in cases of an adverse drug reaction.

It is ironic that the best-fed country in the world, one whose government pays its farmers not to overproduce, that enriches its bread with the vitamin B's and iron, adds vitamin D to its milk, iodizes its salt, and adds vitamin A to margarine, should also have such an enormous, useless sale of vitamin and mineral supplements. Why is it that books advocating the use of "miracle foods" or "health foods" stay on best-seller lists in spite of condemnation by the American Medical Association and leading nutritionists? How does it happen that a country with a highly developed educational system and mass media second to none can be so badly fooled and uninformed in so basic an area? Let us look at some of the factors involved.

The motivations of the food faddists vary. Their actions are stimulated sometimes by ignorance, sometimes by the search for money. Their false claims and stretching of the truth have misled many. Some of their typical approaches follow:

THE HEALTH FOOD–ORGANIC FOOD MOVEMENT

In the last few years consumers rightly concerned over ecology and pollution of the environment have extended their concern to the food supply. This concern about excessive use of pesticides, additives, and chemical fertilizers has overlapped considerably with and been taken advantage of by promoters of various expensive "health foods" and "organic foods." Scientifically speaking, any food that comes from an animal or plant is organic. The popular use of the term usually refers to food that is grown with naturally produced (i.e., animal manures) fertilizers and without the use of pesticides. Foods grown in this manner are perfectly good foods but usually have no different nutrient content from other foods and often are much more expensive.

The added expense of organically grown foods was explained by an interesting study conducted at the Virginia Polytechnic Institute in 1971 and repeated again in 1972.[7] The vegetable yields from two garden plots were compared. In one garden the vegetables were grown organically and in the other, the vegetables were grown with the help of modern agricultural techniques. The chemically protected garden yielded 1,954 pounds of vegetables whereas the organic garden yielded 237 pounds.

Some younger members of society have drastically changed their eating habits. Some use only so-called organic foods while others have become vegetarians. This "counter culture" nutrition is harmless in most cases, but when carried to extreme can be dangerous. For instance, the "Zen Macrobiotic"

[7] Robert C. Lambe, Extension Specialist and Associate Professor in Plant Pathology at Virginia Polytechnic Institute, Blacksburg, Va., 1971.

diet based on the writings of George Oshawa[8] recommends that the diet will help the consumer attain a spiritual state not attainable in any other way. In its extreme form (most desirable, according to the author) nothing but brown rice is to be eaten. This diet could be, and has been on occasion, fatal. Brown rice alone does not supply the nutrients needed for survival, let alone health. There is evidence that macrobiotic children are not growing properly—their birth weight is less than normal, they develop slowly, and they lose their hair.

Most vegetarian regimes, however, can provide adequate nutrition if a *variety* of foods including cereals, legumes, nuts, fruits, and vegetables are consumed. Although legumes (peas and beans), nuts, and soybeans contain some protein, it is difficult to consume the great amounts needed for proper nutrition. If milk and eggs are allowed, then the chances are better that proper nutrition can be achieved. The extreme reaction of some groups to avoid processed foods has been disastrous. In some communes babies have been fed raw milk, resulting in diseases, such as typhoid, which were all but unheard of in this country a few years ago.

As one renowned professor of nutrition has indicated, "We have enough problems as a nation—poverty, ignorance, pollution, racial prejudice, poor planning of our material and intellectual processes, cloudy ethics—without encouraging the creation of new totally unnecessary health hazards."[9]

Unfortunately many manufacturers of health foods and "organic" vitamin supplements (which are no different chemically from synthesized vitamins) have taken advantage of the youthful counterculture for economic gain. Especially disturbing is the fact that some "health food stores" have been noted recently to be accepting food stamps. Surely the low-income person can least afford to spend extra money for food that will give him no more nutrition than the food he can buy in the supermarket.

FOOD ADDITIVES

The old country store is with us no more. Its familiar food odors and cracker barrel are part of a nostalgic past. The crackers are now double wrapped to maintain freshness and crispness for months. The bread on the open shelf is now carefully wrapped and calcium propionate added to prevent it from becoming moldy. The age of the supermarket is upon us. The frozen food sections, with their increasing variety of foods, and the canned and bottled goods departments are part of an era marked by advances in the packaging

[8] George Oshawa, *Zen Macrobiotics: The Art Of Rejuvenation and Longevity* (Los Angeles: Ignoramus Press, 1965).

[9] Jean Mayer, Professor of Nutrition, School of Public Health, Harvard University, Cambridge, Mass. *New York Times,* April 2, 1972.

Food: Claims & Facts

Claim:

Our soil has lost its vitamins and minerals; thus our food crops have little nutritional value.

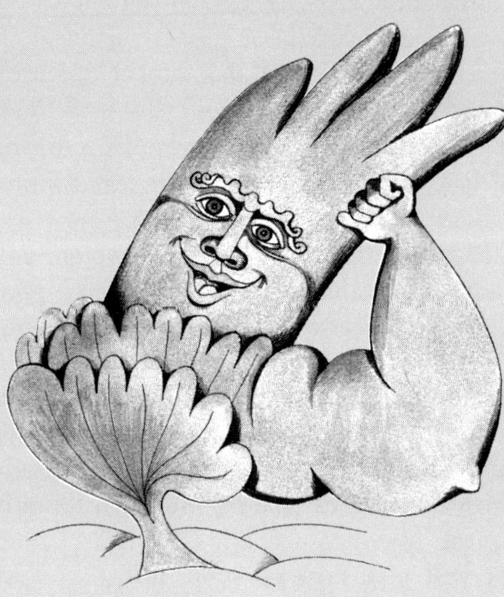

Fact:

Faddists have been hard at work selling the idea that the soil in this country is depleted, resulting in food products lacking in minerals and vitamins. The United States Department of Agriculture, after a great deal of testing, has found that depleted soil, where it does exist, will result in a smaller yield. The food produced, however, will contain the same amount and quality of nutrients. Faddists will often claim that organic fertilizer is the answer to soil depletion, decrying the use of chemical fertilizers as dangerous. There is, of course, no evidence of this. Spreading such ideas usually results in the sale of unnecessary mineral and vitamin supplements by the food faddists. It also spurs the sale of organically grown "health" foods in "health food" stores at many times the normal price.

Claim:

Modern processing removes most vitamins and minerals from foods.

Fact:

While any type of processing, including simple cooking, reduces to some extent the nutrient content or quality of foods, modern processing methods are designed to keep such losses as low as possible. For some foods, nutrients are restored by enrichment after processing.

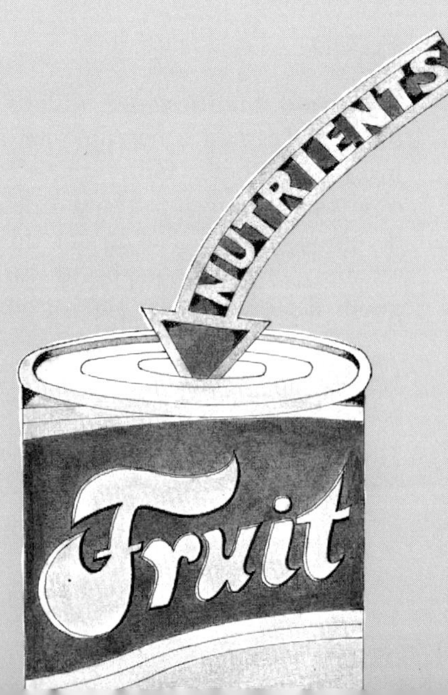

Claim:

If you have an ache or pain or are just feeling tired, you are probably suffering from a vitamin deficiency.

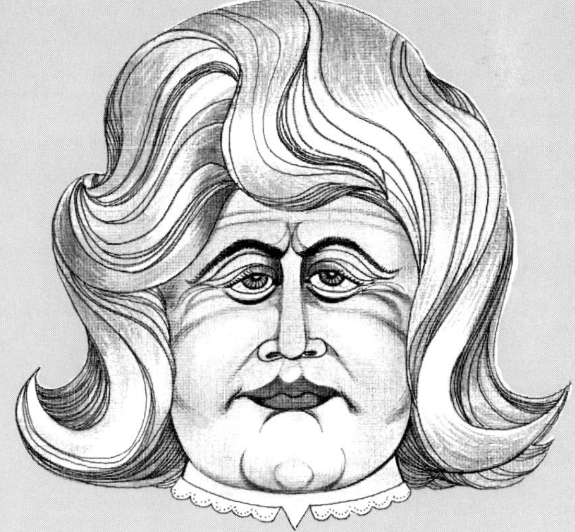

Fact:

Most people feel tired or suffer aches and pains at one time or another. These are symptoms which may be caused by overwork, emotional stress, disease, or lack of sleep, as well as by poor nutrition. If such symptoms persist, you should see your physician. It is difficult for the average person to accurately diagnose the cause of these symptoms.

Claim:

Everyone should take vitamins, just to be sure.

Fact:

The discovery of vitamins was effective in significantly reducing the vitamin deficiency diseases. Enrichment and fortification programs followed, with vitamins being routinely added to foods, so that people could conveniently get adequate amounts of varied vitamins. However, as with many discoveries, an aura of exaggerated effectiveness and function has surrounded the use of vitamins. The faddist has exploited this. The food manufacturer who carefully prints vitamin content of his food, as if it were the only important nutrient it contained, contributes to this exaggerated concept. Pharmaceutical houses have also jumped on the bandwagon with advertisements implying the universal need for vitamin supplementation.

It is common for people to believe that vitamins will give them quick energy. Without their daily vitamin pill they expect to come apart at the seams. Many a college student has his or her suitcase packed for school with the inevitable bottle of vitamins. The idea that the only important nutrients in our foods are vitamins reflects a bit of nutritional misinformation.

Vitamin products have a recognized place as a part of preventive medicine when for some special reason the physician decides this kind of supplementation is needed. The indiscriminate use of vitamins is not only expensive but can in some instances be dangerous and represent a poor substitute for a physician when one does not feel well.

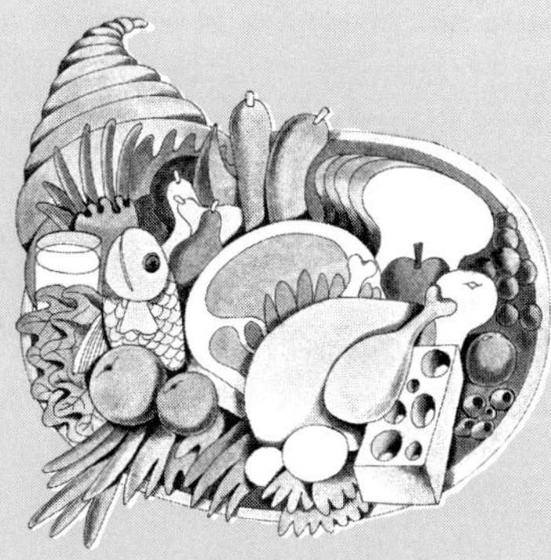

Adapted from FDA *Consumer,* September 1972.

Examples of Food Additives

Antibiotics control microorganism spoilage by inhibiting the growth of molds and bacteria.

Antioxidants, such as vitamin C, are used to prevent fruit from turning brown when being frozen.

Emulsifiers are used so that substances that normally do not mix, such as oil and vinegar, will remain together. Emulsifiers are also used in bakery batters and ice cream to give these products a smoother texture.

Stabilizers and thickeners will thicken and prevent chocolate from settling out of chocolate milk. They are also used in cake mixes and gelatins, where they surround flavor oils and prevent their deterioration.

Neutralizing agents control the degree of acidity or alkalinity in foods which in turn affects their flavor and texture.

Sequestrants are used to separate out certain substances in solutions which in themselves do not cause rancidity, but help the process along. It is used in fats and oils and helps prevent these items from becoming rancid. It is also used in the soft drink industry to inactivate the minerals so that the color and clearness of the beverage are maintained.

Humectants are added to keep moisture in foods such as coconut and marshmallows.

Anticaking agents are used to keep salts and powders free flowing.

Firming agents maintain the texture of processed fruits and vegetables.

Coloring agents are used in a variety of foods to improve their appearance.

Bleaching agents bleach a number of foods, including flour, whose color after milling is yellow. It formerly required months of storage to bleach flour, which led to problems of insect and rodent contamination.

Foaming agents are used in pressure-packed products to facilitate the ejection of the material from the can, as in the case of the many whipped toppings.

Foam inhibitors are used in the canning of liquid foods (e.g., orange juice) where foaming interferes with the canning process.

Nonnutritive sweeteners such as saccharin are used in dietetic foods and beverages.

and preservation of food. In the supermarket are also found maraschino cherries containing a color additive; marshmallows that stay fresh longer, not only because of better packaging, but because an additive helps it to retain its moisture. The poultry and fish have antibiotics added to retard spoilage. An era that has seen rather revolutionary changes take place in food processing and packaging also heralds the coming of age of the food additive, for without them many packaged food products could not be produced.

A food additive is a substance added to food in a variety of ways to make our food better and more abundant. There are two general types of additives. Those that are called *intentional additives* are substances used to perform a specific function, such as nutrient supplements, preservatives, and coloring materials. The others are called *incidental additives* and serve no function in the finished product, but somehow become a part of the food through some production method, processing, or packaging. Examples of incidental additives might be pesticides or chemical fertilizers that are needed to protect our crops from being consumed by insects.

In 1924, iodine was the first food additive used. It was added to table salt to prevent goiter. Iodized salt has been responsible for the practical disappearance of simple goiter in this country. As of July 1972 all salt was required to carry a statement regarding iodine content on its label; for example, next to Iodized Salt the statement "This salt supplies iodine, a necessary nutrient," whereas next to the name Salt, the statement "This salt does not supply iodine, a necessary nutrient."[10]

In the thirties, the fortification of milk with vitamin D was begun. This procedure was developed to prevent rickets in children. Milk is rich in calcium and phosphorus, those minerals that are needed for the proper development of bones. Because vitamin D helps the body to utilize calcium and phosphorus, it followed that milk should be the food selected for fortification with this vitamin. In the early forties the enrichment of flour, bread, and cereal products with several B vitamins (thiamin, riboflavin, and niacin) and iron was begun. This program is believed to be a strong factor in the virtual elimination of pellagra in the southern part of this country. Vitamin A has since been added to margarine to make it the nutritional equivalent of butter. More recently the FDA has decided to increase the amount of iron and B vitamins in the grain products of American consumers. In this way the high prevalence of iron deficiency anemia found by the White House Conference on Food, Nutrition and Health and the Ten-State Nutrition Survey in 1969–1970 might be significantly reduced. Though the early food additives were essentially *nutrient supplements,* those that followed were designed to preserve flavor or color, or maintain texture of processed food.

The control and safety factors in the use of additives have been carefully

[10] "Information on Ingredient Labeling of Standardized Foods," FDA Consumer, March 1972.

worked out. When it is found that a chemical has use as a food additive, it is put through studies to determine if the substance is harmful to living things. These studies are conducted with labaratory animals, some being of a short-term nature while others are long-term studies. When it is determined that the chemical is safe for human consumption, the Food and Drug Administration is petitioned and the test data presented. When the scientists of the governmental agency are convinced of the safety of the chemical, they determine the safe amount and the foods it will be used in and how it will be labeled.

FEDERAL LEGISLATION RELATING TO FOOD IN THE UNITED STATES

Federal Food and Drug Act of 1906

This legislation made illegal the adulteration of food entering into interstate commerce. In this law, adulteration was defined as:

1. The use of poisonous additives of any type.
2. The extraction of valuable constituents from the product. This was aimed at inhibiting manufacturers from utilizing cheaper and less nutritious ingredients in their products.
3. The attempt to conceal inferiority of the product in any way. This legislation was considered to be good for its time, but by 1938, needs for revision became apparent.

Federal Food, Drug, and Cosmetic Act of 1938

This law applied to imports and exports as well as interstate commerce. In it *food* was defined as articles used in food or drink for man or other animals. This legislation again prohibited the adulteration of food. In addition, it made truthful labeling mandatory. Weight and contents of a food package had to be accurately described and not in any way misleading. The name and place of the manufacturer, packer, or distributor needed to be listed on the food package. This legislation also set standards and definitions for foods. It enacted *standards of identity,* which described what the product was. For example, in the identification of fruit preserves, not less than 45 parts fruit or fruit juice needed to be present in the product, with the remaining 55 parts being sugar. If the proportion of fruit or fruit juice is less than 45 percent, then the product must be labeled imitation. This legislation also set *standards of quality,* particularly for canned foods and vegetables, with regard to tenderness, color, and freedom from defects. If a product, for example, is excessively broken, it must

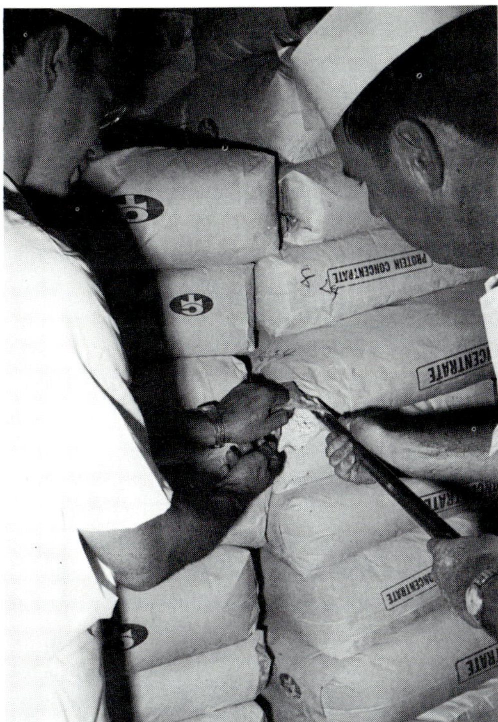

Figure 2–6

FDA inspectors taking a sample of flour to determine its purity and safety for consumer use.

(*FDA Consumer*, November 1972)

be labeled "below standard in quality." The law also established *standards of fill* for a container. This was aimed at preventing deception of the buyer. It was at one time a practice for some manufacturers to place their products in a large container and then only half fill it. This misled the consumer into thinking that he was getting more of the product than he actually received.

Major amendments to the 1938 law have been added. *The Miller Pesticide Amendment* was passed in 1954. The basic provision of this amendment was to set standards for safe amounts of pesticide residue that may be permitted to remain on fruits and vegetables. The *Food Additives Amendment* was passed in 1958. This amendment required proof of safety before a substance could be added to food. It also forbade the use of a substance which was found to produce cancer in man or animals. In 1960 the *Color Additive Amendment* came into being. This legislation placed under control the use of coal tar colors. It required that no coloring matter be approved if it was found to be carcinogenic to man or animal when used in any amounts. If a question arose as to whether a coloring material was carcinogenic, a scientific advisory committee would investigate the matter.

PROTECTING THE PUBLIC FROM THE FADDIST

The question arises, how can we better protect the American public from health food faddists? Education is a key to the prevention of food faddism and the practice of good nutrition. Nutrition education programs in our schools are not as well developed as they might be. They are often too narrow in their scope, concerning themselves only with the nutritional diseases or a recitation of nutrients and their functions. Many elementary teachers, poorly prepared in the area, are often sources of misinformation. In addition, they often use a fear approach and tend to preach instead of teach about nutrition. Secondary school programs are equally in need of review in terms of their content and student coverage. Certainly *all* high school seniors should have basic nutritional facts and be alerted to the public health problems and programs in this area. Public health organizations could then further educate a public that has been given a basis for additional information. The educational task of the public health agency is at present overwhelming. It is time for schools, colleges, and health agencies to coordinate their efforts to achieve adequate nutrition education. Until there are expanded efforts for meaningful nutrition education programs for *all* age groups in the community, problems of nutrition can be expected to increase in scope and severity.

In addition, however, some help is needed from the federal and state governments. Laws concerning food and drugs should be uniform throughout the states. What endangers the public health in Maine will surely be as hazardous in California! Many states take no interest in public health problems and very often these states become handy bases of operation for food quacks. Modernized drug, food, and advertising laws are needed so that the obvious loopholes of the old laws will no longer exist. Along with this modernization should go bigger budgets and larger staffs for the Food and Drug Administration.

PROBLEMS RELATED TO FOOD AND DIGESTION

Food Poisoning

Common types of food poisoning involve *staphylococcal* and *salmonella* contamination. When contaminated foods are ingested, the symptoms of food poisoning appear 2 to 4 hours after eating in the form of nausea, diarrhea, and intestinal cramps, lasting a few hours and usually not more than a day.

Improperly prepared foods, unpasteurized milk and dairy products, contamination of foods by roaches, rodent feces, or infected persons may be some of the ways this condition is transmitted. Some safeguards against food poisoning that can be taken are:

1. Wash raw foods thoroughly.
2. Wash hands *before* handling food, and after handling *raw* foods such as chickens, meats, eggs, and dairy products.
3. Refrigerate all dairy products and leftovers promptly.
4. Keep perishable foods chilled when going on trips or picnics.

In 1972 the American Public Health Association and six other organizations brought a public interest suit against the Secretary of Agriculture. These health organizations did this because of the consistent refusals of the U.S. Department of Agriculture to provide adequate labeling instructions on how to avoid food poisoning from disease-causing raw poultry and meat products.

> Two deaths resulted when 18 people at a Thanksgiving day dinner ate a USDA inspected turkey. Within 18 hours, 17 of the guests developed symptoms of gastroenteritis, including vomiting, diarrhea, fever, and abdominal pain. A 17-year-old boy and a 56-year-old woman died, and the others were hospitalized for between four and twelve days, Sussman reported. Had proper food handling procedures been followed so that this turkey had not come into contact with other foods, and the cook's hands been washed immediately after handling the bird, this incident would never have happened, he said.[11]

Botulism is another form of food poisoning that is highly fatal. The early symptoms of botulism are characterized by double or blurred vision, slurred speech, and difficulty in swallowing. Death due to botulism is usually the result of respiratory and cardiac paralysis, since the poison primarily attacks the nervous system. This occurs in two-thirds of the patients and usually within 3 to 7 days. The symptoms develop in accordance with the amount ingested and appear within 18 hours. Most poisonings in the United States arise from the improper canning of vegetables at home. The botulism organism (Clostridium botulinum) is widely distributed in the soil and is normally harmless when surrounded by air. However, when the organism is in an airtight container, such as a can or a preserving jar, it grows and produces one of the deadliest poisons known to man. When the homemaker is careless or unaware of proper sterilization methods in home-canning, some very serious consequences may be in store. There have been, however, cases of botulism caused by commercially canned products. In July 1971 a death was recorded as a result of botulism from a can of soup. In April 1970 there was a nationwide recall of 80,000 frozen pizzas believed to contain botulism-tainted mushrooms.

[11] *The Nation's Health,* April 1972. (The Official Newspaper of the American Public Health Association.)

During that year 13 people became ill from botulism and 5 died. In 1963, 14 Americans died from infected tuna and smoked fish from the Great Lakes.

Death from botulism need not occur at all since boiling the contents of a can vigorously for 3 to 5 minutes destroys the toxin. This would pertain to soups as well as vegetables—even those green or wax beans to be used for salads and are generally used straight from the can. Never buy cans that are swollen or misshapen and never taste-test a suspicious-smelling food, since only very small amounts of the toxin are extremely dangerous. The treatment for the condition consists of intramuscular injections of botulinus antitoxin only after certain diagnosis of botulism has been made.

Constipation and Laxatives

"No organ of the body is so misunderstood and maltreated as the digestive tract. It has been purged, irrigated, lavaged, massaged, and pummelled, all in the name of that great American obsession, the daily bowel movement."[12] The idea that a daily bowel movement is synonymous with good health has caused a preoccupation with this function. Six out of ten Americans use laxatives, and there are 500 different brands of laxative products on the market. In most instances, the use of these products was completely unnecessary. Most cases of constipation can be relieved without the use of drugs. It must further be recognized that in the great majority of cases where laxative drugs are used, constipation is not even present. Constipation cannot be defined in terms of a daily bowel movement. What is normal functioning here will vary from one individual to another. This variance may be from one or more movements a day to an evacuation only once in two or three days without the slightest of ill effects. Physicians are many times concerned because people overlook the fact that any laxative is potentially harmful and that there is no such thing as a laxative that is natural and harmless in all instances. The theory that a laxative "cleans out" the digestive tract is quite a misleading one. Essentially, what the individual does is to introduce into the digestive tract a cathartic drug which can have a number of harmful effects including dehydration, irritation, and inflammation of the digestive tract. There is a relationship between the incidence of hemorrhoids and fissures of the anus and the habitual use of cathartics. Besides, the very cause of chronic constipation is often associated with the use of these types of drugs. In essence, they may be causing the very condition that they are supposed to be preventing. The best preventive measure against constipation would be for most people to resist taking self-medicative action in the form of laxatives, suppositories, and enemas. A very positive step that can be taken in combating constipation is to add to the diet such foods as fruits, vegetables, and whole wheat grain cereals. These will add roughage to the diet that will maintain proper functioning of the digestive tract. Probably the greatest problem that we have in this country in connection with constipation is the current hysteria related to its supposed existence.

[12] *The Medicine Show* (Mount Vernon, N.Y.: Consumers Union, 1971), p. 47.

BASIC NUTRITIONAL NEEDS

There is nothing more basic to survival than food. The quality of that survival is strongly related to the quality of one's nutrition. What constitutes good nutrition, however, varies with the person, his age, sex, size, his rate of growth, physical activity, or the presence of stress such as disease or fever. Nutrition is thus a science. There are, however, few people who treat it as such. Health motives and knowledge of nutritional needs may play a part, but are hardly the only motives for the selection of foods. What a person eats will be influenced by the season of the year, the amount of money available to buy food, and his geographical location. Within that framework the person will make food choices strongly influenced by his cultural and personal background as well as his tastebuds. Add to this already complex situation misinformation deliberately disseminated by food faddists and some misleading advertisements and it becomes apparent that developing good nutritional practices is a complex process.

The Balanced Diet

In discussing the adequate nutrition we cannot ignore the fact that there are many other reasons for eating besides hunger and health. There has been increasing recognition of the role of emotional factors as related to food intake. The insecure person may choose to eat food as an infant uses a pacifier. Food is frequently offered as a social grace. In many such instances, the person is made to feel awkward if he refuses the offering. Social pressure, therefore, becomes a reason for eating in this case, not nutrition. Food tastes, the manner in which food is prepared, how much time we allow for a meal, and family eating patterns are other factors related to what and how much we eat. The point is that in spite of all these reasons we must keep in mind the basic purposes of food intake. Those who live to eat die early. For those of us who eat to live, let us consider those combinations of foods and nutrients that can help us to do it best.

A varied diet is in itself insurance that we are getting the variety of nutrients needed to maintain health. Using a guide such as the basic four food groups is an easy, yet a fairly specific, check on the nature of our food intake. The basic four food groups include:

1. The Milk Group

Foods included in this grouping consist of milk and milk products, such as cheese and ice cream. The daily amounts recommended for foods in this group include the following: For whole milk, three to four cups for children; four cups or more for teenagers; two or more for adults; four or more for pregnant women; and six or more for nursing mothers. The milk in these cases may be in the form of skim milk, butter milk, evaporated milk, or dry milk. Cheese and ice cream would make adequate replacements for milk. The amounts it would take for either one of these items to replace milk needs to be estimated on the basis of calcium content. A good rule of thumb is that a one-inch cube of cheese will equal $2/3$ cup of milk; $1/2$ cup of cottage cheese is equal to $1/3$ of a cup of milk; $1/2$ cup of ice cream is equal to $1/4$ cup of milk.

The major contribution that these foods make to our diet is that they are good sources of calcium as well as protein, vitamin A, and riboflavin.

2. The Meat Group

This group includes a variety of meats such as beef, veal, lamb, pork, and organ meats. It also includes poultry, fish, eggs, and shellfish. When some of these foods cannot be obtained, alternatives in this group consist of dry beans, peas, lentils, nuts, and peanut butter. It is recommended that a person choose two or more servings each day from the foods found in this group. Each serving should consist of approximately two to three ounces of meat, poultry, or fish. Two eggs, one cup of beans, peas, or lentils, or four tablespoons of peanut butter would count as a serving. The foods in this group are important because they are sources of protein, iron, and the B vitamins (thiamin, riboflavin, and niacin).

3. The Vegetable and Fruit Group

All fruits and vegetables are included in this grouping. It is recommended that four servings each day be included in the individual's diet. Because foods in this group are generally good sources of vitamins C and A, it is recommended that one give consideration to those fruits and vegetables that are rich in these nutrients. Good sources of vitamin C would include the citrus fruits, as well as strawberries, broccoli, and green peppers. Good sources of vitamin A include the dark green or yellow vegetables. These are exemplified by such items as Swiss chard, apricots, broccoli, kale, spinach, pumpkin, sweet potatoes, and turnip greens, among others. Particular attention should be paid to the sources of vitamin C, because of the high incidence of borderline deficiency in this nutrient.

4. The Bread and Cereal Group

This group includes those foods made from grain, namely breads and cereals, cakes, crackers, and other baked products, as well as cornmeal, macaroni, oats, and rice. It is recommended that four servings be chosen daily from this grouping. A serving would be defined for this group as one slice of bread, one ounce of cereal or $1/2$ to $3/4$ of a cup of cooked cereal, cornmeal, macaroni, or rice. The foods in this group, in addition to serving as supplementary sources of protein and iron, are also rich in the vitamin B's and serve as sources of food energy.

Anyone selecting his foods on the basis of the recommendations of the basic four food groups should have a balanced diet. When an individual seeks to lose weight, the recommendation is that the amount of food be somewhat restricted. However, the variety of foods as listed in these four groups should remain consistent if one is to maintain an adequate level of health.

VISION

A pitcher hurls the baseball across home plate. The umpire calls it a ball and the catcher protests. The player and umpire watched the same ball travel the same distance of 60 feet and yet each gave a different version of what they saw. The reason for this is that the eye is a structure that sends images to the brain, and it is the brain that interprets what we see. Very often what we see is influenced by emotions, the kinds of families we come from, our position in life, our friends, or a combination of many reasons. There is no question that many people can see the same thing, yet come up with different explanations of what they saw even though the structure of their eyes is the same. Let us examine the eye for the exacting, marvelous structure that it is. A structure that man has limited ability to repair and can never replace.

Refractive Errors

When someone cannot see clearly, it is said that the person has a *refractive error.* After being examined by an eye doctor (ophthalmologist or optometrist), the refractive error is corrected with eyeglasses. There are several kinds of refractive errors.

In *nearsightedness* (or myopia) the light rays come to focus in front of the retina, so that the person can see things that are near clearly but has difficulty seeing distant objects. This condition tends to develop some time after the fourth year of life. As the eye grows in size, nearsightedness will develop if the focusing apparatus of the eye is not equipped to bring light rays to a focus over this greater distance. As the size of the eye continues to grow with the development of the child, the nearsightedness becomes worse until growth levels off at 18 to 20 years of age. A strong hereditary tendency is involved in this condition. When one parent is nearsighted, 60 per cent of the children can be expected to be nearsighted. Another factor related to nearsightedness is the greater tendency of these individuals to develop detached retinas. For this reason they sometimes are advised by ophthalmologists to avoid contact sports.

In *farsightedness* (or hyperopia), the light rays tend to come to a focus behind the retina, so the person can see distant objects clearly, but has difficulty seeing things up close. This occurs when the eyeball is too short for the focusing mechanism of the eye. Though children are usually born farsighted, they are generally not bothered by the condition because of their great ability to

The Human Eye

The **lens** of the eye is a transparent structure that focuses on near and far objects by changing its shape. This ability is referred to as *accommodation,* and is greatest in childhood. This is why five-year-olds can sit so close to a television set without eyestrain, whereas parents with diminished power of accommodation cannot.

Cornea

Pupil

Iris

Suspensory ligament

Change in the shape of the lens is effected by the action of the **ciliary muscles.** Contraction of the ciliary muscles results in a relaxation of the ligament surrounding the lens, thus causing the lens to thicken. This permits the eye to focus on nearby objects. When the ciliary muscles relax, the reverse occurs and the eye can focus on distant objects.

In a two-eyed person the blind spot of each eye is not significant, because the fields of vision of the two eyes overlap. In a one-eyed person, however, the blind spot could mean not seeing a child at a distance of 30 feet. At twice that distance it could blot out something as large as a car. To demonstrate the presence of the blind spot, close the left eye and stare at the square below with your right eye. Bring the book slowly closer to your eye. At a distance of about 9 inches, the circle will disappear from view. You may repeat this by gazing at the circle with the left eye and closing the right eye.

The **aqueous humor,** found in the forward chamber of the eye, is a clear fluid which carries nutrient material to the tissues of the lens and cornea. It also helps the cornea to maintain its proper curvature.

The **vitreous humor,** found in the chamber behind the lens, is a jelly-like material that gives the eye its shape.

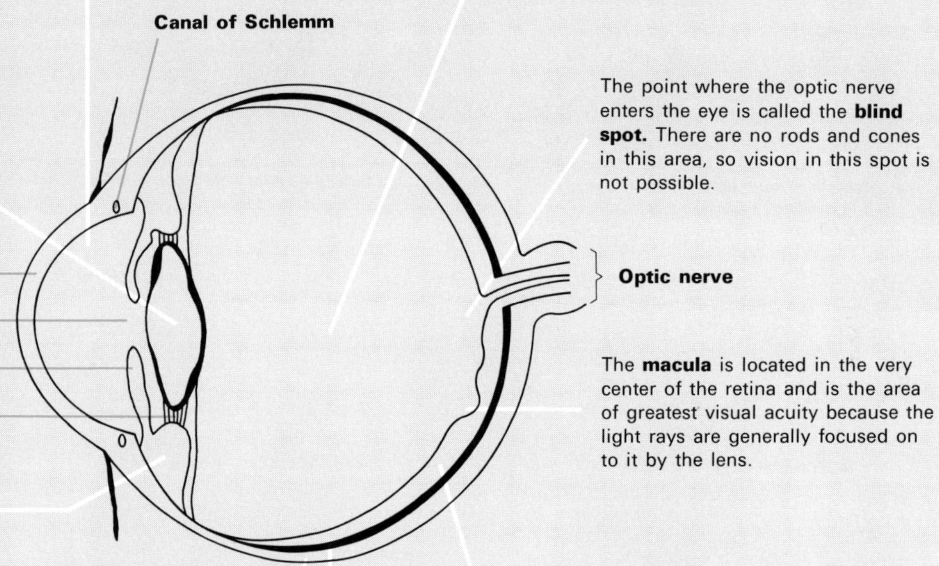

The point where the optic nerve enters the eye is called the **blind spot.** There are no rods and cones in this area, so vision in this spot is not possible.

The **macula** is located in the very center of the retina and is the area of greatest visual acuity because the light rays are generally focused on to it by the lens.

The third layer is the **retina.** Receptors known as rod cells and cone cells make up the retina. The rod cells perceive light while the cone cells perceive color and detail. The cone cells occur in greater numbers in the center of the eye. One effect of this arrangement is that a person needs to look more directly at an object in order to perceive its color. The rod cells are found in greater concentration on the outer parts of the retina. The image picked up by the retina is transmitted by the optic nerve to the visual centers of the brain.

The **choroid** is the middle layer which contains blood vessels, pigment, muscles, and nerve tissue. In front the choroid forms the **iris,** the colored part of the eye which controls the amount of light entering it.

The **sclera** is the outer protective layer referred to as the "white" of the eye. In the front of the eye the sclera is transparent and is called the **cornea.**

The Normal Eye

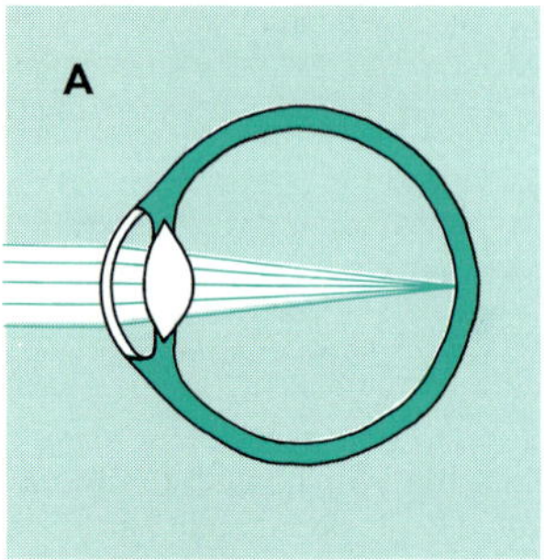

Parallel rays of light (from a distant object) are focused on the retina

The Nearsighted Eye (Elongated Eye)

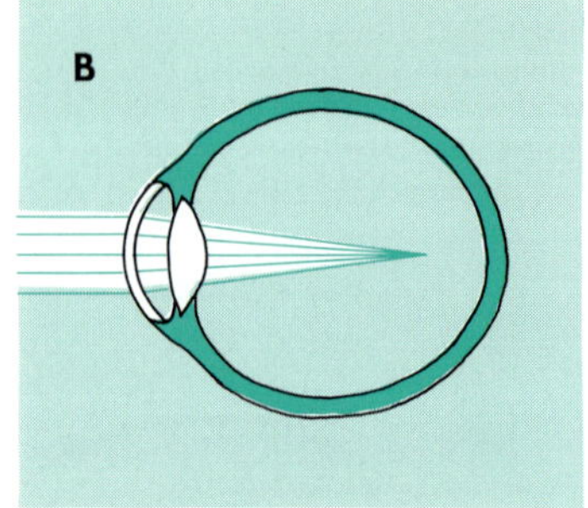

Parallel rays of light focus in front of the retina (distant objects are not in sharp focus)

The Farsighted Eye (Short Eye)

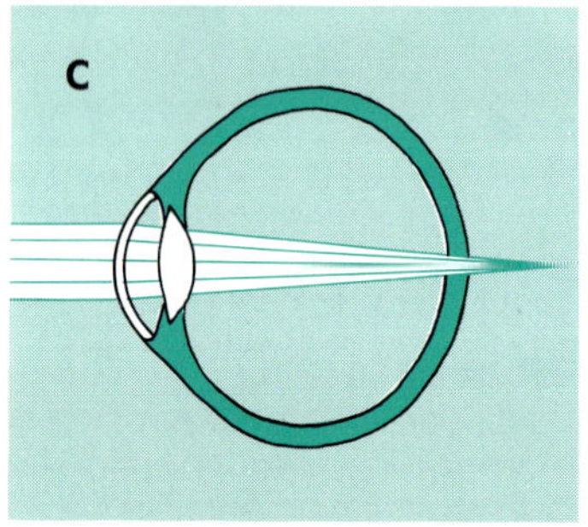

Parallel rays of light come to a focus behind retina

The Farsighted Eye—Accommodating

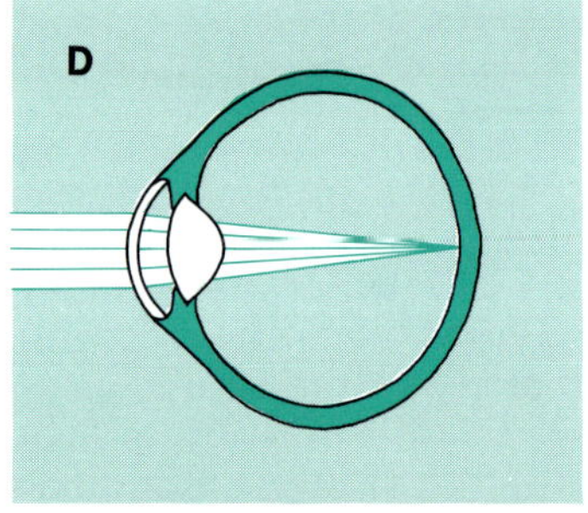

Parallel rays of light are brought to a focus on the retina by accommodation (lens becomes thicker, thus increasing its refractive power)

Figure 2–7

accommodate.[13] The need for glasses in farsightedness would therefore depend on whether the continuous use of accommodation is causing discomfort and fatigue. Dislike of close work, complaints of dizziness, headache, and nausea are some of the symptoms that might appear.

In most cases, as the child grows, the eyeball lengthens and the focal point in the eye returns to the retina.

In *presbyopia,* the lens loses some of its elasticity and thereby its ability to focus, particularly on near objects. This condition is often associated with middle age. The person usually finds that he has to hold the newspaper or phone book farther and farther away in order to read it. The inflexibility of the eye lens and its resultant inability to focus on objects is thereby compensated for by the bifocal eyeglasses. Bifocal lenses are used to correct the condition with the upper lenses in these eyeglasses used for viewing distant objects and the lower lenses used for reading or other close work.

Astigmatism results in the blurring of vision because of an improper curvature of the cornea or the lens, and represents the most common type of refractive error. The improperly shaped cornea or lens creates visual distortions, such as those seen in wavy panes of glass. Astigmatism can occur in combination with hyperopia or myopia, although its causes are not related to these

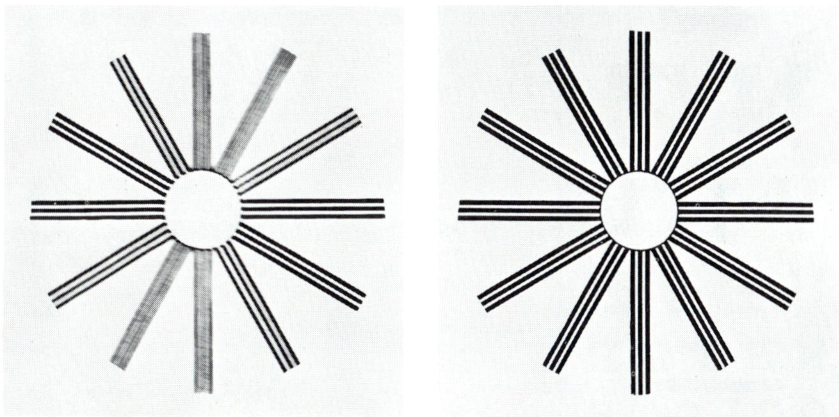

Figure 2–8

The test for astigmatism is positive if the spokes of a wheel are not straight or look gray. If the spokes are straight and all of the same black intensity, the person is not astigmatic.

---

[13] By changing its shape, the lens of the eye focuses on near and far objects. This ability is known as accommodation. The ability of the eye lens to accommodate is greatest in childhood and decreases with age.

conditions. It can be corrected by specially ground lenses that will eliminate the distortions arising from this structure defect.

Vision Testing

Three main types of professional men specialize in matters concerning the eye; the optometrist, the ophthalmologist and the optician. The *optometrist* is a graduate of a school of optometry. He is licensed in all fifty states to measure how well one sees, to prescribe glasses, and to perform other non-medical measures. He is not a medical doctor and is therefore not trained to treat diseases of the eye.

The *ophthalmologist* (oculist) is a medical doctor who has specialized in ophthalmology. He is qualified to treat all conditions of the eye. He is licensed not only to measure how well one sees, but to treat diseases of the eye and to perform eye surgery.

An *optician* is the craftsman skilled in the grinding of lenses according to

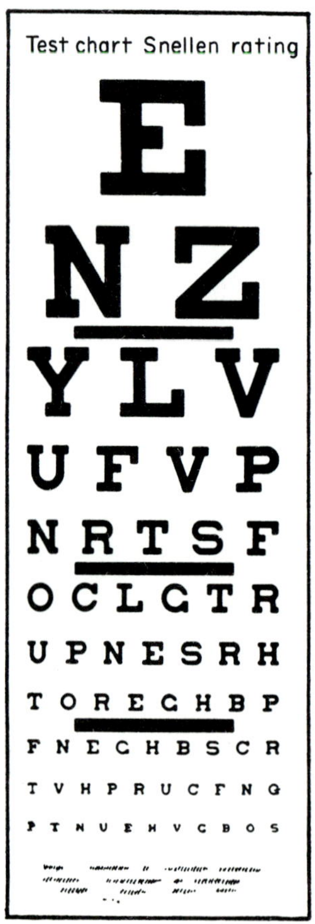

Figure 2–9

A Snellen chart.

(Bausch and Lomb Optical Co.)

the prescription of the ophthalmologist (oculist) or optometrist and in setting these lenses properly in frames.

The most common screening test used is the *Snellen Visual Acuity Test.* 20/20 vision on this test indicates normal vision and the ability to read letters of a given size at 20 feet. 20/40 vision refers to the ability to read letters of a larger size at 20 feet that the normal eye can read at 40 feet. Therefore, 20/200 vision represents the ability to read a letter of an even larger size at 20 feet when the normal eye can read it at 200 feet. This test can identify myopia when the individual's vision indicates visual acuity of 20/40 or more. It must be emphasized that the Snellen Visual Acuity Test is merely a screening device and for a complete eye examination one should see one's opthalmologist or optometrist.

Eyeglasses

Eyeglasses correct refractive errors to varying degrees while they are worn. A person who does not wear his glasses will not ruin his eyes any more than a person wearing them will cure his refractive error. The fact that you can see more clearly with them on seems to be reason enough to wear them.

Safety lenses are eyeglass lenses that have been heat-hardened by being exposed to a temperature of 1300 degrees F. The result is that the lenses will not break as easily, and should they be broken the edges of the broken lens will not be as sharp.

In 1970 the Food and Drug Administration announced its new regulation that all eyeglass lenses be made of either heat-tempered glass, laminated glass, or plastic. This regulation removed from the market lenses made of crown glass that shatters when broken into potentially blinding slivers. The thousands of cases of eye injury or blindness because of such lenses is well documented.

A further safety need that still remains is the production of flame-resistant eyeglass frames. While American manufacturers produce flame-resistant frames, foreign-made frames often are made of cellulose nitrate, a highly flammable material. Eyeglass frames made of this material can explode into flames by the person lighting a cigarette or merely leaning over a gas stove burner or barbecue.

Contact Lenses

The idea for the contact lens dates back to 1887, when an artificial eye manufacturer made a simple glass shell to fit over an eye whose lid had been removed. It was later discovered that a phenomenon known as surface tension could hold a properly shaped, moistened glass disk against the surface of the eye. Early experimentation with contacts was directed primarily to the scleral lenses. This larger type of contact lens covers not only the cornea, but most of the sclera (white of the eye). Scleral lenses are used by some individuals whose occupations might lend to the easy dislodging of the smaller corneal lenses. The corneal type contact lens covers the cornea and the iris that lies behind it (covering only the colored portion of the eye). Though the scleral lens has been greatly improved, the corneal lens is by far the more popular. These lenses have also been reduced in thickness to 4/1000 of an inch. With the advent of plastics in the early 1950s, and the concept of an individualized curved lens, comfort has increased and the popularity of contact lenses has soared.

The motivation for the use of contact lenses is usually to improve appearance. Contact lenses also offer advantages in certain occupations and activities. Surgeons, actors, musicians, policemen, and other outdoor workers may find them better than eyeglasses because they do not fog up or get wet in the rain or reflect stage lights. Contact lenses can also provide a better correction for severe nearsightedness than regular eyeglasses. They also correct corneal astigmatism more effectively because they replace the distorted surface of the cornea with a properly shaped one.

Research conducted by the Food and Drug Administration in 1964 and several independent studies published in medical journals have noted that numerous eye injuries result from the use of contact lenses. The difficulties are caused basically by improper fitting of lenses, unsanitary practices by the wearer resulting in infections, and wearing of the lenses for too long a time. A moment of forgetfulness, as in going to sleep without removing the lenses, can result in permanent damage to the eyes.

Because properly fitting lenses are of utmost importance if eye injury is to be avoided, identifying the skilled practitioners in this field is essential. The two kinds of professionals qualified to prescribe contact lenses are those selected ophthalmologists or optometrists who do a good deal of work in this area. These should be individuals who have had specific training in the fitting of contact lenses. When in doubt, a person may write to the Contact Lens Association of Ophthalmologists, 40 West 77th Street New York, New York 10024, or the American Optometric Association, 7000 Chippewa Street, St. Louis, Missouri 63119, for the name of an experienced practitioner in his area.

Regardless of how well a person may be fitted with contact lenses, not all people can wear them. People with chronic infection or inflammation of the eyes or eyelids are poor candidates. People with allergies or other disorders that make the eyes water would also do well to avoid them. There is a period of discomfort and adjustment that the wearer must go through in being fitted for these lenses. Contact lenses are, after all, foreign bodies that are placed in the eyes and they take some getting used to. It is during this initial period of use that close professional supervision is necessary. Pain that the wearer may experience can be normal reaction to the lenses or may be indicative of a poor fit, damage to the cornea, or a given person's inability to wear such lenses.

Sanitary handling of contact lenses is essential to avoid infection. Before each insertion, the wearer should wash his hands carefully and wash the lenses in a wetting agent and under tap water. After each removal, the lenses need to be stored in a special case.

The appearance of the *soft* contact lens in 1971 promised new hope.[14] The soft lens is made from a water-absorbing plastic that is soft and pliable when moist and hard and brittle when dry. They are slightly larger than the hard contact lenses (soft lenses range in diameter 12.3–15.5 millimeters; hard lenses range in diameter 8–10.2 millimeters) and are invisible on the eye. The soft lenses are more comfortable to use, particularly at the beginning. They do not fall out as easily as the hard contact lenses and they allow the individual to switch back to regular eyeglasses with little or no blurring of vision. They have been highly effective in treating diseases of the eye, either in using them as "bandages" for the cornea or by impregnating them with medication for the treatment of glaucoma. They have also been successfully used on infants and young children who underwent cataract surgery and could not tolerate the hard contact lenses.

The cost of the soft lens is about $100 more than the hard contact lens and up to $300 more than for regular eyeglasses. A major drawback with the current soft lenses is the nightly 15-minute sterilization procedure to keep the lenses free of bacteria. Another concern is the possibility that soft lenses might absorb harmful vapors or fumes from paint sprays, tear gas, smoke, hair spray, or industrial chemicals. If an individual without glasses came in contact with these harmful substances normally the flow of tears would quickly wash them away. However, with the soft contact lens, chemicals may be absorbed and held against the eye until the lens was removed.

Strabismus (Cross-eye)

The eyeballs are coordinated in their movements by a set of six muscles for each eye. When a muscle of the eye is not of balanced strength with its counterpart, it will cause a cross-eyed condition (strabismus). There is a hereditary factor associated with the condition. Strabismus occurs in varying degrees of intensity. In some instances, the condition is noted only when the eyes are tired, resulting in a slight wandering of one eye out of position. In the more severe forms, an eye is in a fixed inward or outward position, although there are other possibilities. As a result the person sees double or is said to have double vision. In order to avoid this annoying double vision the individual suppresses the vision of the crossed eye. Eventually, this will result in the loss of sight in this eye. Experience has shown that children do not outgrow this condition and that it should be treated early. If it is ignored until after eight years of age, considerable, if not complete, visual loss can be expected in the crossed eye. Strabismus can be corrected by prescribing special glasses, by exercising eye muscles, by placing a patch over the good eye (forcing the crossed eye to straighten), or by performing surgery on the eye muscles. When the child fails to receive early medical attention for strabismus, the resultant loss

[14] The following discussion of soft contact lenses has been adapted from "Soft Contact Lenses: They Have Their Limitations," *Consumer Reports* (Mount Vernon, N.Y.: Consumers Union, May 1972), pp. 272–278. Copyright © 1972 by Consumers Union.

of vision in one eye handicaps the individual in several ways. He will have a narrowed field of vision, a blind spot in the good eye that cannot be compensated for, and the inability to judge the distance of objects from oneself. Our depth perception, or the ability to judge distances is the result of two-eyed vision. To demonstrate this, one need only to place a book on its side. Closing one eye, attempt to bring the forefinger down on the front edge of the book. You will find that you can perform this task more accurately with both eyes open. In the late teens, some people have crossed eyes straightened for cosmetic reasons. This does not, however, correct the visual loss, which is usually considerable by this time, if not complete.

Detachment of the Retina

A conservative estimate is that one person in 20,000 suffers from a detachment of the retina. Two out of three cases occur in persons with a high degree of myopia. Blows to the head are also recognized as contributing factors.In the past, a detached retina meant blindness in the eye or eyes affected. At the present time there are several methods of treatment available. So-called "shallow" detachments may be treated by using the xenon arc or the laser beam. In more extensive detachments a variety of surgical techniques may be used. Critical to the success of any treatment procedure is the length of time that elapses from when the detachment occurs to when treatment is sought. The retina is basically made up of nerve tissue and constantly needs a source of nourishment if it is not to degenerate further.

Diseases of the Eye

Trachoma is a chronic infection of the lids caused by a filterable virus. This is the most widespread infection of the eye and the leading cause of blindness in the world. It is not prevalent in the United States, but can be found in countries with low standards of living and unsatisfactory sanitary conditions. It responds readily to sulfonamides and antibiotics. In the absence of treatment, the virus attacks the conjunctiva and cornea of the eye. The World Health Organization has been active in combating this disease by establishing community clinics, dispensing antibiotics, and educating the people in the endemic areas.

"Pink-Eye" is an infection or inflammation of the conjunctiva. It is an acute, highly contagious infection. It readily responds to treatment and can be cleared in two days or linger for two weeks if untreated, thereby remaining a source of infection for an extended period of time. Dust, smoke, and powders can also cause the inflammation of the conjunctiva. Because of its highly contagious nature, the use of a separate face towel is recommended.

Styes are caused by bacterial (staphylococcal) infections of the small glands on the margin of the eyelid. Repeated styes reflect a poor state of general health. Medical attention should be sought in such repetitive cases or when the stye becomes quite painful.

Cataract is the development of an opacity (cloudiness) of the eyelens or the capsule in which it is enclosed. It is *not* a growth. The disease often progresses slowly, and when the lens can no longer be seen through, vision is restored by the surgical removal of the lens. Eyeglasses are then used to replace the removed eye lens. Cataracts may be caused by injury or by diseases such as glaucoma, diabetes, and prenatal exposure to German measles. Two-thirds of occurring cataract conditions, however, are from unknown causes.

Glaucoma. There are two types of glaucoma: the acute type and the chronic. The acute type is characterized by sudden onset and extreme pain, with the eyeballs becoming stony hard. Surgery for this type of the disease must be performed promptly, usually within 24 to 48 hours in order to prevent blindness. The chronic or insidious version of the condition is the more common type. Symptoms include headaches, nausea, and the seeing of colored halos around lights. The symptoms are frequently vague and go unnoticed until irreversible damage to the retina has occurred. In glaucoma, increased fluid develops pressure within the eyeball which can cause the destruction of the retina and the optic nerve. This disease is a leading cause of blindness in the United States, despite the fact that we know how to detect the condition, treat it, and prevent the ensuing blindness. Early detection of glaucoma is important, because the progress of the disease can be arrested through treatment with drugs or surgery. It is estimated that 2 per cent of the population over 40 years of age has developing glaucoma. The incidence tends to rise sharply in the 50- to 60-year-old age groups. Periodic examination of the eyes by an ophthalmologist should include the testing of fluid pressure with a tonometer. This is recommended as a preventive measure, particularly for people over 40.

Color Vision

Defective color vision (color blindness) results from the inability of the cones of the retina to perceive all colors. The degree of this inability varies from complete color blindness to difficulty distinguishing one shade of color from another. The defect is hereditary, with 1 male out of every 25 and 1 female out of every 200 affected. There is no way of correcting the defect. Color perception tests are usually administered in schools to determine if defective color vision is present and to what degree. The most common color vision defect found is the inability to distinguish red from green; blue-yellow defective perception is the next most common. Defective color vision can be an inhibiting factor where employment is concerned. Occupations in which the ability to identify color accurately is important are best avoided by people with this defect.

Sunglasses

Sunglasses may be worn to diminish discomfort from sunlight of high intensity. They should not be worn to eliminate headlight glare, because when they are worn at twilight or in darkness they can blot out enough vision to

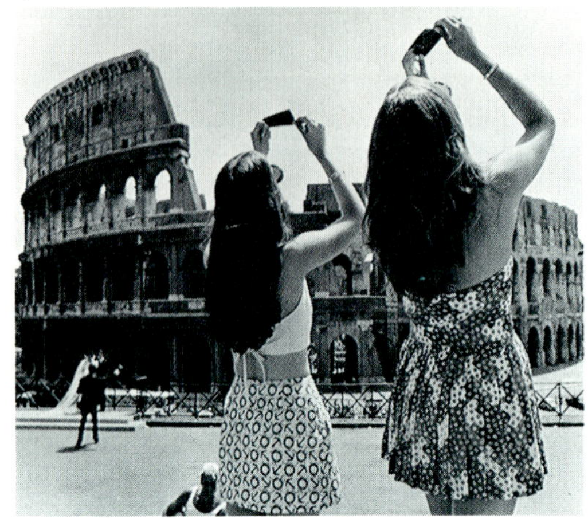

Figure 2–10

Viewing an eclipse through sunglasses, film negatives, or smoked glass does not protect the eyes from the damaging rays of the sun.

[United Press International (UPI)]

constitute a safety hazard. The constant use of sunglasses can limit one's ability to tolerate light. Should a person develop the symptoms of photophobia (the inability to tolerate light), it is an indication that medical attention is needed, not sunglasses. Looking directly into the sun even with sunglasses can result in serious damage to the eyes. In spite of warnings via the mass media before each eclipse of the sun, a number of persons do damage to their eyes by looking at the sun through sunglasses or smoked glass. The safest way to watch an eclipse of the sun is via the television set.

The Visually Handicapped

A person whose vision is 20/70 or less in the good eye after correction (i.e., with eyeglasses) is considered to be visually handicapped. Children whose visual acuity falls into this category are often placed in special classes. They are provided with books with larger print, are taught to use a typewriter early, and in all ways provided a setting that will best facilitate learning.

Blindness is often regarded as the complete loss of sight. *Legal blindness,* however, is commonly defined as 20/200 vision in the good eye after correction, or loss of 80% or more of the visual field. The latter condition is often referred to as tunnel vision. Though a person with tunnel vision may have 20/20 vision in his narrowed visual field, he is considered to be blind.

The adjustments of the blind to their handicap need to be made so they may function adequately. Even everyday tasks such as preparing meals and moving about one's home require learning. The ability of the blind to travel on foot or via public transportation is important if the blind person is to travel, to work, shop, or visit friends. The blind must also be taught work skills so they can successfully compete on the job market. The handicap of blindness should not be permitted to extend into the ability of a person to maintain financial and personal independence.

Though a great deal has been written and said about the blind and their adjustment to their handicap, little has been said about the poor adjustment made by seeing people to the blind. People often seem to be so overwhelmed with the handicap that they become "blind" themselves to the personality before them. The greatest loss of the blind is often not their vision, but normal interrelationships with "normal" people.

Eye Banks

Eye banks have significantly contributed to the reduction of blindness due to damaged corneas. People wishing to contribute their corneas to a blind person need to register with an eye bank sometime during their lives. After the death of a donor, the cornea is removed and within a matter of a few days transplanted to the person in need. Not all transplant operations are successful. A bodily response to injury is to grow small blood vessels in the area to heal the wound. When the "wound" is corneal surgery, the small blood vessels that occasionally grow into the area will cover the new cornea, thus blocking the vision once more. This reaction is called vascularization.

A corneal transplant whereby a clear, healthy cornea replaces a damaged one will restore vision to an affected person. This act literally becomes the gift of sight. Donating one's eyes in a will is not recommended because by the time the will is read, tissues of the cornea are beyond use. Registration with an eye bank is the recommended procedure.

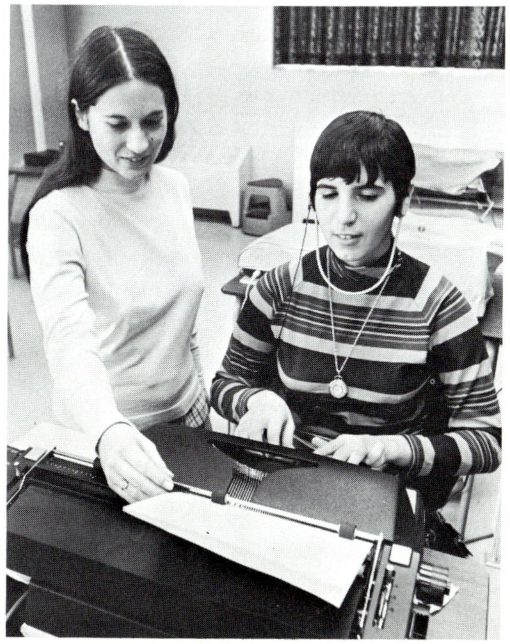

Figure 2–11

A blind student, with her instructor looking on, is typing a letter being transcribed via a dictaphone. Being a typist is one of many occupational skills a blind person can learn.

(The Northeastern Rehabilitation Center for the Blind and Visually Handicapped. Albany Association of the Blind Inc.)

HEARING

The sense of hearing, though obviously valued by people, is probably underrated in its importance. Our ability to communicate with others depends on it more than on any other of our senses. The loss of hearing immediately transforms the world around us into one of silence and isolates the individual. If one were to sit quietly and listen to all the background noises in the environment (whether in an office of a busy city or sitting on a stump in a wooded area), one would become aware of the many noises one hears but is often not conscious of. We live in a world of sound—sound that is not only a means of communication, but may be a warning of danger, a gauge of emotions, or a spark of humor. The familiar sounds often envelop us in a cloak of security. The ear is the mechanism that serves as the vehicle for this major means of communication. Let us examine its care and functioning.

Noise and Hearing Loss

Noise pollution is best described as unwanted sound. Besides being annoying, loud noise over a period of time can cause permanent and irreversible damage to the auditory nerve. Federal and state health and safety codes have set 90 decibels as the maximum level of noise that workers should be exposed to without wearing ear protection. To maintain a lower noise level, industry has in many instances redesigned machinery or modified manufacturing processes. When noise levels exceed 90 decibels, ear protection in the form of earplugs or earmuffs are worn.

Concern in recent years has been expressed by hearing specialists with regard to hearing loss caused by electronically amplified music. Rock music groups can produce sound at the level of 120 decibels if you are 4 to 6 feet from them. This is well above what is considered a safe level of sound. It is estimated that 10 per cent of those who expose themselves to music of that loudness will not have their hearing effected. Ninety per cent will suffer from significant hearing loss at least temporarily. Permanent hearing loss will occur for some listening to loud music for a week or two. For others it may take a year of exposure before permanent damage is effected. Tests show that hearing losses occur in the high frequency speech range. This is similar to the hearing losses experienced by older people who urge others to stop mumbling and to speak up!

The Nature of Hearing Loss

The usual concept is that people either have the ability to hear or are deaf. The many gradations of hearing and types of hearing loss are generally overlooked.

Sound is measured in terms of two basic qualities: its loudness, measured

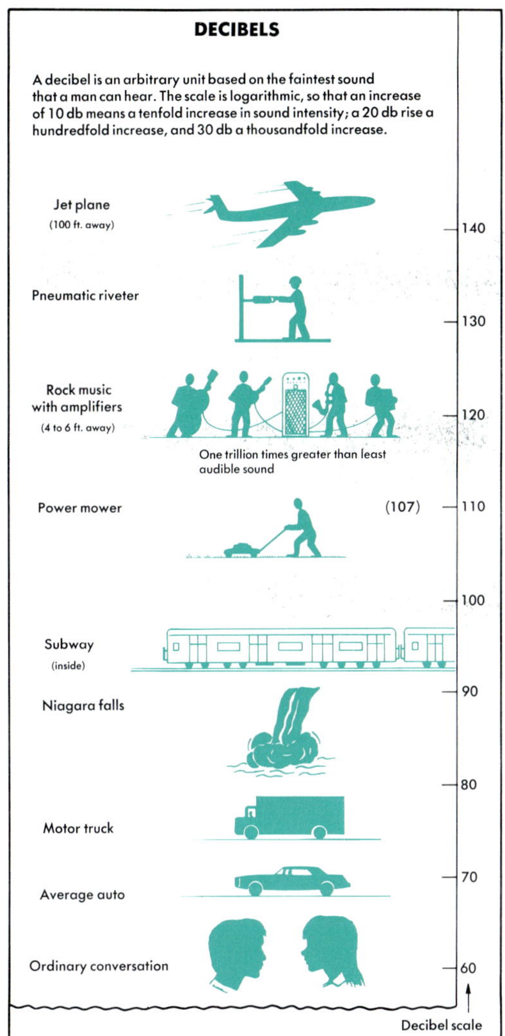

Figure 2–12

Human hearing: schematic representation of intensity and frequency characteristics of the human ear and loudness of sounds.

in terms of *decibels* of sound; and its pitch, measured in terms of sound wave *frequencies.* In measuring one's hearing acuity, an instrument called an audiometer is used. Its function is to detect a person's ability to hear sounds of various frequencies (pitches). When a sound of a given pitch cannot be heard at normal decibel (loudness) level, then the audiometer measures how much louder that sound must be before it is heard. In effect, the person's hearing can be measured and then charted in a diagram known as an audiogram. Specific types of hearing loss are thus identified.

A *conductive hearing loss* is due to a malfunction of one of the conductive

The Human Ear

The **middle ear** consists of the eardrum (or tympanic membrane), the three ear ossicles or bones (hammer, anvil, and stirrup), and the eustachian tube. The function of the middle ear is to carry sound waves received from the auditory canal to the inner ear.

The pinna, the external part of the outer ear, serves to catch sound and send it into the auditory canal.

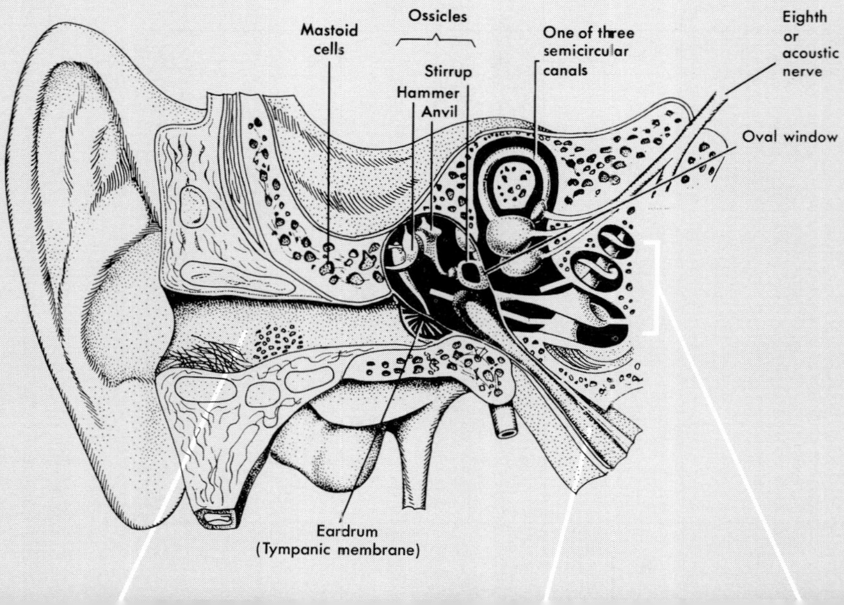

Mastoid cells
Ossicles
Stirrup
Hammer
Anvil
One of three semicircular canals
Eighth or acoustic nerve
Oval window
Eardrum (Tympanic membrane)

The **inner ear** is made up of the semicircular canals and the cochlea. The semicircular canals do not have a hearing function, but serve to give us our sense of balance. They can be troublesome when overstimulated by plane, car, or boat travel causing motion sickness. Drugs such as dramamine are available for the control of this ailment.

Hearing loss due to inner ear malfunction can be precipitated by a number of causes. Diseases such as measles, scarlet fever, and syphilis (congenital or acquired) can damage the inner ear, as well as circulatory disturbances and loud noises.

Inside the **auditory canals** are the glands that produce cerumen, or ear wax. The cerumen not only helps to keep inquisitive insects out of the ears but also has an antiseptic action. Sometimes an oversecretion of ear wax may affect the hearing ability of an individual. In such cases, it should be removed by a physician. Attempts to remove excess ear wax with hairpins or matchsticks may not only push the wax further back into the canal, but may result in damage to the walls of the auditory canal and possible puncture of the eardrum.

The **eustachian tube** connects the middle ear to the back of the throat and keeps the air pressure on the inside of the eardrum equal to that on the outside. This permits the eardrum to vibrate properly when sound waves strike it. Anything inhibiting the vibration of the eardrum will affect hearing. Because of the position of the eustachian tube, throat infections can migrate up through it to the middle ear. Blowing of the nose too vigorously when one has a cold can force infectious material into the middle ear, with resulting fuzzy sensation in the ears. Blow gently with both nostrils open!

The second structure of the inner ear, the **cochlea,** is a snail-shaped structure that is filled with fluid into which project nerve endings. Vibrations received from the stapes (stirrup) of the middle ear set this fluid into motion which in turn stimulates the nerve endings. Some nerve endings pick up high-pitched sounds, while others are sensitive to low-pitched sounds. These thousands of nerve endings come together to form the auditory nerve carrying the sound to the brain for interpretation. Damage to the auditory (eighth) nerve is sometimes due to the side effects of drugs such as salicylates, quinine, and streptomycin. Physicians are, of course, aware of these drug side effects and prescribe them judiciously.

Middle ear infection (otitis media) is a leading cause of hearing loss in young people. Infection can damage the ear ossicles, and in some cases completely destroy them. Infectious fluid can also build up in the middle ear cavity. If this is not relieved by medical attention, it may break through the eardrum and result in a draining or ''running'' ear. A good rule to follow is to have all earaches checked by a physician. The self-medicating use of heat, oils, or other things may relieve the pain but not the infection, and does not prevent ensuing damage.

Damaged eardrums can now be replaced surgically. A surgeon may use the eardrum of a donor as well as the ear bones if necessary and replace the damaged parts of the middle ear. This procedure has been highly successful in restoring hearing to the normal range.

parts of the ear (outer or middle ear). It usually results in the person's having difficulty hearing the low-pitched sounds (vowel sounds).

In the *neural (nerve) type of hearing loss,* the nerve endings in the inner ear are damaged, and the person usually has difficulty hearing the high-pitched sounds (consonant sounds).

There are instances of a *mixed hearing loss,* where both a conductive and a neural loss are present, with the result that the person has difficulty with both high- and low-pitched sounds.

When emotional problems affect a person's hearing, it is said that the individual is suffering from a *psychogenic hearing loss.* This would be part of a neurotic behavior pattern and is not to be confused with inattentiveness. Although there is nothing organically wrong with the ear, the person does not hear. Distinguishing a psychogenic hearing loss from a loss faked by a malingerer seeking disability compensation poses problems for specialists who measure hearing. A number of effective tests, however, have been developed for this purpose.

Hearing Specialists

An Otologist is a medical doctor who specializes in the care and treatment of disorders of the ear and hearing.

The Audiologist is a highly specialized technician trained to measure hearing acuity with the use of such instruments as audiometers and is usually certified by the American Speech and Hearing Association (ASHA).

The Otorhinolaryngologist is a medical doctor who specializes in the care and treatment of disorders of the ear, nose, and throat.

When hearing loss is suspected, competent professional help should be sought. One should start with the family physician or seek out an otologist. Speech and hearing centers are available in some larger communities. The audiologist will many times be called in by the physician for additional diagnostic help. Some confusion arises between the ASHA (American Speech and Hearing Association) Certified Audiologist and the Hearing Aid Audiologist. The latter is either a hearing aid salesman or works for one and does not have the in-depth training and education that the ASHA Certified Audiologist has. Only after careful examination and testing can an accurate diagnosis and possible course of treatment be prescribed. Treatment may include a wide variety of possibilities: medication to clear up an infection; a stapes mobilization operation; speech reading (lip reading); speech therapy (particularly where hearing loss has affected the speech development of young children); or the use of a hearing aid.

Hearing Aids

Hearing aids should be purchased on prescription very much the way eyeglasses are. They should be prescribed by an otologist with the possible consultation of an audiologist. The type, cause, and severity of the hearing loss will help determine the nature of the hearing aid prescribed.

Hearing aids are of two basic types and work on the principle of air conduction or bone conduction. *Air conduction* hearing aids send sound through its normal route via the auditory canal. *Bone conduction* hearing aids send sound directly into the inner ear usually via the mastoid bone located behind the ear. They are used when the conductive parts of the ear are not functional. Hearing aids also vary with regard to their power. Small hearing aids, such as the type that can fit into the ear canal, are usually adequate for moderate hearing losses. They are not powerful enough, however, for the more severe losses. Some people are inclined to shout at those who wear aids, overlooking the obvious fact that the hearing aid is already amplifying their voices.

A major objection to the use of hearing aids used to be their size and weight. With the introduction of transistors, these instruments can now be placed in eyeglass frames, or even be worn as a barrette in a woman's hair. The tendency is still to hide the hearing aid. We have, to a very great extent, overcome this negativism with regard to the use of eyeglasses, and it is to be hoped the acceptance of hearing aids will soon follow.

The Psychological Aspects of Hearing Loss

Those who have severe hearing loss or deafness have more than just an auditory loss to deal with. Their relations with others can be seriously affected. While blindness evokes a sympathetic reaction, deafness many times stimulates an opposite kind of response in people. Severe hearing loss or deafness tends to cut off the major means of communication and serves to isolate the individual. The person sometimes becomes suspicious of the motives of others, with ensuing effects on personality and sociability. The person who does not hear cannot use his ears for cues to danger in the environment, such as a siren, a whistle, or a car horn. He uses his eyes for this purpose and must be ever alert to changes in light and movement. We have a responsibility to help those with hearing losses to make good adjustment to their handicap by contributing when possible to the emotional security of these individuals.

To Hear or Not to Hear

A flute player impressed with his own music, claimed that even wild animals could be tamed by his tunes. To test his ability he went to the wilds of Africa, where his playing delighted the natives assembled in the small village. He was convinced his tunes would have a calming effect on the wild beasts and despite the warnings of the village natives he went forth into the jungle.

He soon met a hyena, ravenous for food. Just as it was about to spring upon him, a few melodious flute notes turned the animal into putty. Down it sat to listen.

Next came an elephant charging with fury. But the strains of music stopped the beast in his tracks. He sat down beside the hyena enraptured by the music.

Then came a great ferocious killer, the king of all jungle beasts. The natives fled in horror. The lion licked his chops as he approached the

> flute player, who, overconfident from success, played with a talent greater than ever.
>
> With the hyena and the elephant watching, the lion pounced on the flute player and devoured him forthwith. Looking with scorn on the other two animals, the lion sat down to digest his meal.
>
> The elephant was the first to speak: "Why did you do such a thing? Didn't you see how we were enjoying the wonderful music?"
>
> Whereupon the lion raised his big paw to his ear and bellowed: "What did you say?"
>
> —Adapted from *Hearing—A Handbook for Laymen,* by Norton Canfield, M.D. Doubleday & Co., 1959, p. 213.

Perhaps the moral of the story is that blindness tends to evoke sympathetic reactions from others because the handicap is obvious to them. A cane, dark glasses, or a seeing eye dog is evidence of the handicap. Hearing loss or deafness is often not visible. When someone with a severe hearing loss does not respond to speech or sound, we are surprised, or annoyed . . . and sometimes devoured!

DENTAL AND ORAL HEALTH

Dental and oral disease is an almost universal problem. By the age of 16, the average youth has seven to 8 decayed, filled, or missing teeth. By 45 years of age, the average adult has lost half of his teeth. The American Dental Association has reported surveys estimating that there is a backlog of 700 million unfilled cavities among Americans. There are over 100 million people who have suffered tooth loss because of diseases of the gum or supporting structures.

There are many factors related to tooth decay. Controlling the intake and frequency of refined carbohydrates is particularly important if tooth decay is to be minimized. Children should *not* be rewarded with lollipops, hard candies, or caramels whose sugary influence remains in the saliva and on the teeth for a long time. It would also be wise to break the habit of continuous eating. It is of little value to brush one's teeth after lunch and then accept some chocolate candy five minutes later. Another factor in tooth decay is the individual's heredity or the composition of one's saliva that makes up the environment surrounding the teeth. The degree of decay proceeds at different rates in different people.

In addition, tooth decay has been related to the presence of oral bacteria which react with carbohydrates (particularly refined sugars and starches). This interaction results in the production of organic acids that will dissolve the enamel of the tooth and thus start cavities. Dental plaques, a gelatinlike film that sticks to the teeth, can act as protective mediums for oral bacteria. Proper cleaning of the teeth will help temporarily to remove dental plaques.

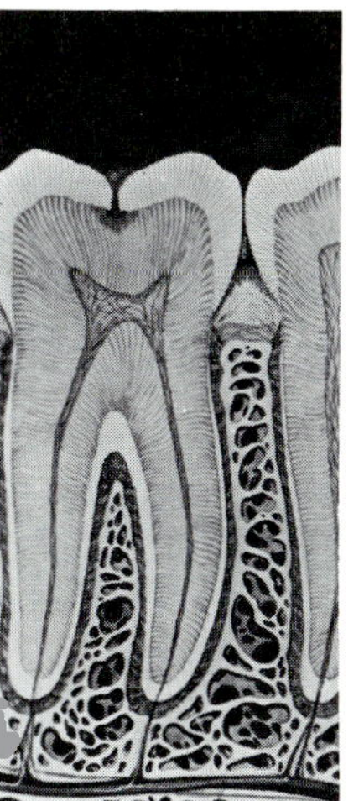
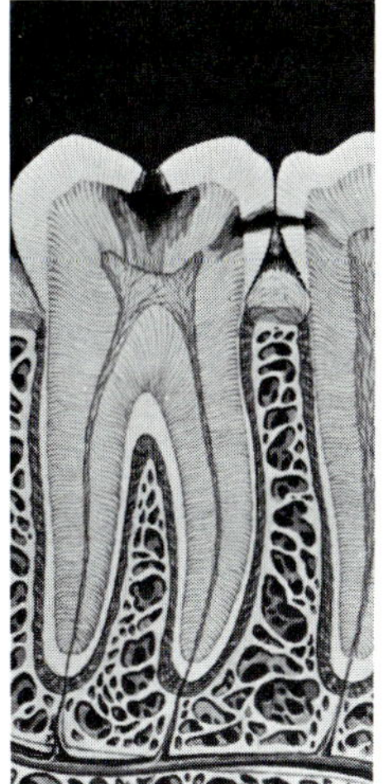
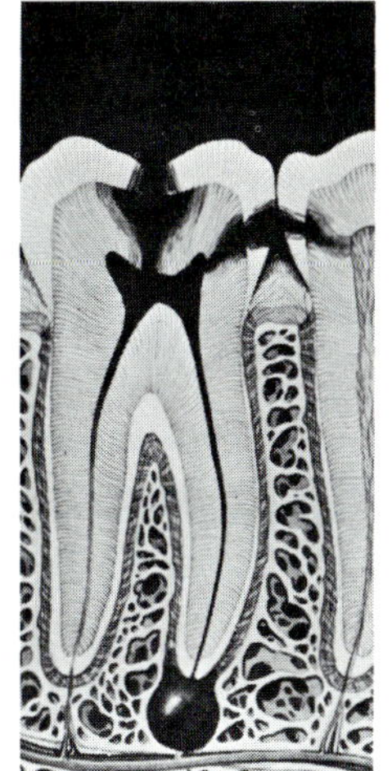
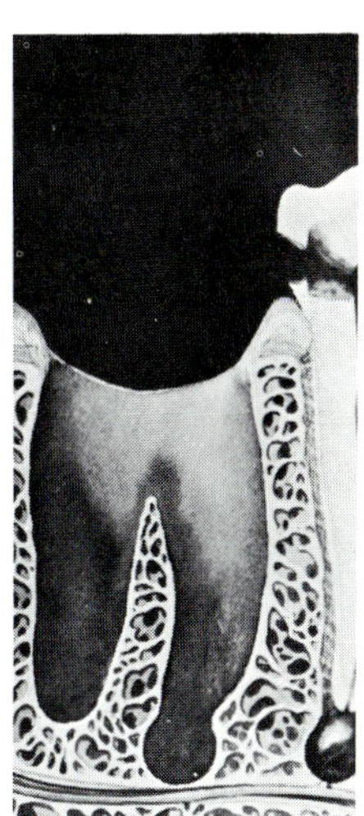

Figure 2–13

Progress of tooth decay.

(Copyright by the American Dental Association. Reprinted by permission.)

Probably the most important factors in tooth decay are the level of oral hygiene (brushing and flossing) one maintains and the quality of professional dentistry he seeks. In situations where one cannot brush after eating, particularly sweets, rinsing the mouth with water might help prevent cavities. In addition to brushing one's teeth correctly and using dental floss to get into the crevices between teeth, it is advised to have a dentist or dental hygienist remove tartar that may form on the teeth. This cleaning or prophylaxis should take place at the interval suggested by the dentist.

Periodontal Diseases

These diseases of the gums represent the major cause of tooth loss in adults over 35. More than 70 percent of all Americans suffer from these disorders by the age of 50, with almost all being affected by the age of 75. A number of factors can contribute to disease of the gum; among them are malocclusion (malocclusion by irregularly positioned teeth can often precipitate periodontal disease by causing undue pressure on some teeth, entrapping food debris, and creating a chronic gum irritation), bacteria and their products, dental plaque, and vitamin C deficiency. Its major cause is usually tartar (calculus) that accumulates on the teeth. Tartar is a crusty deposit that can irritate the gums. The chronic irritation of the gum tissues leaves them prone to infection which attacks the periodontal membrane and bone which support the tooth. The tooth is then without support. Some people who have had little or no tooth decay lose their teeth to periodontal disease.

Through early diagnosis by the dentist, and *proper,* daily brushing of teeth, periodontal disease is minimized. If periodontal disease has developed, the dentist may refer the patient to a periodontist. The periodontist will treat the infected gum tissue and recommend home care. He may utilize gingivectomy (surgical removal of gum tissue) as a treatment.

Malocclusion

The irregularity of tooth position or a "poor bite" (improper fitting together of teeth when the jaw is closed) is malocclusion. There are two general types of causes for this condition, namely those that are hereditary in nature and those that are acquired.

Hereditary factors include dental arches of inadequate size and primary teeth that are shed too early or retained too long. Acquired malocclusion may result from thumb-sucking or the early loss of primary or permanent teeth with the resultant drifting of some teeth out of position. The prevention of early tooth loss can prevent malocclusion and subsequent periodontal disease. Early dental care is therefore important to long-term dental health.

The *orthodontist* is the dental specialist who treats malocclusion. Through a variety of treatment methods, he brings teeth and jaws into proper relationship. Malocclusion can be corrected even in adults, although there are advantages to treating the problem at an earlier time.

Figure 2–14

Malocclusion before and after treatment.

(Copyright by the American Dental Association. Reprinted by permission.)

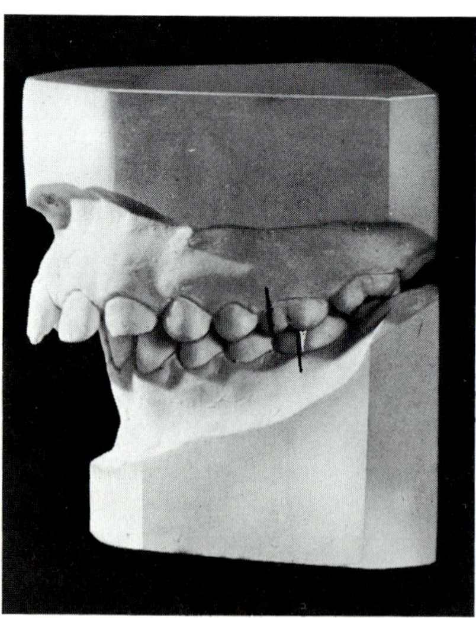

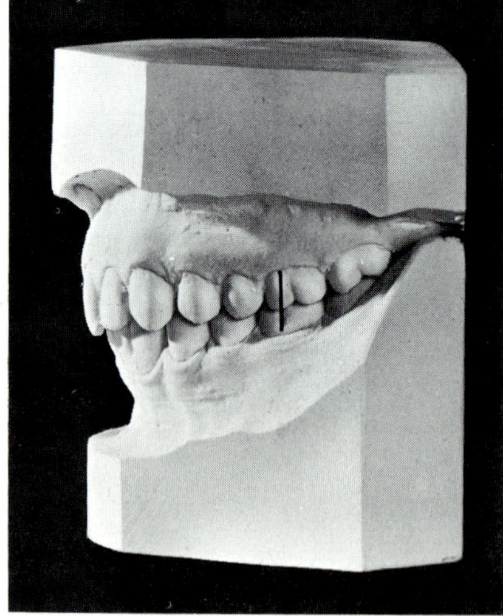

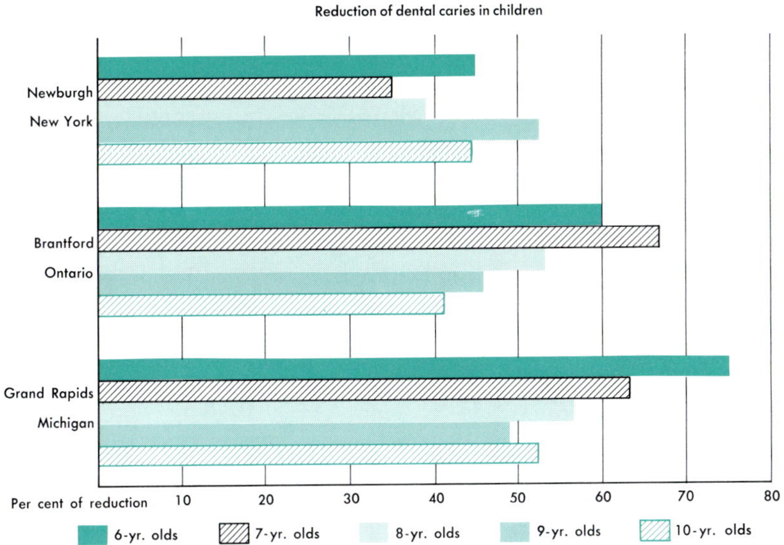

Figure 2–15

Reduction of dental caries in permanent teeth of children in continuous residence in three areas after ten years of fluoridation.

(Copyright by the American Dental Association. Reprinted by permission.)

Fluorides and Tooth Decay

Minute amounts of fluorides used in various ways have been found to be remarkably effective in preventing tooth decay. When one part fluoride is added to every million parts of drinking water, dental caries experience is reduced by about 65 per cent in children who drink fluoridated water from birth. Several fluoridation programs have been in effect for more than twenty years, consistently substantiating their contributions to dental health. Over 1300 communities in the United States have now had programs of this type for over ten years.

The manner in which fluorides work is not completely understood. It is generally believed that they combine with the tooth enamel to make it harder and more resistant to decay.

Where communities do not yet fluoridate their drinking water, other means may be utilized to give children the benefits of fluorides. The dentist can give topical applications of a fluoride solution. Tablets that contain appropriate amounts of fluoride can also be given to children from birth up to completion of the development of the second molars. A fluoridated dentifrice can also be used. Although these methods of fluoride use are helpful, they do not decrease the amount of tooth decay as effectively as fluoridation of the water supply. In addition, research has shown a beneficial supplemental effect of fluorides when added to those obtained in the water supply.

Almost all of our major cities use fluoridated drinking water. This public health measure is strongly endorsed by the major health organizations in the United States. In spite of this, there is still opposition by sincere, but misinformed people to proposals for the fluoridation of drinking water. Those in the community who are uninformed with regard to the safety and effectiveness of fluorides are often confused by the opposition. The result is usually a delay in the implementation of a much-needed public health program.

PROBLEMS OF THE FOOT

The layman's concept of foot problems usually starts with corns and callouses and ends with bunions and ingrowing nails. However, problems related to feet stem from many and varied causes. They can be congenital, hereditary or neurogenic in nature, as well as metabolic, infectious, traumatic, or environmental.

It seems ironic that about 99 per cent of us are born with perfect feet, but all too soon develop foot problems. It is documented that many of our schoolchildren already are plagued with foot ailments. During childhood the foot is a pliable structure reacting to many stresses and strains. As the child grows, the foot becomes sturdier. It is during this period that the child's feet must be carefully observed and protected, for they can be distorted, made weak, and deformed. Very often these deformities are imposed by well-meaning, but uninformed mothers and shoe salesmen. Some babies spend their entire infancy in stretch suits that could serve as a toe-curling device if the size of the garment is not checked periodically. Booties and socks on infants should be loose and floppy. Some physicians are convinced that crooked shoes are being put on straight feet. In one instance a toddler toed in when walking in his "high, sturdily built, good supporting, expensive shoe." When the shoe was removed the child walked straight. The shoe's structure was such that although it looked straight, the forefoot pointed inward. The physician's advice was for the child to walk barefoot where there was no danger of injury to his feet, but if protection was needed, for the child to wear a soft shoe or sneaker. The misconception that the lace-up oxford-type shoe will prevent foot deformities still persists, even though most physicians feel that if the foot is normal there is no need for rigid special supports.

Clubfoot is a congenital malformation (that is, a baby is born with it) in which the tendons of the foot are misplaced and turn the foot in at an awkward angle. Years ago, a person born with this affliction went through life with an unattractive limp. Today, when the condition is recognized at birth a plaster cast is applied to the foot soon thereafter. The casts are changed frequently as the foot assumes a more normal position. In some cases where the foot does not respond, surgery may be performed by an orthopedist to correct the condition. An orthopedist may also treat pigeon toes (or metatarsus adductus) early in a child's life when the bones are still soft and pliable. Here again casts are used to urge a more correct position of the foot.

Those Environmental Factors

Foot troubles can also arise from *environmental factors* such as overweight, overwork, ill-fitting shoes, tight hosiery, and abuse or neglect of the foot. A great offender of these environmental factors seems to be ill-fitting shoes. Since 80 per cent of podiatry patients are women, one would suspect that women are driven by the dictates of fashion into shoes that are incorrectly shaped for their feet. The habitual use of high-heeled shoes shifts the body weight forward to the metatarsal heads, almost completely eliminating the heel as one of the weight-bearing points. The foot is also pushed forward so that the toes are shoved into the narrow toe area. An additional result of the constant wearing of high heels is that the calf muscles will shorten and the person experiences discomfort in the calf of the leg when wearing flat shoes or goes barefoot.

Sneakers have finally been redeemed. The idea that sneakers caused flat feet has been a part of our culture for too long. Likewise the idea that arch supports will *correct* flat feet has flourished from generation to generation. Actually very little is known as to the causes of a flattened longitudinal arch (officially known as pes planus). Many people with flat feet suffer no foot pain and have full range of use. After many years of treating flat feet with steel arch supports (now plastic) some physicians are beginning to question this form of treatment for fallen arches.

The rule of thumb on shoes is comfort, not price. A soft shoe with low heal and a wide space in front for uncramped toes is what most podiatrists and physicians are recommending.

The new phenomenon of not wearing any shoes among our teenagers and young adults has stirred some mixed feelings. Some shopkeepers feel compelled to publicly display signs prohibiting the entrance of bare footed individuals for "sanitary" reasons. The barefoot ones themselves see and feel the disadvantages of bare feet on city streets. The pounding of the pavements on an unprotected sole is very tiring, to say nothing of the fungus infections, the cut toes, and the burning from hot pavements. Many physicians contend, however, that "walking barefoot on softer surfaces—sand and earth—is still considered the best of foot exercises for young and *old*."[15] With some reservations, physicians welcome the barefoot trend as the end of years of foot constrictions that led to bunions, hammer toes, corns, and aching feet.

[15] "Shooting Out Myths About Footwear," *Today's Health* (May 1971), p. 34.

REVIEW QUESTIONS

1 What appear to be the answers to our declining levels of physical fitness?

2 Why is hyperopia in children a lesser problem than myopia?

3 Eyeglasses are corrective, but do *not* cure visual defects. Explain.

4 What are some of the dangers involved in the use of contact lenses? How may these difficulties be minimized?

5 What kinds of visual problems are associated with strabismus? How can this condition be corrected?

6 Why is glaucoma an unnecessary cause of blindness?

7 What are some of the limitations that should be observed in the use of sunglasses?

8 Describe the operation of an eye bank. What kind of blindness does it serve to correct?

9 What are the common causes of hearing loss in the middle ear?

10 How do various types of hearing loss differ? What implications do these differences have for hearing aids used to correct them?

11 Define: (1) otologist, (2) audiologist, (3) otorhinolaryngologist.

12 What are the sociopsychological implications of hearing loss?

13 What have been the contributions of fluorides to the prevention of tooth decay?

14 What are the relationships of malocclusion to periodontal disease?

15 What are some of the environmental factors that contribute to foot problems?

16 What changes have been taking place in the nature of our nutritional problems? To what extent are some of our new nutritional problems the result of overcorrecting for some of our former problems?

17 What are some of the typical approaches used by the modern-day food faddists?

18 What protection is provided the public from the food faddist? Evaluate the effectiveness of this protection.

19 What is the role of education as a means of combating food faddism?

20 Describe the dramatic changes that have been brought about by the introduction of food additives.

21 How did the purposes of the early food additives differ from those of the most recent ones?

22 In what way does the Federal Food, Drug and Cosmetic Act protect the health of the consumer? What are the provisions of the major amendments to this law?

23 What are the factors that make the problem of weight control difficult and complex?

24 Why do so many attempts at dieting fail?

25 Why has quackery in the area of weight control been so successful?

26 What particular nutritional problems do poor Americans face?

3. Disease Prevention & Control

SINCE HIS EARLIEST DAYS man has always been plagued with the trauma of disease. With the discovery of the microbe, he has made significant progress in counteracting these diseases caused by "germs." To date, man has been less successful with those disorders referred to as the chronic and degenerative diseases. Such maladies as heart disease, cancer, genetic diseases, and arthritis among others have emerged as the leading causes of death and disability. Their causes are more related to one's life-style, environmental factors and one's genetics rather than to microorganisms. The rapidly developing knowledge with regard to these disorders has become a challenge to the individual and society to use this new information so that we may live better and longer.

THE COMMUNICABLE DISEASES

In spite of the success against communicable diseases that man has achieved, he has failed to eradicate a single disease. Every communicable disease ever known to man still exists today in some part of the world. Though man's progress with this kind of health problem cannot be measured by his ability to eradicate disease, there are other means of measuring his success.

A comparison of long-term mortality rates from selected communicable diseases illustrates the dramatic downward trend in the number of deaths from these diseases. Similarly, a decreasing incidence of a particular illness suggests that a measure of control has been achieved. Smallpox is perhaps the most vivid example of a communicable disease that has been effectively controlled in our country. Widespread immunization programs and increased public awareness are undoubtedly the essential factors in the changing status of smallpox in the United States. In 1972, the U.S. Public Health Service issued a historic recommendation that routine smallpox vaccinations be discontinued in this country. This decision was based on the fact that the risk of complications from the vaccinations now outweigh the probability of a person contracting the disease.

To emphasize further the point that control of a disease does not imply eradication, one need only glance at the morbidity and mortality data relative to poliomyelitis over the past few years. In 1954 there were 38,476 cases of poliomyelitis reported and 1,368 deaths resulting from the disease. Following the development of the first successful vaccine in 1954–55, by Dr. Jonas Salk, and the perfecting of the first live-virus vaccine by Dr. Albert B. Sabin in 1961, an abrupt change in the poliomyelitis patterns became evident in this country. By 1963 the number of cases of this disease was reduced to 449, with only 27 deaths. A milestone was reached in 1969 when for the first time no fatalities due to polio were recorded and with only 21 cases of the disease reported in 1971. A surprise outbreak of polio occurred in 1972 at a school in Greenwich, Connecticut.

> The private coeducational school—whose 129 pupils are for the most part Christian Scientists—was the scene of the most serious outbreak of paralytic polio in the United States in the last seven years. Eleven students are suffering the symptoms of the disease, and at least four have been partially paralyzed. And all the stricken youngsters—as well as most of the student body—had never been immunized against polio because of their parents' religious beliefs. . . . After parents agreed to have their children vaccinated in an emergency mass immunization session, the health officials decided not to quarantine the school, and classes continued in a relatively relaxed atmosphere.[1]

The American Academy of Pediatrics has warned that immunization efforts are lagging. They estimate that 50 per cent of inner-city children have not been vaccinated against polio. Obviously, if we are to continue our remarkable control over poliomyelitis, efforts to encourage mass immunization of the public must be continued.

Despite these impressive achievements, a number of diseases such as hepatitis, influenza, and pneumonia are still taking their toll. Venereal disease in recent years has become epidemic, even though effective treatment for these diseases was discovered over a quarter of a century ago.

[1] "Polio: The Price Paid by Believers," *New York Times,* October 29, 1972.

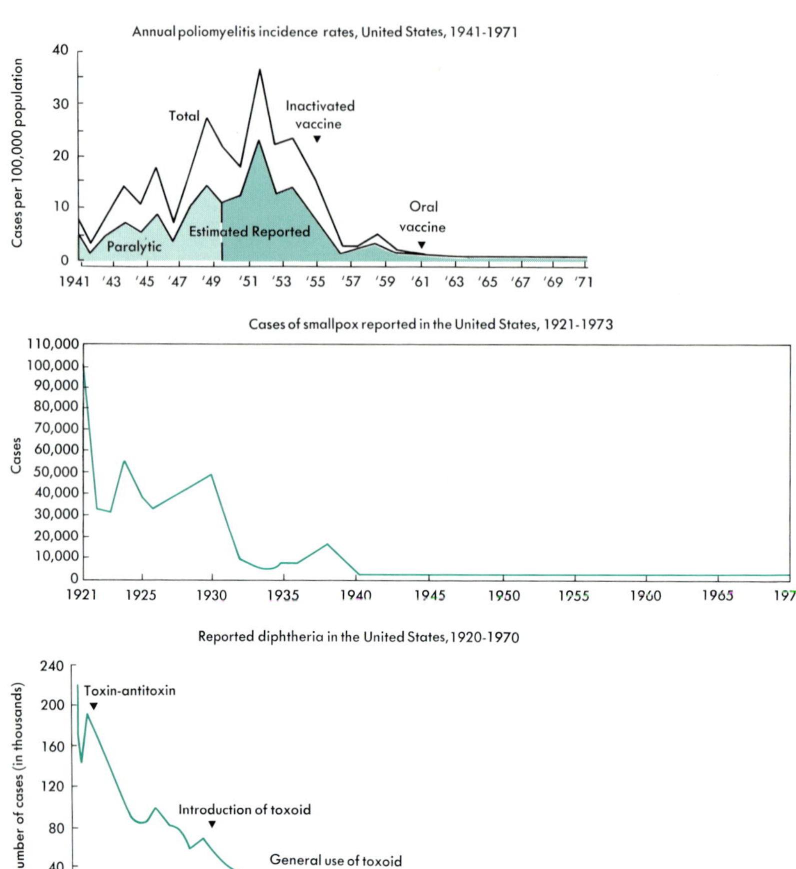

Figure 3–1

Vaccines have nearly eliminated these major diseases in the United States.

(Center for Disease Control)

If one takes a broader view of communicable diseases and considers their international significance, it becomes apparent that in many regions of the world, smallpox, plague, cholera, and other diseases persist as leading causes of death and human misery. These diseases prevail in areas where the scientific knowledge which would enable them to understand, control, and change their environment is lacking. National and international efforts are being made to eliminate these communicable disease conditions the world over. However, our concerns here are primarily with those diseases of a communicable nature which appear to be most prevalent and/or problematical in our nation today. Attention will be directed toward that group of diseases that presents the most serious threat to the young adult.

TERMINOLOGY OF THE COMMUNICABLE DISEASES

Familiarity with terms frequently used in any formal discussion of diseases is essential if the student is to develop understanding of the subject. These terms may at first seem cumbersome, but will soon prove to be invaluable as your acquaintance with the subject broadens.

Communicable disease is illness caused by some infectious agent (or pathogenic organism) or its poisonous products. It can be transmitted to a person directly or indirectly. Use of the term *communicable disease* is favored by the health scientist; lay people frequently employ the term *contagious* when referring to the same group of diseases. These two terms may be used interchangeably.

Morbidity statistics are used to indicate the number of cases of a disease in a given population. Generally, these data are expressed in terms of the case-rate per 100,000 population per year.

The *mortality rate* refers to the number of deaths attributed to a specific disease for a given population. The size of the reported population may vary, depending largely on the nature of the disease and the characteristics of the group in question. Often, mortality rates are given for specific diseases, age-groups, sexes, and other significant differentials which may be appropriate in statistical reporting.

Endemic refers to those diseases that are prevalent or common in certain geographic areas. For example, cholera is endemic in parts of India.

An *epidemic* is an outbreak of a disease in a community or region where the numbers of ill persons from the disease is clearly higher than the normal expectation for that disease.

Pandemic refers to disease outbreaks that cover entire countries, continents, or large areas of the whole world. Pandemics of influenza occurred in 1889, 1918, and 1957.

Epidemiology. The science of epidemiology started with Hippocrates back in the Golden Age of Greece. He recognized that disease outbreaks were not haphazard occurrences. Some diseases were seasonal; others affected certain groups such as children, adults, and so on. At one time this study was confined to communicable diseases only. Now, a broader definition includes the study of factors that influence the health of people.

Through epidemiologic studies it has become possible to determine that people with certain characteristics are more susceptible to a given disease than people without those characteristics (e.g., people with high cholesterol levels in their blood are more susceptible to cardiac disease). Epidemiology has also helped to identify reasons for illness in certain groups (e.g., cigarette smoking is related to a higher incidence of lung cancer). In Chapter 9, "Living Safely," the *epidemiology* of the automobile accident will be discussed.

ORGANISMS THAT CAUSE DISEASE

Bacteria are one of the lowest forms of plants. While most of these microorganisms are helpful or harmless (decomposing organic matter, making cheese) some can cause disease. These organisms take three basic forms, being rod-shaped (bacilli), round (cocci), or spiral (spirochetes). They cause such diseases as tuberculosis, typhoid fever, whooping cough (pertussis), or "strep" throat, among others.

Figure 3–2

A body membrane infected with herpes simplex virus.

(Center for Disease Control)

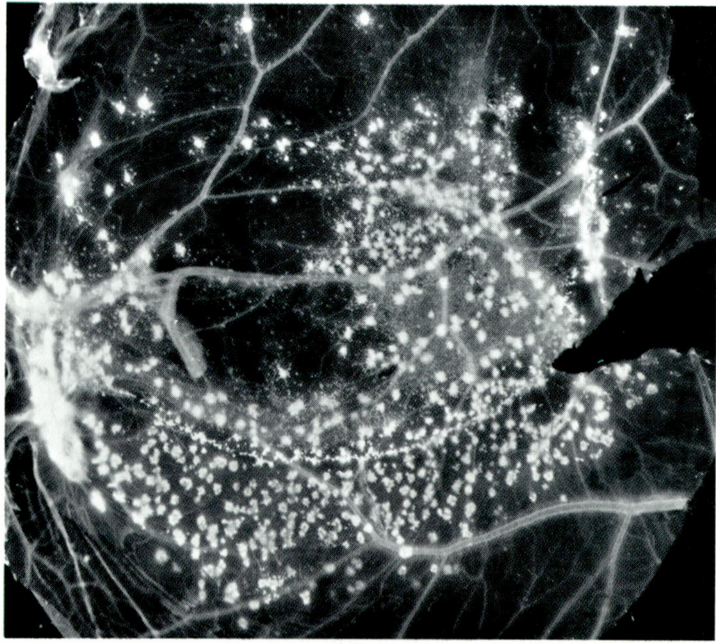

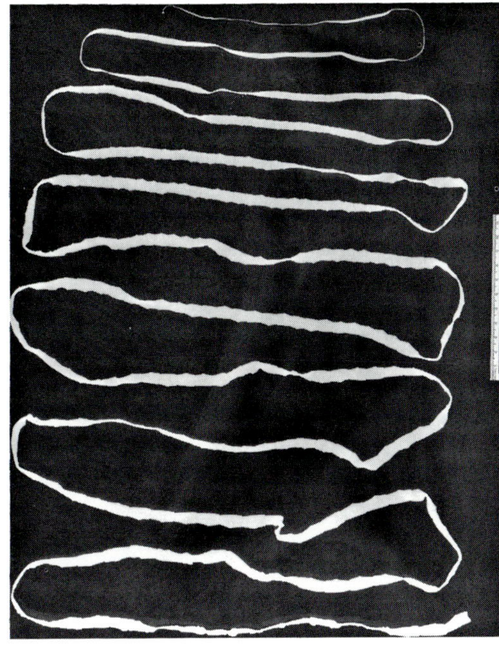

Figure 3–3

A tapeworm, a parasitic worm found in the intestinal tract.

(Center for Disease Control)

Viruses are the smallest of the disease-producing organisms and can be seen only under the electron microscope. They require living cells for their growth and reproduction. Poliomyelitis, the common cold, measles, mumps, and hepatitis exemplify diseases produced by them. Drugs that are effective against viral diseases are rare. The main means of combating these diseases are prevention via those vaccines that are available, or avoidance of the sources of infection.

Fungi are plant forms that include yeast and molds. Infections that come under the category of "athlete's foot" or "ringworm" are caused by fungi. "Ringworm" gets its name from the ringlike appearance that the fungal growth often takes in scalp infections.

Protozoa are one-celled animals and represent the simplest form of animal life. Some protozoa are parasitic to man and can cause such disorders as malaria, amebic dysentery, and African sleeping sickness.

Parasitic Worms take varied forms and can produce a number of human diseases. These organisms can vary in size, with many being visible to the naked eye. Hookworm, tapeworm, pinworm, and schistosome (the agent causing schistosomiasis) are examples.

Rickettsia are organisms smaller than bacteria and are barely visible under conventional microscopes. They are responsible for such conditions as Rocky Mountain Spotted Fever, typhus, and Q fever.

Spreading Diseases

There are many ways these disease organisms are transmitted from a source of infection to a susceptible person. Transmission can be accomplished through *direct contact* with an infected person, as in touching, kissing, or sexual intercourse. Transmission of infectious agents can also take place through *indirect contact,* that is, through the touching of contaminated articles such as eating utensils, clothing, food, and so forth. *Droplet infection* takes place when the agents are carried by small droplets through the air, usually a matter of a few feet. This represents a type of contact infection because of the close proximity of the people involved. Coughing, sneezing, or talking can serve as means of facilitating droplet infections.

Vectors are insects or animals that serve to transmit disease. The mosquito that carries the protozoan that causes malaria from an infected person to the uninfected acts as a vector. Mosquitoes that carry the virus that causes encephalitis perform a similar function as do the ticks that carry the rickettsia that cause Rocky Mountain Spotted Fever. Vectors often serve as reservoirs of infection. Control of a given disease frequently depends on effectively diminishing the population of the vector.

RESISTANCE AND IMMUNITY TO DISEASE

What course of action can one take to protect oneself from communicable diseases? If your childhood learnings have carried over into early adulthood, your response to this question will probably reflect parental teachings relative to the "theory of disease resistance." Most young adults tend to support the concept that by following basic hygienic principles it is possible to maintain a reasonably high level of resistance to disease. The protection thus attained is general in nature and is not specific for any disease. On the other hand, any single element of a healthful regimen does not constitute a panacea of disease prevention. That is, healthful exercise does not guarantee protection from disease any more than either proper diet or recommended amounts of sleep can be expected, in themselves, to provide ultimate resistance. Yet, it is not uncommon for some individuals to engage in rigid dietary programs or weight-training plans designed supposedly to protect them from infectious disease. When an individual is obsessed by such health fads, practices, or beliefs, it is apparent that his concept of disease resistance is limited and that his efforts to maintain a desirable state of mind and body are misdirected.

Disease Immunity

Protection from specific communicable diseases is spoken of in terms of *immunity* to these illnesses. Immune persons possess substances called *antibodies* which provide varying degrees of protection from different diseases. When certain foreign substances (almost always protein in nature) are introduced into a person's body, complex protective reactions may result. The foreign substance, perhaps a virus, is the *antigen* and its presence stimulates the production of substanccs (antibodies) having the capability of destroying the antigen. An important characteristic of antibodies is that each particular type is effective in destroying only one variety of organism. Thus, measles antibodies protect only against measles virus, and mumps antibodies are specific only for mumps.

It is important to note that not all disease-producing organisms provoke this body response. Modifications of this defensive mechanism are apparent in diseases such as the common cold, where immunity, if at all present, is of short duration (probably a few days).

Immunity resulting from antigen-antibody reactions never provides total protection from the disease that originally triggered the reaction. Experience has demonstrated that antibody levels which have proven to be effective under

Figure 3–4

Peanuts cartoon by Charles M. Schulz.

PEANUTS
ALL RIGHT, NOW COUGH!
10-10
COUGH! COUGH! COUGH!
STOMP! STOMP! STOMP! STOMP!
THERE'S A BATCH OF COLD GERMS THAT WILL NEVER BOTHER ANYONE AGAIN!
SCHULZ

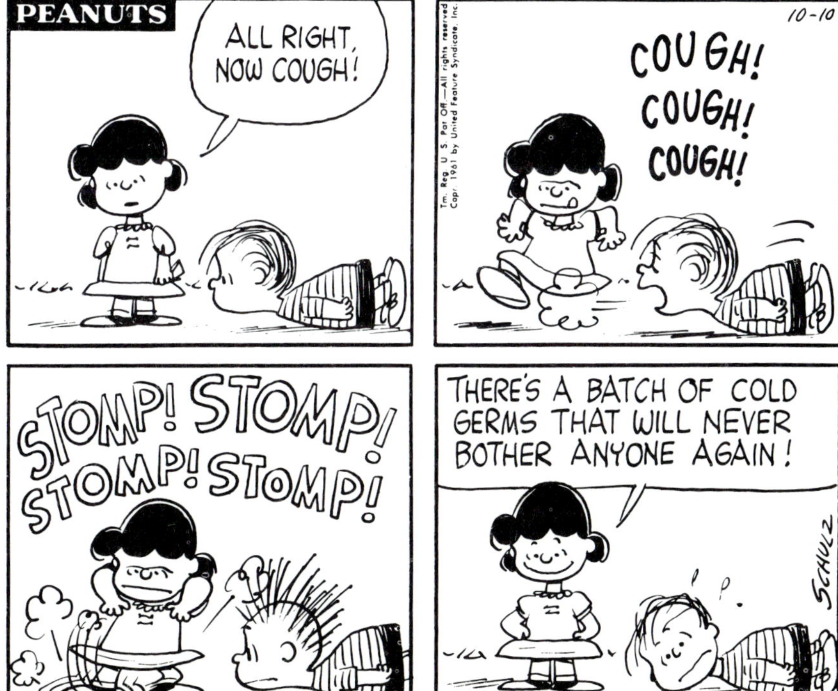

normal living conditions may be overwhelmed by unusually high concentrations of antigenic material.

Clearly, the ultimate purpose of all varieties of antibodies is essentially the same—to destroy antigens. A closer examination of the manner in which they perform this function is fascinating. Some antibodies, classified as *agglutinins,* cause a clumping of bacteria. As a consequence of this agglutination, the mobility of the bacteria is reduced and they are more easily devoured by leukocytes (white blood cells). Other antibodies, the *bacteriolysins,* possess the peculiar ability to form a solution (lysis) of bacteria, thus destroying the organisms. *Opsonins* are yet another antibody type that cause bacteria and other antigens to be more attractive to white blood cells.

Types of Immunity

An active immunity occurs when the body's own efforts are involved in the development of protective antibodies. This would occur when a person has a disease or when he receives a vaccine containing a weakened form of the disease organisms. Having the disease or a weakened form of it (vaccine) stimulates the body to produce its own antibodies against the disease organisms.

A *passive* immunity can be effected by injecting into the person ready-made antibodies produced in another person or animal. For example, the antibody for German measles can be isolated from the blood of those people who have had the disease. The injection of these antibodies (in the form of gamma globulin) will produce a temporary immunity. Because these antibodies were "borrowed," the immunity is considered passive. Passive immunization may be advised in response to the need for protection after exposure, or in cases where one anticipates exposure to a disease. Such might be the case when an expectant mother, in her first few months of pregnancy, is exposed to German measles. In an effort to protect the fetus from harm, the physician may recommend the administration of immune serum in the form of gamma globulin.

Whether artificially induced or the result of actually being ill with a disease, active immunity provides more lasting protection than passive immunity and in many instances is lifelong.

Vaccines

Suspensions of dead or weakened disease organisms or their toxic products, are classified as *vaccines*. Recognized as a vital factor in reducing the threat of communicable diseases, vaccines are capable of starting antigen-antibody reactions with little or no discomfort to the recipient of the antigenic material. Whenever the vaccine consists of bacterial toxins rather than the bacteria themselves, the resultant vaccine is known as a *toxoid* (denatured toxin).

The extent to which the threats of smallpox, pertussis (whooping cough), diphtheria, and poliomyelitis have substantially lessened is indicative of the importance of vaccines to human well-being. In the middle 1920s, for instance, more than 55,000 cases of smallpox were reported in the United States. By 1971, largely as a result of mass immunization programs, not a single case of smallpox was reported in this country. While this dreaded disease has been largely eliminated in the United States and Europe, there are still areas of the world—India, Bangladesh, Pakistan, and Ethiopia, for axample—where smallpox persists as a threat to health and life.

The recent history of diphtheria is striking. During the 1930s more than 30,000 cases and 3,000 deaths were recorded in a single year. Since this period, widespread use of diphtheria toxoid has greatly reduced the incidence of this infection. In 1973 about 210 cases of diphtheria were identified in the United States, and indications are that the disease will continue to decline.

Although it is true that periodic outbreaks of poliomyelitis have occurred since the development of a successful vaccine, most of the victims have proved to be those who had never received a full series of inoculations. Apparently,

Figure 3–5

Cataracts are one of the main physical defects of children who are impaired at birth because their mothers had German measles during their first three months of pregnancy. Other defects from this cause include hearing loss, crippling, heart malformations, small head size, mental retardation, and blood disorders.

(Merck, Sharp & Dohme, West Point, Pa.)

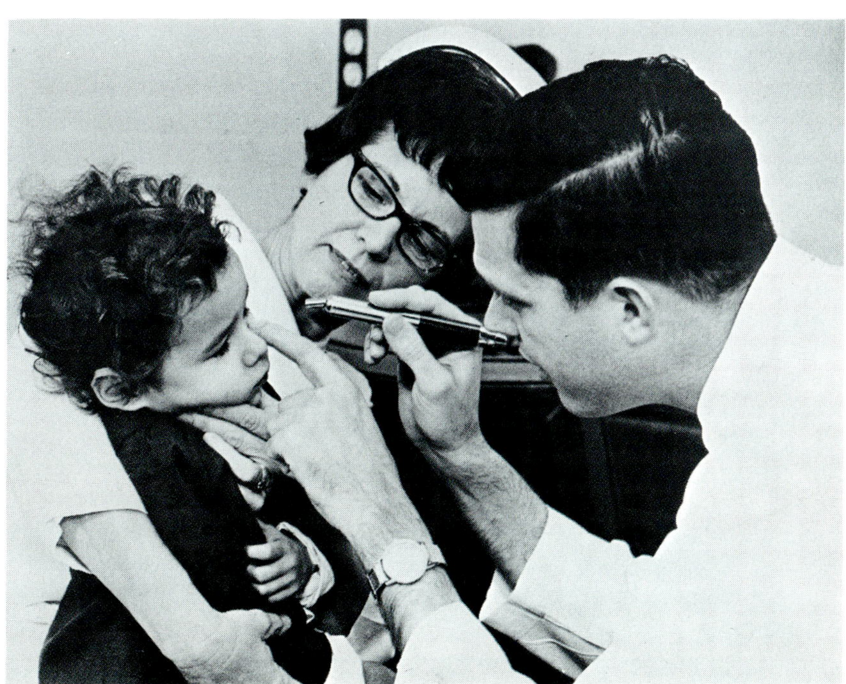

one of our nation's major concerns should be to make people aware of how they may protect their health by the utilization of vaccines. Furthermore, the medical facilities and services essential for such protection should be made available to all people. Experience has demonstrated that in those areas where intensive immunization programs are underwritten and conducted, the disease is virtually nonexistent. It is entirely possible that the conscientious and determined use of oral polio vaccine will, within the next generation, practically eradicate this disease throughout the world. The introduction of the Enders measles vaccine in 1963 is producing similar results.

Rubella epidemics occur in the United States about once every ten years. The disease is usually over in three days and there are no lasting effects—unless the patient was a woman early in her pregnancy. Then the effects of the disease

TABLE 3–1

Standard Immunizations

Here are the recommendations of CU's medical consultants. Included as a reminder is the tuberculin test. Consult a physician about your individual immunization. Some people are prone to side effects, and immunization practices may vary according to local needs.

When	Immunization needed	Comments
2–3 months old	1st diphtheria-tetanus-pertussis (DTP) 1st oral polio	Usually given together
4–6 weeks after 1st DTP 6–8 weeks after 1st polio	2nd DTP 2nd oral polio	Can be given together
4–6 weeks after 2nd DTP	3rd DTP	
1 year old	Tuberculin test	At least 2 days before measles vaccination.
	Measles Mumps Rubella	Can be given together.
8–12 months after 2nd polio	3rd oral polio	
1 year after 3rd DTP	4th DTP	
5–6 years old	Diphtheria tetanus booster	On beginning school, and every 10 years thereafter.
	Polio booster	On beginning school.
Up to 15 years old	Measles	If not immune. (Little danger of getting measles after 15.)
15–16 years old	Diphtheria-tetanus booster	And every 10 years thereafter.
All adults	Diphtheria-tetanus booster	Repeat every 10 years.
All adults	Mumps	If not immune (by having had disease or vaccine).
All females before puberty	Rubella	
All females after puberty	Rubella	If a blood test determines you're not immune. Must not be pregnant and must not become pregnant sooner than 2 months after immunization.

Source: *Consumer Reports,* August 1974, p. 605.

on her unborn child can be devastating. As a result of the 1964–1965 rubella epidemic 50,000 children either died in the womb or were born with a loss of hearing, impaired vision, congenitally damaged hearts, or mentally retarded. Very often these children have several of these impairments and are multi-handicapped. The need for protection was met in June 1969 when the first rubella vaccine was licensed. This vaccination program, like the others, is based on the well-established principle of "herd immunity." The herd immunity approach calls for vaccinating enough people of the community to produce a large percentage of immune persons so that a disease would be unable to spread in epidemic fashion. Children are targets of the vaccination program since 90 per cent of cases occur among children in the lower grades.

The "success story" in modern medicine is exemplified by these figures indicating that in 1972, 25,507 cases of rubella were reported—some 50 per cent fewer than the numbers reported between 1967–1971. In 1972 only 33 cases of congenital rubella syndrome were reported—again, a 50 per cent drop from the previous year.

There has been some question as to the long-term effectiveness of the program. One study suggests that periodic serological surveys of children vaccinated should be implemented to determine whether or not these children remain safe from rubella as they approach their childbearing years. Outbreaks of rubella are now most common among unvaccinated high school students.

Artificial immunization is presently available for many more diseases than our discussion would indicate. Pertussis, tetanus, influenza, typhoid fever, and tuberculosis are examples of other diseases for which prophylaxis (a vaccine) is used in the United States. The American Academy of Pediatrics has suggested an immunization schedule which, in its judgment, represents the soundest course of action for those seeking artificial immunizations.

SOME COMMUNICABLE DISEASE PROBLEMS

Influenza and Pneumonia

The United States Public Health Service and other official health agencies combine the data on influenza (flu) and pneumonia when reporting on the incidence and severity of either disease. Both of these conditions affect the respiratory system and are commonly referred to as "clinical companions." That is to say, an attack of the flu can and does lead to pneumonia, especially if the victim represents a high-risk group. Influenza predisposes the lungs to later bacterial infections, including pneumonia, and whenever a flu epidemic strikes there is a corresponding increase in pneumonia deaths.

Though these diseases are not the killers today that they were in past years, they are the only acute diseases remaining among the major causes of sickness and death in the United States. Both usually take their heaviest toll among infants and the elderly. As the percentage of citizens age 65 and over increases, we can expect influenza and pneumonia to continue as major health problems. This will, in fact, be the case, unless effective control measures are developed and applied in our society.

Influenza is an acute, highly infectious disorder of the upper respiratory tract resulting from invasion by one of several filterable viruses. At least three virus types (Types A, B, and C) have been identified and are classified in the myxovirus group. The symptoms usually begin 24 to 72 hours (incubation period) after the virus has entered the host. The early symptoms mimic those of the common cold, with accompanying chills, achiness (especially in the back and limbs), and weakness. Influenza is a self-limiting disease and typically runs its course in two to three days. In many cases, however, a nonproductive cough and general feeling of fatigue persist long after the disappearance of other symptoms.

Those who are afflicted with more than one attack of influenza in a given season are very likely to be victims of more than one virus type. To date, effective vaccines are available for the prevailing strains of Type A and Type B viruses. The periodic emergence of new virus strains has resulted in the presently available inoculations' being only partially successful in controlling the disease.

Special risk groups, including the very young and the elderly, and those suffering from chronic cardiac, respiratory, metabolic, renal, and neurological disorders, are commonly advised to receive inoculations. There is some evidence that pregnant women show a greater tendency to develop pulmonary complications following influenza, and many medical authorities consider these individuals as a risk group.

For the young adult the major dangers from influenza do not involve serious illness. Bed rest is recommended for a quicker recovery, with many physicians sometimes prescribing additional therapy, depending on the needs of the individual.

Infectious Mononucleosis

Known popularly as "mono" and the "kissing disease," mononucleosis affects an estimated half a million young people each year. The majority of these cases are found in the 15- to 30-year-age group, with a slightly greater incidence among males. Mononucleosis is not a new disease. As early as 1889, Emil Pfeiffer described an epidemic of "glandular fever," a disease remarkably similar to that now known as mononucleosis. This term was first used to describe glandular fever in 1920.

In spite of the fact that medical personnel have known about this curious disease for more than three-quarters of a century, it remains largely a medical mystery even today. For example, the causative organism is generally believed to be a virus, though none has been identified. Its unknown etiology is further complicated by the fact that attempts to transmit the infection from one person to another via blood, stool samples, and nasopharyngeal secretions have not been very successful. The term "kissing disease" implies that mononucleosis is transmitted by way of respiratory discharges. Yet, medical research has not determined that this is the actual mode of transmission.

The mononucleosis syndrome is variable and the common symptoms include enlargement of lymph nodes (usually the cervical nodes are involved), sore throat, headache, and irregular fever (commonly ranging from 100 degrees to 103 degrees, or higher). Frequently these symptoms increase in intensity during the first week of the illness and will be severe enough to convince the patient that a medical consultation is advisable. Examination by a physician may reveal noticeable enlargement of the spleen. In some cases, a chaotic condition of lymphocytes is noted and is helpful to the physician in diagnosing mononucleosis. A new diagnostic test has been developed that utilizes blood serum from suspected mono victims and blood from horses. Reportedly, blood serum from an infected individual causes a clumping of red blood cells in horse blood. This diagnostic technique is still being studied, and researchers are encouraged by its effectiveness and simplicity. Because of the dangers of liver or spleen involvement, mononucleosis should be treated by a physician. Typically, the discomforts of mononucleosis persist from two to eight weeks. In many cases, the individual does not feel acutely ill, but his physician should prescribe a daily regimen.

Hepatitis

Hepatitis (inflammation of the liver) is an acute infection and its symptoms commonly include fever, loss of appetite, nausea, malaise, and abdominal discomfort; sometimes followed by jaundice. Jaundice, a yellowish tinting of the skin and sclera, results from the appearance of certain bile salts in the

Figure 3–6

Viral hepatitis cycle—a high incidence of hepatitis appears to recur periodically.

(Center for Disease Control)

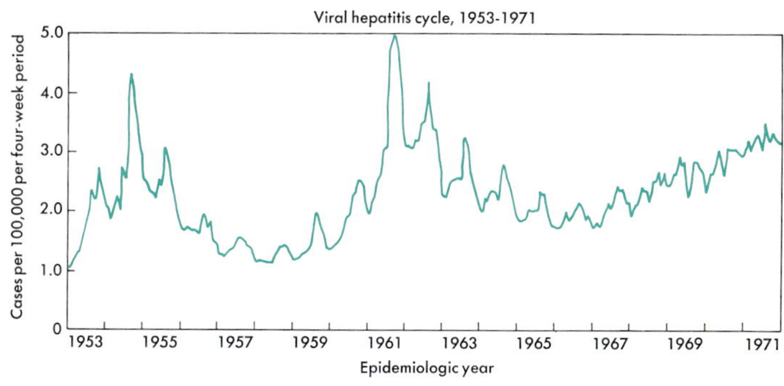

blood. The discoloration lasts for varying lengths of time. There are, however, many cases of hepatitis in which this symptom does not appear. Whether jaundice is or is not present, the convalescent period may extend for weeks or months.

The presence of antibodies found in gamma globulin of pooled blood suggests that the majority of adults have probably had this type of infection and not even been aware of its presence. Although its effectiveness is questioned by many authorities, immune serum globulin may be administered to those who have had contact with the disease. There is some evidence that these inoculations may provide passive immunity lasting from six to eight weeks.

A distinction must be made between infectious hepatitis and its close relative, serum hepatitis (homologous serum jaundice).

Infectious Hepatitis has a reputation as one of the most serious communicable diseases in the United States. Actually, it is not a new disease, but has only in recent years gained public attention. It is known variously as "yellow jaundice," "camp jaundice," "infectious jaundice," and "catarrhal jaundice."

In temperate zones, infectious hepatitis becomes more prevalent in the late summer months and typically reaches its peak in late fall or early winter. It is essentially a disease of children and young adults and often causes prolonged incapacitation.

Complete information on this disease is lacking because of the inability of virologists and other researchers to adequately identify and cultivate the causative agent. To date, most experimental work has had to be done on human volunteers because of the difficulty of artificially transmitting the disease to laboratory animals. The exact manner by which infectious hepatitis is transmitted is poorly understood, though the medical community generally agrees that it might possibly be transmitted via respiratory discharges. Curiously enough, efforts to demonstrate virus A in nasopharyngeal secretions have been largely unsuccessful. The most common source of infection is contaminated fecal material, and the usual mode of transmission is via the intestinal-oral route. Perhaps the reason why the disease appears to be most common in children is that many in this age group have not yet formed basic hygienic practices such as washing the hands after using the bathroom and washing before meals. A further reason for our lack of total control of hepatitis is that contaminated food, water, and milk have been known to be reservoirs of infection responsible for epidemics.

Serum Hepatitis is caused by a virus (Virus B) that is different from infectious hepatitis (Virus A) and appears to be transmitted only by subcutaneous, intramuscular, and intravenous injection. The incidence of serum hepatitis was on the decline until recent years. The drug abuse problem with its widespread injected use of heroin and amphetamines has caused a resurgence in the incidence of this disease. The prevalence had been reduced largely through routine screenings of individuals who donate blood and as a result of intensified efforts to sterilize instruments used when various kinds of injections are administered. The relatively recent use of disposable hypodermic syringes and needles has undoubtedly reduced the number of those who might otherwise have been infected by contaminated equipment.

Venereal Diseases

Ironically, the incidence of venereal diseases has been rising throughout the world. The increased incidence started about 20 years after effective treatment in the form of penicillin was discovered in the mid-1940s. There was a significant spread of venereal disease in the early 1940s during World War II. With the discovery and introduction of penicillin as a form of treatment, both syphilis and gonorrhea receded in incidence. The expected demise of these diseases was not to occur, however. Starting in the late 1950s there has been a steady and alarming increase of venereal disease. There has to date been little understanding of the significance and consequences of this unnecessary scourge. Positive efforts, however, to eliminate this ignorance are currently being made, as many school systems are becoming involved in instructional programs to familiarize young Americans with the nature of the venereal diseases.

All of the venereal diseases are highly infectious and spread by direct contact with an infected individual. The nature of this contact nearly always involves intimate sexual relations. Chancroid lymphogranuloma venereum, granuloma inguinale, syphilis, and gonorrhea make up this group of dreaded diseases. Because the latter two venereal infections are most common and present the greatest challenge to public health authorities in the United States, the discussion here will be limited to them.

Syphilis. Syphilis is caused by treponema pallida, a corkscrew-shaped organism (spirochete) that requires both moisture and body temperature to grow and reproduce. These critical requirements are satisfied by the warm, moist surfaces of the mucus membrane of the oral cavity and the genitourinary system. Syphilis is also known to enter the body when infectious material is introduced into cuts or other breaks in the skin. Conditions of temperature and moisture are so vital to the survival of the spirochete that direct contact is almost always the manner by which the infection is transferred. It is quite unlikely that the organism could live for more than a few seconds on inanimate objects such as toilet seats. It is generally agreed that almost all cases of syphilis are transmitted as a result of direct contact during sexual intercourse or other intimate sexual activities whether they be heterosexual or homosexual.

Shortly after contact with the treponema, the newly infected individual harbors the organisms in his lymphatic system. Before the primary symptoms appear, the infection reaches the bloodstream. Usually the symptoms of primary syphilis are evident in about three weeks, but may not appear for three months following contact.

A certain element of risk is involved whenever one attempts to describe a classical disease syndrome. Deviations from the pattern described herein are

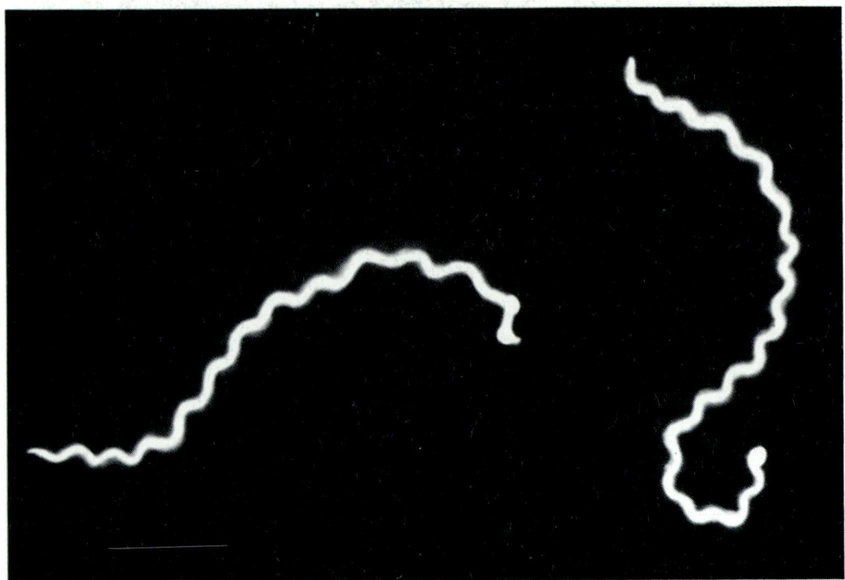

Figure 3–7

Treponema pallidum, the causative organism of syphilis.

(Center for Disease Control)

common and certainly should not be reason for a person to postpone medical attention at the first suspicion of venereal disease. As a rule, venereal diseases are most easily cured in the early stages and become progressively less responsive to therapy as the infection persists.

The development of the syphilis infection may be conveniently divided into four major stages:

PRIMARY SYPHILIS. The initial symptom is oftentimes a chancre. This lesion is usually a hard, painless papule, although some may be soft and irritating. The chancre is a highly communicable source of the disease and is usually located in the ano-genital region, but many appear on the lips, tongue, finger, or wherever the spirochete first entered the body.

Many syphilitics pass through the primary phase of their infection without being aware of their condition. The presence of the chancre is not always detected by the infected person. The chancre appears as an open sore usually on the surface of the body. Even when the chancre is noticed, it quickly heals even without treatment. Spontaneous disappearance of the chancre misleads many into believing that they must be rid of the infection. This assumption is most unfortunate, because the infection is permitted to continue to develop at a time when antibiotic therapy would be most effective.

During the primary stage, the organisms may not be present in the blood in sufficient force to show a positive reaction in a blood test. It is, therefore, possible to harbor an early syphilis infection and still react negatively to blood tests. If the physician and patient suspect that this is the case, frequent blood tests are recommended until a firm diagnosis has been made. Needless to say, the patient should refrain from intimate sexual contact until his physician is convinced that syphilis is not present.

SECONDARY SYPHILIS. Secondary symptoms may appear as soon as three weeks or as late as six months after the appearance of primary symptoms. The nature of these more advanced symptoms varies greatly from one patient to another, but those appearing most commonly are a non-itchy rash covering the entire body or confined to the hands and feet, head-ache, mild fever, sore throat, and alopecia (hair falling out in patches). Infectious lesions may appear on the ano-genital surfaces, and mucous patches may be evident on the membranes of the mouth. The disease is highly contagious in this stage of its development, and it is possible to spread the infection to others by kissing or other intimate contact. It should be noted that the symptoms associated

Figure 3–8

Infectious syphilis outbreak. Fort Worth, Texas 1971.

(Today's VD Control Problem 1972. Published by American Social Health Association.)

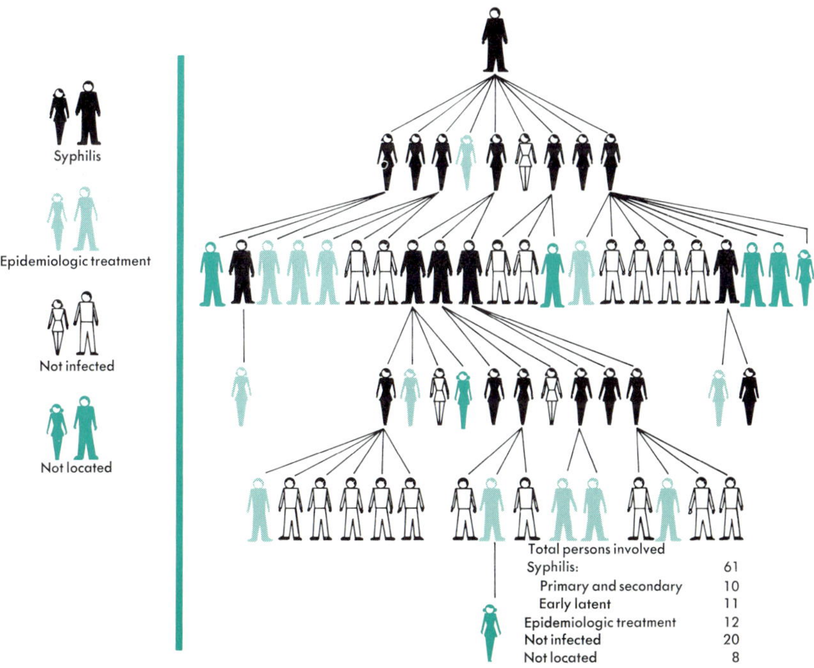

with this period may be confused with those of other diseases. For this reason syphilis is sometimes referred to as the "great imitator." Sometimes the rash, sore throat, and other discomforts are so mild as to go unnoticed. Whatever the case, these symptoms will eventually disappear even without treatment, and the infection will continue on its course of destruction.

Blood tests are highly reliable in diagnosing syphilis that has progressed to this point, and antibiotic therapy is very effective in curing secondary syphilis.

LATENT SYPHILIS. Because the treponemae pallidae settle down in clusters in various parts of the body, no symptoms are evident. The syphilitic may feel perfectly normal during a period that extends from five to twenty years or longer. As is true in the secondary stage of syphilis, blood tests are reliable in detecting the disease during the latent period. Because the patient is symptom free during the latent period, it does not mean he has been cured of the disease. In fact, it is during this period when most damage to the internal organs, the central nervous system, bones, and other structures is taking place.

LATE SYPHILIS. When syphilis is permitted to go untreated, the victim eventually may develop the tragic, chronic, and disabling conditions associated with long-term syphilis infection. The United States Public Health Service has reported that of untreated syphilitics, approximately 7 per cent will suffer cardiac disorders, 4 per cent will be crippled or paralyzed, 2 per cent will experience severe mental disturbances (paresis), and nearly 1 per cent will be blinded. These unfortunate afflictions, as well as the deaths resulting from syphilis, have made this the most devastating of the venereal diseases.

Although syphilis cannot be inherited, if a woman with syphilis becomes pregnant it is possible for her unborn child to develop congenital syphilis. Whenever the conception of the child occurs at approximately the same time the mother becomes infected with syphilis, it is likely that the child will be harmed unless treatment is administered. Occasionally, a woman becomes infected rather late in her pregnancy and the symptoms go unnoticed. Under these circumstances the child may exhibit symptoms of syphilis at birth or at some later date. Ordinarily the symptoms of congenital syphilis resemble those of secondary syphilis. Many children are stillborn or born with severely handicapping conditions such as blindness, skeletal deformities, and neurosyphilis.

The most effective way of reducing the frequency of congenital syphilis is to require blood tests of pregnant women. In fact, the majority of states require such measures. This is apparently not the final solution to the problem, for even today thousands of pregnant women do not receive adequate prenatal care. Perhaps in years to come, legislation, education, and better distribution of medical personnel and facilities will result in the eradication of this tragic form of syphilis.

Penicillin remains the preferred medication for treating all stages of syphilis. In those few cases in which patients are allergic to penicillin, other equally effective antibiotics may be prescribed by the physician. The objective of antibiotic therapy is to maintain a high level of penicillin in one's bloodstream to destroy all of the syphilis microorganisms and eliminate the infection. The goal is more easily attained when treatment is begun early, preferably during the primary stage of the disease. When the infection is untreated and allowed to progress, increasing doses of antibiotics are required over longer periods in order to eliminate the disease.

Even individuals suffering from advanced cases of syphilis may benefit from antibiotic treatment. Central nervous system disorders, syphilitic heart, and other organic damage resulting from late infection cannot, however, be repaired by even the best antibiotic therapy.

Unlike most other communicable diseases, syphilis can strike the same individual more than once. Apparently, a person does not develop an immunity to syphilis as one does with measles, chickenpox, and mumps.

Following the isolation and identification of treponema pallida by Schaudinn and Hoffman in 1905, Wassermann and his colleagues developed (in 1906) the first satisfactory serologic test for detecting syphilis infections. Wasserman's original procedure was rather complex and it has since been simplified and improved upon. Today the Wassermann Test is still of great value in the diagnosis of syphilis. Of course, additional diagnostic laboratory tests have been in use in recent years.

Gonorrhea. In both sexes, gonorrhea is essentially a disease of the genitourinary system. Since 1957 there has been an accelerating incidence of the disease from a reported incidence of 216,476 to an excess of half a million. Estimates are that actual incidence is far in excess of a million cases. The group with the highest venereal disease rate is the 15–24-year-age group. Some health authorities have described venereal disease as being "out of control" . . . others have described it as being "epidemic." Suffice it to say that only the common cold exceeds it in terms of incidence. Better public understanding and community health programs to counteract the devastation of gonorrhea are now in order.

The microorganism responsible for gonorrhea is the gonococcus, a bacterium discovered by Neisser in 1879. Intimate sexual contact (nearly always sexual intercourse) is the manner by which the causative agent is transmitted. The disease remains communicable until it is cured.

Unlike syphilis, gonorrhea is usually an infection of the sex organs and their adjacent structures. In women, the infection ordinarily starts in the vagina, and if untreated, progresses to the uterus and fallopian tubes, where it may cause inflammation and adhesions, blocking the passage of ova from the ovary. Obviously, in such cases sterility may be the consequence. Gonorrheal infections in males begin in the urethra, causing widespread inflammation and irritation. If allowed to progress, the infection may eventually involve the testes and convoluted tubules, resulting in sterility. In those relatively uncommon cases where untreated gonorrhea invades the circulatory system, the gonococci may invade the body's connective tissue. The result of this is inflammation of joints,

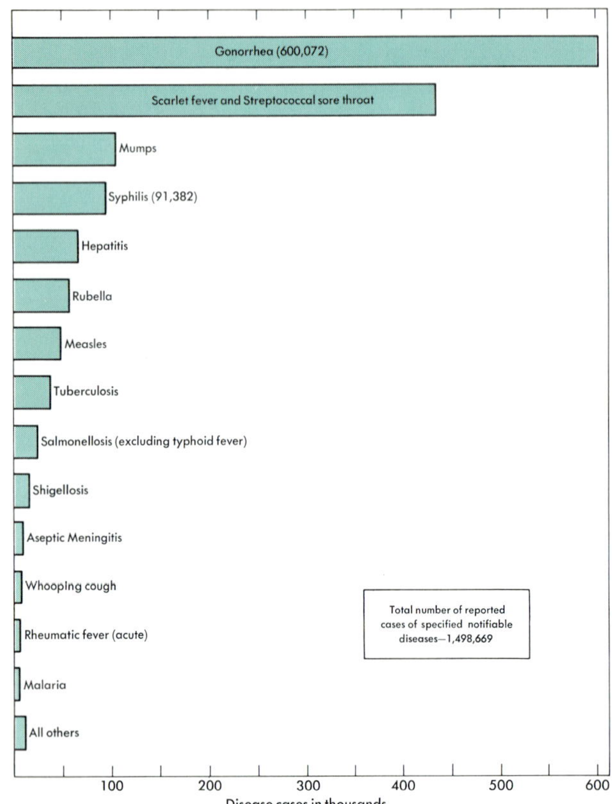

Figure 3–9

Communicable diseases—number of reported cases in the United States, 1970.

(U.S. Public Health Service)

which may lead to gonorrheal arthritis, or inflammation of cardiac tissue. The latter condition may lead to severe heart disorders. Generally speaking, however, the total impact of untreated gonorrhea is much less damaging to the individual than is untreated syphilis.

The incubation period of the disease is short, with initial signs and symptoms usually developing within three to four (at times 9 days or longer) days following contact. Men often experience burning sensations, especially when voiding urine, as soon as three days following contact, and a puslike discharge from the penis may be observed. This discomfort is apt to intensify upon urination as the inflamed urethra (urethritis) is irritated by urine. Females, however, often do not experience such early discomfort. The inflamed vagina is somewhat less sensitive than the penis and obviously is apart from the female urinary system. Therefore the burning irritation so common in males in early gonorrhea is typically absent in females. Furthermore, the internal reproductive system of the female makes the discharge of pus less obvious than in males. In one sense, these sexual differences are unfortunate because they so frequently lead to delayed diagnosis and treatment of the infection.

Women usually experience their first discomfort from gonorrhea several months after contact, when the fallopian tubes become inflamed. The usual symptoms at this time are pain in the lower abdominal region.

There are many causes of urethritis in males and vaginitis in females. By no means does the presence of a viscous discharge necessarily indicate a gonorrheal infection. Any abnormal discharge should be referred to a physician so that accurate diagnosis can be made. Sometimes discharge in males accompanies a bladder infection that should be treated immediately. Vaginitis, with an accompanying discharge, is indicative of an abnormal condition not necessarily gonorrhea. Improper hygienic practices are a common cause of these infections.

A positive diagnosis of gonorrhea results when gonococci are detected in samples of secretions from the reproductive system. Very often the organisms are not observed in a routine microscopic examination of the samples. In such cases the culture should be incubated for three or four days and reexamined. Even this procedure may not yield positive results, and it is sometimes necessary to take several cultures. Recently a new blood test for gonorrhea was developed. It represented a major breakthrough in the worldwide battle to combat the gonorrhea epidemic because of its potential use for mass screening. This new blood test can be performed in two hours and necessitates only a blood sample thus enabling more specimens to be processed. If the blood test is positive, then final diagnosis must still be made through the bacteriological culture procedures. It is hoped that the test will prove helpful in detecting gonorrhea especially in women who experience no symptoms. More than 80 per cent of all women infected are asymptomatic and act as carriers of the disease without knowing it.

One very important difference between gonorrhea and syphilis is the extent to which their respective causative agents respond to penicillin therapy. In discussing syphilis, it was mentioned that penicillin therapy in syphilitic control appears to be as effective today as it was when penicillin was first used to treat syphilis in 1943. Gonorrheal infections, on the other hand, are "fast becoming refractive [resistant] to penicillin. It is not known whether this is due to the nature of the organism, which closely resembles the meningococcus and which organism is also becoming resistant, or whether the use of long-acting antibiotics in the treatment of venereal disease has produced a type of organism which now requires, in some instances, high blood levels to destroy it."[2] Medical authorities have become alarmed over the increasing amounts of penicillin required to cure some gonorrheal infections. Perhaps one day, if

[2] *Control of Communicable Diseases in Man,* 10th ed. (New York: American Public Health Association, 1965), p. 24.

present trends continue, gonorrhea will not respond to any program of penicillin therapy. The implications of such a development would require the use of other antibiotics for our venereal disease control programs.

Whenever a case of gonorrhea is diagnosed, the physician should also perform routine serological examinations for syphilis. Experience has shown that these two venereal diseases often infect an individual simultaneously. Were the gonorrheal diagnosis positive and no serological studies initiated to determine the presence of a syphilis infection, the routine antibiotic therapy for gonorrhea might obscure the symptoms of syphilis. In past years, this occurrence was fairly common and a concurrent syphilis infection was allowed to progress in the unsuspecting patient. Physicians are quite aware of this possibility now and routinely conduct blood tests for all individuals infected with gonorrhea.

Years ago, gonorrhea of the newborn was not uncommon. Infected mothers were responsible for infection of their infants because the infectious material was introduced into the child as it passed through the birth canal during delivery. In most cases, these infant infections involved the eyes, and a condition known as gonorrheal ophthalmia often led to blindness. Today, with our increased understanding of gonorrheal infections, solutions of silver nitrate or penicillin are routinely administered to the eyes of infants to prevent infection. This control measure has greatly reduced the incidence of gonorrheal ophthalmia and blindness in infants.

Controlling Venereal Diseases

In response to the resurgence of venereal disease, public health leaders have suggested several measures to control and finally eliminate the venereal disease problem. They follow:

1. Increased local, state, and federal funds to expand present control efforts.
2. Enactment by state legislative bodies of laws requiring the reporting of all cases of venereal disease by all laboratories.
3. Required serological tests on all routine hospital admissions.
4. Support of venereal disease education programs in school and colleges.
5. Initiation and expansion of courses in venereal disease management in medical schools.
6. Intensification of research efforts to develop effective gonorrhea and syphilis vaccines.
7. Expansion of behavioral science research that will contribute to the control of venereal diseases.
8. Encouragement to physicians to report all cases of venereal disease.

Those working in public health VD programs find that individuals with VD are often inhibited from seeking treatment or reporting who their sexual contacts were out of concern that moralistic judgments may be made with regard to how they contracted the disease. This is also a factor with physicians who do not report cases of VD in order to "protect" their patient.

Physicians and public health personnel recognize that venereal disease must be treated as a disease with moralistic judgments left to others if they are to handle this problem effectively. A number of state legislatures recognizing this aspect of the problem have passed legislation making it possible for minors to seek VD treatment without requiring that the physician inform the parent. In essence, it is essential that treatment personnel and facilities be easily and comfortably approached if the VD problem is to be reversed. These measures are realistic and attainable and the key to their success is largely an aroused and concerned public. It is entirely within the realm of possibility to eliminate venereal disease as a blight on our society.

THE CHRONIC AND DEGENERATIVE DISEASES

It is a common misconception that the study of chronic and degenerative diseases is of interest to the older members of our populace because only they are affected by them. Though these diseases are more prevalent among our older population, their incidence is higher among our children and youth than is generally recognized. Many times, the incidence of chronic or degenerative conditions later in life can be prevented by a change in living patterns at an earlier age.

The chronic and degenerative diseases are of increasing public health concern since they have become the major cause of death in the country. In the 1900s tuberculosis, pneumonia, diarrhea, and enteritis were the leading causes of death. At the present time, heart disease, cancer, stroke, and accidents top the list. As we have gained greater control over the communicable diseases, people have survived to those ages when heart disease, cancer, and stroke are more prevalent.

Research effort and increased medical services are being focused on these leading causes of death. The acceptance of premature death from disease is being tolerated less and less. The term "died of natural causes" is rapidly becoming obsolete. Those "natural" causes are now being identified as diseased entities, with treatment procedures being developed to correct them and, more important, preventive measures used to eliminate or forestall them.

CARDIOVASCULAR DISEASES

Cardiovascular diseases, which are responsible for more than half of all deaths that occur in the United States, deserve our primary attention. These are diseases relating to the heart (cardio) and the blood vessels (vascular) of the body. There is an increased incidence of cardiovascular disease in those countries that have raised their standards of living and have gone from malnutrition to overnutrition and from rural to urban living with its stresses, sedentary life, and pollution. Cardiovascular disease is increasingly being recognized as an "affliction of civilization."

Artery Diseases

Arteriosclerosis is commonly referred to as hardening of the arteries. Changes take place, as a result of this condition, in the middle layer of the artery wall, which causes a loss of elasticity and contractility. Atherosclerosis, which is the most common form of arteriosclerosis, is a condition in which fatty substances are deposited on the inner lining of the artery. These individual deposits are referred to as atheromas. As more and more of the atheromas are formed, they tend to increase in size and gradually narrow the channel through which the blood flows. The roughening of the lining of the artery through this process facilitates the forming of blood clots. The accumulation of fatty tissues in the lining of the arteries may ultimately result in the blocking of these blood vessels. This is particularly important when it happens to the coronary arteries of the heart or the cerebral arteries of the brain.

There are a number of factors associated with artery diseases:

Heredity. There seem to be family tendencies to develop high cholesterol levels which would increase the possibility for atherosclerosis.

Age. Atherosclerosis and arteriosclerosis affect middle-aged and older people, with significant increases in the 45- to 54-year-age group.

Figure 3–10

Atherosclerosis, known to be one cause of heart attack, has been associated with elevated levels of cholesterol in the bloodstream. Here is a human artery plugged by an atherosclerotic lesion, an important component of which is white fatty cholesterol.

(National Institutes of Health)

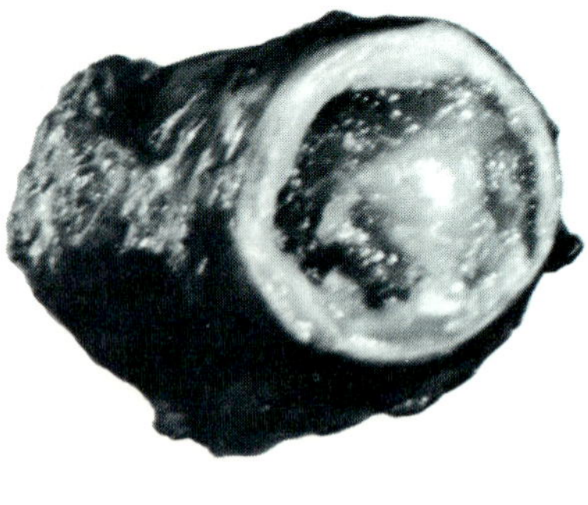

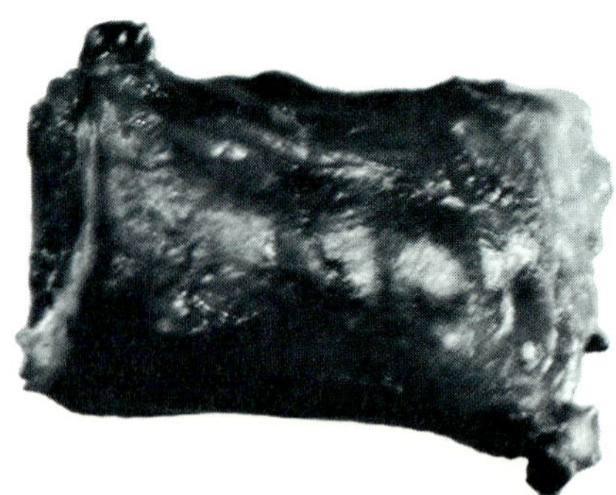

Sex. The incidence of artery disease is lower in younger women than in men. After menopause (or change of life), women become as susceptible to the disease as men.

Cholesterol level. High levels of cholesterol and other serum lipids in the blood increase the chances of developing this disease.

Obesity. Overweight persons increase their chances of developing artery diseases.

Lack of exercise. Those individuals who are inactive in their jobs and leisure time activities suffer higher rates of heart and/or artery disease.

High blood pressure. The incidence of artery disease for people with high blood pressure is greater than in those with normal pressures.

Smoking. Smoking accelerates arteriosclerosis.

Heart Attack

The coronary thrombosis, or heart attack, may be caused by a blood clot in a coronary artery. Such a blood clot would be known as a thrombosis. A closure of the artery may also be effected by an accumulation of atheromas. Closure of an artery by either one of these causes will deprive that part of the heart of blood. The muscle tissue of the heart is thus deprived of oxygen and nutrient material necessary for maintaining its life. Fortunately, most closures of coronary arteries occur in the smaller vessels. The result is that most heart attacks are not fatal.

Symptoms of a heart attack will often include painful sensations of pressure in the chest. These sensations sometimes spread to the arms, throat, or back and may persist for long periods of time. Sudden and intense shortness of breath will often accompany the condition, along with sweating and possibly loss of consciousness. Nausea may sometimes be a symptom that can be mistaken for acute indigestion. Only a physician should make the diagnosis.

Complete rest is usually prescribed following a coronary, whose duration may last from several weeks to months, to permit the healing process to take place. A new supply of blood is also sent into the area around the injury through the development of new blood vessels that branch out into the affected part. This growth of new blood vessels into the injured area is known as *collateral circulation*. Loss of excessive weight and a modification of the diet is usually part of the therapy for a coronary patient. Such a patient is usually advised to stop smoking. Anticoagulants (heparin) are sometimes used to prevent the formation of additional blood clots. A deadly combination of three risk factors—high cholesterol, high blood pressure, and heavy smoking—greatly increases one's chances for a heart attack.

Angina Pectoris

Angina pectoris is really not a disease but a symptom. It is an indication of an inadequate blood supply to the heart muscle. The person usually experiences a feeling of tightness or pressure in the chest and sometimes pain or a tingling sensation that extends to either shoulder or upper arm. These symptoms usually occur following exercise or emotional excitement; they reflect the inability of enough blood (carrying oxygen and nutrient material) to reach the muscle tissues of the heart in order to feed it properly. During the intervals between the angina attacks, the patient is not aware of any discomfort and claims to feel fine. X ray and listening with a stethoscope reveal no abnormality. Even an electrocardiogram will be normal in one-third of the patients with angina. However, the electrocardiogram will sometimes show nontypical irregularities or abnormalities suggestive of coronary insufficiency. In these cases the patient might be given a controlled exercise tolerance test which will in all probability bring on an angina attack. The angina patient is, in essence, forewarned that he has an atherosclerotic condition of the arteries of his body. Management of this condition is generally through loss of weight, exercise, and controlled diet. Because present evidence suggests that there is a cause-and-effect relationship between smoking and atherosclerosis,[3] this patient is usually advised to stop smoking. Nitroglycerine or other forms of nitrate are often prescribed before exercise to dilate the coronary arteries and prevent an angina attack.

STROKE (CEREBROVASCULAR DISEASE)

A stroke occurs when the blood supply to a part of the brain is significantly reduced or completely cut off. As a result, nerve tissue in the brain is not able to function. Those parts of the body which this brain tissue controls will also cease functioning. A stroke, therefore, can result in a variety of effects including loss of speech or memory, or paralysis of various parts of the body. There are several causes of stroke as shown in Figure 3–11.

There are sometimes warning episodes that will lead a doctor to suspect a developing stroke condition. Numbness, dizziness, and confusion are many times indicative of small strokes that precede more significant episodes. Approximately one-third of all strokes can be traced to blood vessels of the neck that have become clogged due to the formation of atheromas. Surgical removal of this material will correct the condition.

The American Heart Association states, ". . . for the first time, suggestive evidence linking cigarette smoking and strokes was shown. The stroke death rate was 40 per cent higher in men aged 55–64 who smoked cigarettes, as compared with nonsmokers. In this same disease category, incidentally, the risk proved unexpectedly greatest for women. Female smokers in all age groups had up to twice the stroke death rate of nonsmoking women."[4]

[3] Jack P. Strong, M.D., "More Artery Hardening Found at Post-Mortem in Coronaries of Cigarette Smokers" in American Heart Association *Heart Research Newsletter,* Vol. XI, No. 4 (Fall 1966).

[4] "AHA Highlights Heart Risks of Smoking," *The American Heart,* Vol. XVII, No. 2 (Spring 1967).

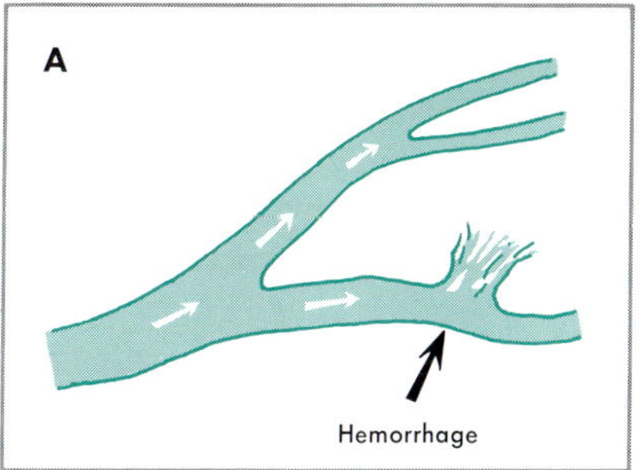

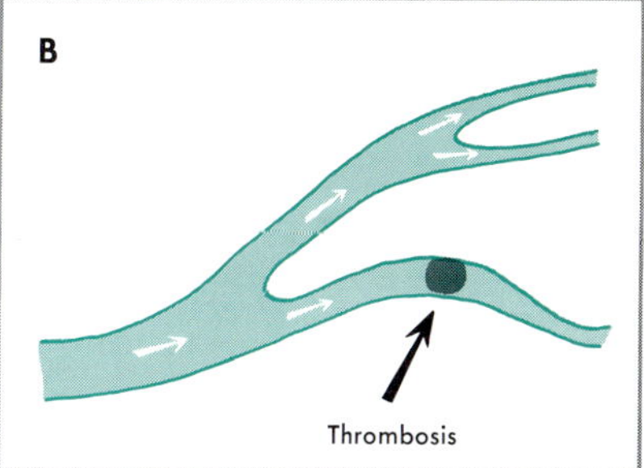

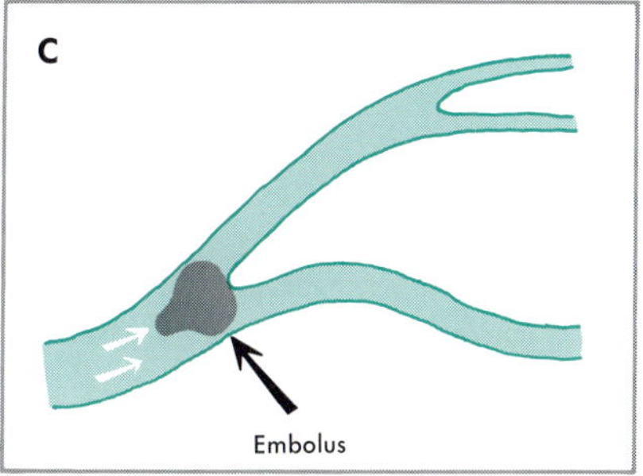

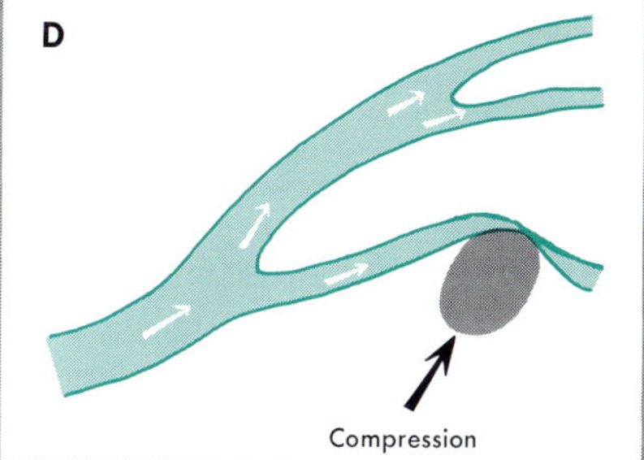

Figure 3–11

Causes of a stroke. (A) Hemorrhage, or bleeding. If an artery wall breaks down as a result of injury or inherent weakness or disease, blood seeps into the surrounding tissue instead of flowing in its normal channels. Although the most dangerous, this kind of stroke is less frequent. (B) Thrombosis, or clot formation. Because of a diseased condition in an artery or vein, a clot of blood may form at some point, and grow in size until it finally plugs the vessel completely. (C) Embolism, or traveling clot. A blood clot formed somewhere else in the arterial system (most commonly in a diseased heart) may break loose, be pumped into a brain vessel and block it. Thrombosis and embolism are frequent and the most common causes of strokes. Fortunately they are also the conditions doctors now have good prospects of controlling. (D) Compression. A tumor or swollen tissue may press upon a blood vessel to the point where it stops the flow of blood. Since brain tumors, however, are relatively rare, this condition is the least common source of a stroke.

(American Heart Association)

An individual's susceptibility to stroke increases noticeably when the person suffers from hypertension. Their risk is four times greater than those individuals with normal blood pressure. This is also supported by a study done in Washington whereby 88 per cent of the hypertensive deaths below the age of 60 were blacks. Hypertension appears at a younger age, is more severe, and results in a higher mortality rate, more commonly from stroke rather than coronary artery disease in the black population.

The presence of diabetes also increases the risk of stroke in man. It follows, then, that a combination of diabetes and hypertension is an extremely dangerous one and makes individuals six times more prone to having a stroke than normal persons.

It becomes obvious that stroke or cerebrovascular disease is merely a small part of the larger problem of cardiovascular disease. A new preventive approach to this disease seems imperative, for once the brain is damaged, recovery or return to normal is difficult, if achieved at all. If the stroke-prone individual is identified early and preventive measures are pursued, it is probable that many strokes could be forestalled or prevented completely. The measures for the prevention of stroke seem to be the same as those indicated for the prevention of coronary heart disease.

HIGH BLOOD PRESSURE

Blood pressure is the force exerted by blood against the walls of the vessels. This force or pressure is measured by a sphygmomonometer and consists of two readings. The higher reading is the systolic pressure recorded during the heart's pumping stroke. The lower reading is the diastolic pressure recorded when the heart is relaxed and refilling between beats. Blood pressure readings vary with individuals and the physician considers all factors before labeling a reading normal or high.

The causes of primary hypertension (or essential hypertension) are generally unknown. It is more common and less serious than secondary hypertension but if left untreated can become a more serious problem. In secondary hypertension the causes are known and usually involve a renal (kidney), vascular (blood vessel), or endocrine malfunction. One of the contributing factors to primary hypertension appears to be hereditary. For example, it has been documented in numerous scientific studies that the incidence of hypertension among the black population is far higher than among whites. A family history of hypertension is a common finding. Though these findings suggest it is an inherited characteristic, there are familial patterns of living that could be making entire families susceptible, not solely owing to the genetic makeup. Another contributing factor is the emotional makeup of the individual. The tense, nervous person who consistently overreacts to stressful situations is highly susceptible to hypertension.

There is a close relationship between arteriosclerosis and heart attacks with hypertension. Uncontrolled hypertension hastens the development of atheromas which in turn increases the risk of heart attacks and stroke from blocked vessels. Uncontrolled hypertension also forces the heart to pump harder, and in extreme cases the strain may cause heart failure. Though we can neither prevent nor cure hypertension, enough is known about the many facets of the disease that reasonable control over the condition is possible.

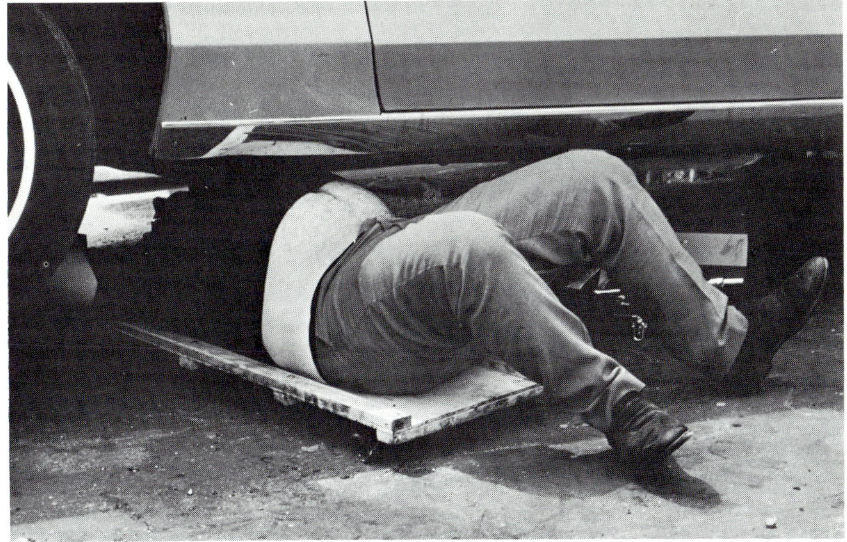

Figure 3–12

In addition to predisposing one to high blood pressure, obesity can be an occupational hazard.

(Dennis Chalkin)

Hypertension can sometimes be treated successfully by diet control. Very often the overweight person who diets successfully and returns to a normal weight will also return to a normal blood pressure. When hypertension does not respond to changes in living patterns, the physician today has at his disposal a myriad of drugs or combinations of drugs designed to lessen tension, dilate blood vessels, encourage the kidneys to excrete salt, or block nerves that prevent the reflex that constricts the vessels. As a result of improved diagnostic and treatment techniques the death rate from hypertension has decreased by nearly 50 per cent during the past ten years.

RHEUMATIC FEVER AND RHEUMATIC HEART DISEASE

Rheumatic fever is a disease that sometimes follows a streptococcal infection. It is estimated, however, that 90 to 97 per cent of streptococcal infections do not develop into rheumatic fever. Rheumatic fever, in turn, may or may not result in rheumatic heart disease. Rheumatic heart disease, however, does develop often enough to account for much of the cardiovascular disease among the young people of this country. It is estimated that approximately 500,000 children between the ages of 5 and 19 have this condition.

The etiology of this disease is not completely understood. It is recognized that a streptococcal infection precedes a rheumatic fever attack. Prevention of the disease is therefore aimed at preventing recurrent streptococcal infections through the administration of antibiotics, because the body, instead of developing a resistance to the streptococcus, seems to become more vulnerable to each recurring attack. The damage to the heart in this condition is done by the scarring of the valves between the auricles and the ventricles. The bicuspid or mitral valve on the left side of the heart is the one that is usually most seriously affected. The disease may also cause damage to the endocardium, which is the inner lining of the heart. Surgical procedures have been developed that permit the cutting of the scar tissue which inhibits the proper functioning of the valves. Now, with the heart-lung machine, surgeons are given a dry field to work in and can replace entire valves with artificial ones.

Because there is no specific cure for rheumatic fever, drugs such as penicillin and cortisone are used to relieve symptoms and inflammation. The amount of bed rest that would be required varies with individual patients. It may be a matter of weeks or sometimes months. How much activity a person with rheumatic heart disease may be permitted will depend on the amount of damage done to his heart. Many rheumatic fever children recover and will live normal lives, provided that they receive proper medical care. Because rheumatic fever can be prevented through the utilization of penicillin or sulfa drugs, it is at the present time the only major form of cardiovascular disease that we have the specific knowledge to prevent.

CONGENITAL HEART DEFECTS

Congenital heart defects represent malformations that occur in the structure of the heart or the large blood vessels associated with it. Although these defects may be present at birth, they are many times not detected until childhood or even adulthood. The causes of congenital heart defects are generally unknown. There appears to be a hereditary factor associated with some. Others are believed to be caused by viral diseases such as German measles during the first trimester of pregnancy. In a study conducted by Dr. Aloss J. Beuren, of the University of Gottingen, Germany, it was found that vitamin D in excessive amounts during pregnancy could severely damage the functioning of the fetus heart by narrowing the aorta and thereby obstructing blood flow.

A blue baby is one that has a malformation of the heart or of the major blood vessels near the heart. These conditions prevent his blood from getting enough oxygen, resulting in the skin and lips taking on a bluish tinge (cyanosis). These malformations are varied. In some cases a congenital heart defect may involve openings between walls of blood vessels or of chambers within the heart itself. It may involve a narrowing or constriction of a blood vessel or a valve inhibiting blood flow. Sometimes several of the above-mentioned malformations combine to form a more serious problem.

The development of the heart-lung machine has made it possible to operate more effectively on the heart. The machine permits the blood to bypass the heart, giving the surgeon a dry field to operate in. Stopping the heart by cooling it with ice is another new technique that permits the surgeon to operate on the organ when it is not in motion. Of the 30,000 to 40,000 children born each year with heart defects, it is now estimated that 75 to 80 per cent of them can be helped by surgery.

HEART RESEARCH

Since cardiovascular disease remains the number one killer of our adult population there is an intensive effort in research activities. One such investigation is The Framingham Study which began in 1949 and continued for twenty-five years. Five thousand persons participated in the study which centered in the Framingham Union Hospital in a Boston, Massachusetts, suburb. The study uncovered vulnerable persons on their way to coronary attacks through the use of a coronary risk profile. Information for the profile was gathered from laboratory findings, physical exercise information, personal habit reports, and electrocardiogram readings. The subjects were followed as they aged and acquired disease conditions and were compared with themselves at an earlier age. The advantage of such a long-term study is that most participants now range in age from 50 to 70 plus and their profiles for other chronic diseases is of considerable scientific value. Children and spouses of the original study group (now numbering 3,927) are also being studied to help determine whether there is an inherited factor that determines fat levels in the blood. A new Framingham Eye Study has evolved, studying patients from the original Framingham Study about whom vast amounts of information have already been collected. The Eye Study will explore diseases such as cataracts, glaucoma, and diabetic complications of eye disease. Another new study evolving is the Multiple Risk Factor Intervention Trial (or Mr. Fit) where *intervention* (i.e., actually changing nutrition and smoking habits and lowering blood pressure with drugs) rather than observation will hopefully get more conclusive answers concerning the connection between heart attacks and high cholesterol, high blood pressure and smoking.

Researchers working on the development of an artificial heart believe that the replacement of a diseased heart by a mechanical substitute will be routine in the future. Various models are currently in the animal experimentation phase and have maintained life in animals from 18 to 51 hours. Some are run on

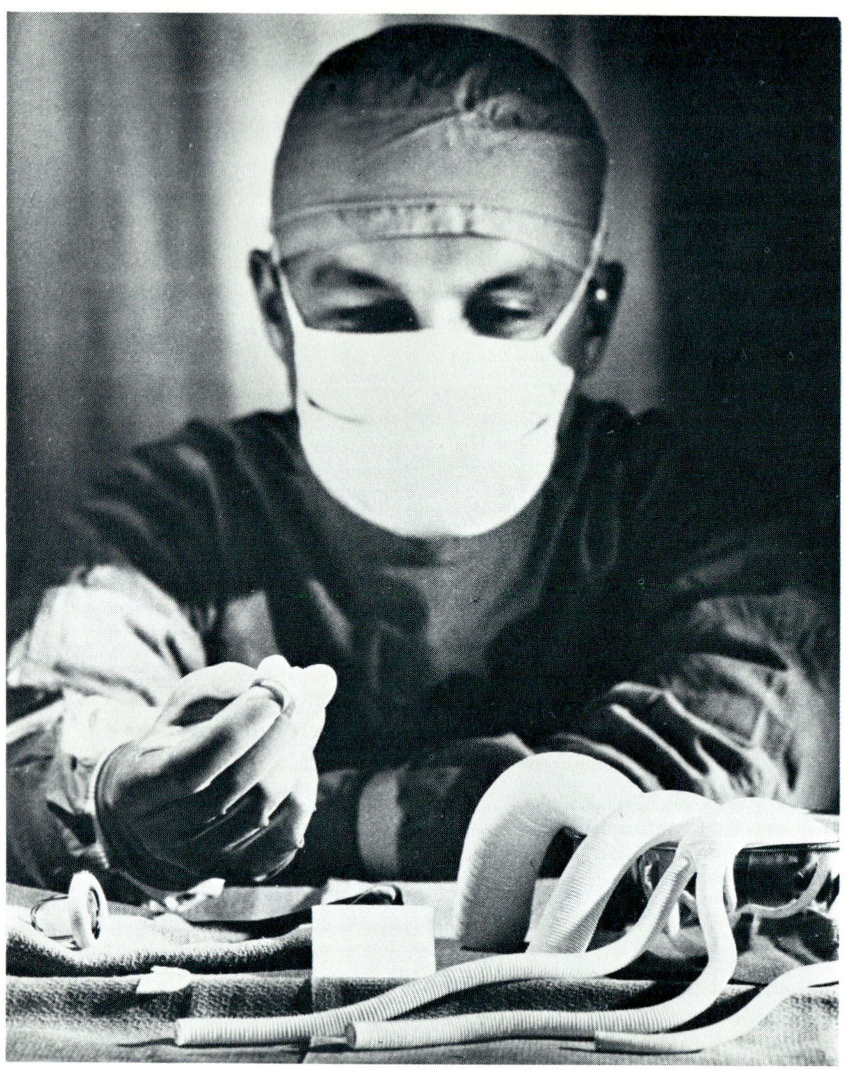

Figure 3–13

Artificial spare parts—valves, vessels, and patches—are used by heart surgeons to repair many once fatal or disabling defects in the heart and blood vessels.

(Photo Jerry Hecht N.T.H.—WHO)

compressed air, others on fluid or electricity. Scientists are even thinking in terms of atomic-powered hearts. This work is laying the groundwork for the ultimate use of permanent heart-assist devices and ultimately a total mechanical heart replacement.

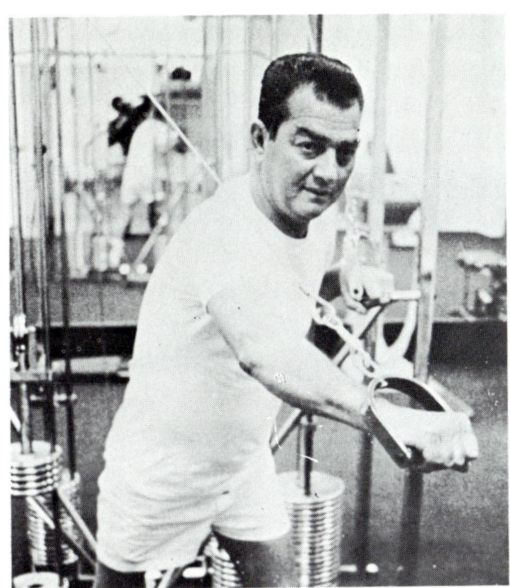

Figure 3–14

On October 15, 1970, Mr. Richard Cope received the heart of a 17-year-old motorcycle accident victim. Mr. Cope is shown exercising his new heart.

(Suffolk Heart Association, Inc.)

The years of 1968 to 1969 will go down in history as the era of the heart transplant. The startling news from South Africa that Dr. Christian Barnard had transplanted a human heart from a *dead*[5] man to the heart-diseased dentist Philip Blaiberg resounded around the world. The floodgates had been thrust open and in the year 1968, 102 heart transplants were performed.

The initial enthusiasm for this procedure began to wane when it was realized that though the surgical techniques were sound and successful, physicians could not prevent the patient's rejection of the new "foreign" heart. It had been assumed that the heart would be initially struggled against, but with the aid of medications be tolerated and finally accepted, as had been demonstrated to a greater degree with kidney transplants. The year 1969 saw only 48 transplants and by 1970 the number dwindled down to 16. As of July 1974, of the 240 persons receiving donor hearts, there were 37 survivors, 5 of whom will be celebrating their fifth anniversary. The physician who has had the most success with the heart transplant procedure is Dr. Norman Shumway of Stanford University, who has 26 survivors out of 76 cases. His success has been attributed more to his ability to control rejection of the heart by the body than to unusual surgical technique. One of the significant gains made

[5] "dead"—As a result of the era of heart and other organ transplants legislatures in more than 40 states developed laws establishing new definitions of death. The American Medical Association has also developed guidelines for physicians contemplating transplants. In June 1972 a jury in Richmond, Virginia, returned the verdict that death occurs with the cessation of brain function and not pulmonary or heart function. It gave legal sanction to the concept of brain death.

from the transplant era was that for the first time in history fresh human heart tissue as well as newly removed diseased hearts were available for microscopic and biochemical examinations. In one study it was found that a chemical imbalance was present in all diseased tissue. Further study of diseased hearts in dogs and rabbits revealed the same imbalance. The development of drugs or hormones to prevent this imbalance is now being studied. The moral, legal, sociological, and medical questions raised during this period will keep the philosophers, lawyers, sociologists, and physicians pondering for many a decade.

As organ transplants become more routine the problems related to supply and demand inevitably begin to surface. Such has been the case with kidney transplants. The increased expertise in this transplant area has resulted in a shortage of kidney donors. A letter to the editor of *Today's Health* magazine offers a possible solution.

New Source of Kidney Donors?

> In your December, 1972 issue Dr. Belding Scribner ("Health Criticism: An Action Plan to Help Kidney Patients,") mentioned that no country in the world gets more than 30 percent of the kidneys it needs for transplants.
>
> Passing out donor cards for people to fill out and carry in their wallets apparently isn't working, probably due to the inertia we all have.
>
> The best source for these donor organs would be the many thousands of healthy people who die every year in auto accidents. Why can't our state motor vehicle departments perform a public service by printing a donor agreement on the backs of all new drivers' licenses to be filled out by those people wishing to donate organs after their deaths?
>
> *Donald Lieberman, M.D.*
> *Santa Clara, California*[6]

The suggested plan may result in increased numbers of donated kidneys as well as other needed organs. It might also result in more careful driving.

Synthetic tubing is now being used to replace diseased arteries. Where large aneuryisms (dilation of the blood vessel due to the weakening of the arterial wall) are found in major arteries such as the aorta, extensive Dacron or Teflon tubing is used to replace the damaged portion of the blood vessel. Artificial heart valves have been successfully implanted in thousands of people. There has also been the successful transplant of heart valves from cadavers to cardiac patients. The implantation of these valves has been made largely possible by the development of the remarkable heart-lung machine.

Artificial pacemakers have been successfully implanted to maintain a regular heart rhythm in those persons whose natural pacemaking mechanisms have been impaired. Many of these battery-powered electronic devices are implanted under the skin of the abdomen with the wiring connected internally to the

[6] *Today's Health* (March 1973), p. 72.

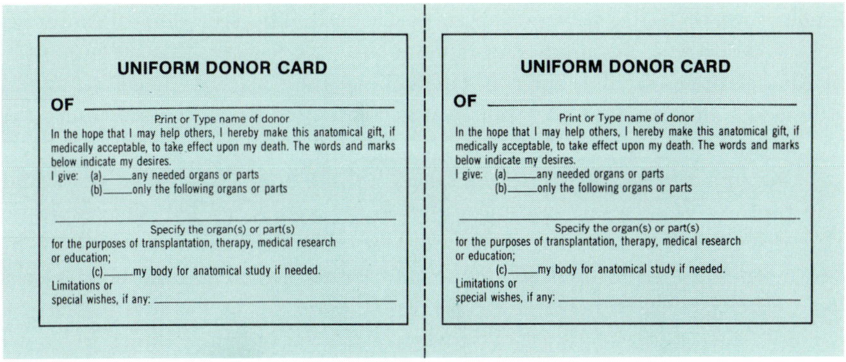

UNIFORM DONOR CARD

OF ______________________________

Print or Type name of donor

In the hope that I may help others, I hereby make this anatomical gift, if medically acceptable, to take effect upon my death. The words and marks below indicate my desires.

I give: (a)_____any needed organs or parts

(b)_____only the following organs or parts

____

Specify the organ(s) or part(s)

for the purposes of transplantation, therapy, medical research or education;

(c)_____my body for anatomical study if needed.

Limitations or special wishes, if any: ______________________________

UNIFORM DONOR CARD

OF ______________________________

Print or Type name of donor

In the hope that I may help others, I hereby make this anatomical gift, if medically acceptable, to take effect upon my death. The words and marks below indicate my desires.

I give: (a)_____any needed organs or parts

(b)_____only the following organs or parts

____

Specify the organ(s) or part(s)

for the purposes of transplantation, therapy, medical research or education;

(c)_____my body for anatomical study if needed.

Limitations or special wishes, if any: ______________________________

Figure 3–15

An authorization card to donate body parts after death.

(American Medical Association)

heart. Before the two- to three-year life of the battery runs out, it can be replaced in a doctor's office under local anesthesia. Most pacemakers have a fixed-rate (usually 80 beats per minute); however, some of the newer, more sophisticated models make allowance for faster rates to meet the body's needs during exertion. These are highly reliable mechanisms; however, to date their failure has come from breaks in the stainless steel or platinum iridium wires that convey the pacing pulses to electrodes implanted in the heart. A new alloy developed (Elgiloy) may prove to withstand prolonged stresses better than any previously used. The need for wire electrodes is completely eliminated by a radio-frequency pacemaker developed at Yale University. A transmitter worm outside the body beams radio energy through the intact chest wall to a tiny receiver implanted in the pericardium, thus eliminating the need for minor surgery to replace worn-down batteries.

CANCER

Cancer is best described as a group of diseases that have a characteristic of abnormal cell growth. Cancer is not so much a disease of the body as it is a disease of the cells. The cells of any living organism are under the control of a regulating mechanism that permits its birth, life, ability to reproduce, and death. The rate at which this happens is carefully controlled. When something goes wrong with this controlling mechanism, and cell division becomes much more rapid, tumors then develop. When these tumors are malignant, their atypical cancer cells can erupt into the blood and lymphatic systems and be carried to various parts of the body. This spreading of cancerous cells is known as *metastasis* (me-TAS′-ta-sis). The cancer cells are not only produced more rapidly but are different in their nature. Their structural differences are such that they can in many instances be recognized under the microscope.

Although the specific causes of cancer are unknown, a number of related contributing factors and possible causes have been identified. Overexposure to radiation has been found to be a predisposing factor to the development of cancer. A higher incidence of leukemia has been found among those infants who were X-rayed in prenatal life. Excessive exposure of the skin to the sun is also a factor in the increased incidence of skin cancer. A more judicious use of medical and dental X rays has resulted. For high-incidence groups in which tuberculosis is being sought, a simple tuberculin test is recommended as a first procedure. If the results of this test are positive, then a chest X ray is recommended.

A good deal of research is now going on to explore the relationship of viruses and cancer. A number of animal cancers have been identified as having been produced by viruses. There is suspicion that these microorganisms also play a role in the development of some human cancers.

The relationship of hormones to cancer has become suspect. There have been spontaneous recoveries from terminal cases of cancer which were attributed to changes in the hormonal environment. The use of hormone treatment in cancer of the breast, uterus, or prostate is already well established. At the other end of the spectrum there is some belief that vaginal cancer in young women up to age 22 may be a direct result of the administration of estrogenic hormones to their mothers during pregnancy. Though cancer as a disease cannot be inherited, with the exception of retinoblastoma,[7] it appears that a predisposition to some types of cancer may be. A physician's study of recent family history may give some clues as to preventive measures that one might take. Certainly, where a parent or grandparent has been claimed by lung cancer, one should view cigarette smoking with a jaundiced eye.

Various chemicals have been identified as being carcinogenic (cancer-producing) in nature. Coal tar colors that were used as color additives at one time have been identified as among these types of chemicals. Chimney sweeps in England, for instance, have a higher incidence of skin cancer, which is related to their contact with soot. A high incidence of cancer of the bladder among dye workers has been traced to aniline dyes. Studies have also shown arsenic to be a cancer-producing agent, particularly cancer of the skin. Chronic irritations of various types have also become suspect as possible cancer-producing factors. Even omissions in the diet have been demonstrated to be related to

[7] "Retinoblastoma" is usually found in children under the age of four and is considered to be a congenital tumor. The aim of treatment is to save not only the life of the patient but the vision of at least one eye.

the incidence of cancer of the liver in communities of South Africa and Java, where vitamin B is lacking in the diet. The incidence of leukemia is 20 times as frequent in patients suffering from Down's syndrome (mongolism) as in the normal population. An abnormality of chromosome 21 appears in patients with a certain type of leukemia, though it is not the same as found in Down's syndrome (mongolism). The riddle of the relationship between this type of cancer and this genetic abnormality remains unsolved.

While the research scientists are looking for the specific causes of cancer, the epidemiologist can perform the function of identifying those factors that are responsible for triggering certain cancers. The identification of these factors and where they occur in our environment can play a very significant role in the prevention of this disease.

SITES OF CANCER

Lung Cancer has assumed epidemic proportions among men. The recovery rate from this disease is very low, with only approximately 7 per cent of the males and 8 per cent of the females recovering. The incidence of lung cancer among women has doubled in the last 22 years. The lung cancer death rate among American men has increased more than 14 times in 40 years and partially accounts for the general increase in the male cancer death rate from 280 per 100,000 population in 1947 to 304 deaths per 100,000 population in 1970.

Diagnosis of this condition is difficult and often too late. Heavy smokers may take 15 years to develop a lung lesion or tumor, after which time it becomes lethal in a matter of months. The early morning cough and sputum may be ignored for too long and the clear cut symptoms of chest pain and blood tinged sputum that follow may be the indicators of lung cancer.

Cancer of the Colon and Rectum Together, cancers of the colon and rectum make up the second leading cause of cancer death in the United States. Approximately 93 per cent of cancer of the colon or rectum occurs in people over 45 years of age. Three out of every four of these afflicted people can be saved, for it is a highly curable disease when detected early. Digital and proctoscopic examinations should be routinely included in annual physical checkups as a means of early detection.

Breast Cancer lends itself to early detection through breast self-examination, mammography (a special breast X ray), and thermography (a heat sensitive photograph of the breast). Hopefully a newly devised test involving cell examination of fluid extracted from a breast will reveal early irregularities of cell growth similar to the Pap smear for cervical cancer. Approximately 95 per cent of all breast cancers have been detected by women themselves. For this reason it is important that all women be properly instructed with regard to this procedure. Lumps or thickenings in the breast are sometimes sympto-

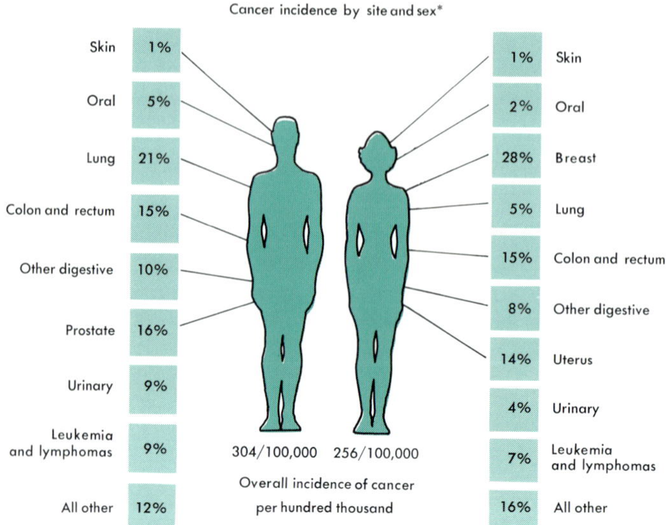

Figure 3–16

Cancer incidence by site and sex.

(American Cancer Society. *'74 Cancer Facts and Figures*)

matic of this disease. It must be remembered, however, that most lumps appearing in the breast are not cancerous in nature. Nevertheless, all irregularities should motivate the individual to confirm this with a medical opinion. Bleeding from the nipple and swollen lymph nodes under the arm pit are also possible signs of this disease. It is the leading cause of death among women.

Cancer of the Skin is easily detected, diagnosed, and treated. This is a site of cancer that a physician can view easily. He can check telltale signs of the disease such as moles and skin blemishes that change in size or color, or a sore that does not heal. Construction workers, sportsmen, and farmers seem to be more prone to the development of cancer of the face, neck, and hands because of their greater exposure to the sun. Fair-skinned people are also more susceptible.

In spite of the fact that this type of cancer can be easily detected, diagnosed, and treated, approximately 5,000 unnecessary deaths per year can be attributed to it.

Cancer of the Stomach. There has been a 40 per cent decrease in the last twenty years in cancer of the stomach, for reasons that have not been determined. Persistent indigestion and bloody discharge with bowel movements are the prime symptoms related to this condition.

Cancer of the Uterus. Uterine cancer is a malignancy that can occur in the cervix (neck of the uterus) or the body proper (corpus) of the uterus.

Most uterine cancers occur in the cervix, and there seems to be no age limit. After age 45, however, cancers of the body of the uterus tend to be most prevalent. Deaths due to cancer of the uterus have been significantly reduced since the introduction of the Pap (Papanicolaou) test. The test consists of removing and examining cells from the vagina and from the cervix of the uterus. The microscopic examination of the cells will indicate whether cancer or precancerous cells are present. The cure rate for this type of cancer is exceedingly high, provided it is detected early enough. Entire communities have organized for action to bring the women in for their yearly Pap smear. Some hospitals have initiated the policy of doing a Pap smear on every female admitted regardless of the reason for admission. The importance of early detection and prompt treatment has been substantiated by the fact that the cure rate has risen from 38 per cent to 50 per cent in the last 25 years.

Cancer of the Prostate. The function of the prostate gland is to secrete a thick alkaline fluid which aids the sperm cells to get through the acid environment of the urethra. Incidence of cancer of the prostate is highest in men over 55 years of age. Black men are 65 per cent more likely to suffer from cancer of the prostate than whites. Frequent, thorough rectal examinations in men over 40 are helpful in detecting the disease early. Blood in the urine or in the ejaculate are significant signs. These symptoms, however, may be indicative of a number of other conditions including the bacterial infection of the prostate, bladder, or other related structures. Treatment for prostatic cancer, where the cancer is limited to a small nodule or hard area in the gland itself, is usually surgical removal. However, when the cancer extends beyond the prostate gland itself, alteration of the hormonal balance is carried out, either through surgical removal of the testes (orchiectomy) and possibly the administration of female hormones (estrogens).

Cancer of the Blood, or Leukemia. Leukemia is the leading cause of nearly half of the deaths due to cancer in children between the ages of 3 and 15. This is a cancer of the blood-manufacturing organs, the bone marrow, spleen, and lymph glands. Its presence is detected by large numbers of white blood cells or the presence of immature blood cells. The acute form of leukemia occurs in younger people, and the survival period of this form of the disease is now five years or more. This has been made possible with the use of a barrage of drugs. Some of these drugs are called inducers and bring about a remission of the disease, with a second group of drugs used to help maintain the remission. The chronic type of leukemia occurs usually after 25 years of age. The patient with this disease may survive for ten years or more. Through the use of drug therapy, physicians have managed to obtain some control over leukemia. Steroid hormones and cytotoxic drugs are among those used in chemotherapeutic procedures. Blood transfusions are also utilized as a means of controlling anemia. Optimism has been expressed that effective drug therapy will soon be possible for the control of this condition.

Cancer of the Lymph Glands is a cancer that arises in the lymphatic system and is characterized by enlarged lymph glands. Hodgkin's disease is one of several malignant disorders of the lymphatic system that affects adults between the ages of 20 and 40. It is a relatively uncommon type of cancer.

If lymph glands should remain enlarged for three weeks or more, a physician should be seen so that a biopsy (the microscopic examination of body tissue to determine the presence of cancer cells) may be performed. The progress of the disease is slow and the person affected may live a normal life for many years, provided he is under treatment with drugs and/or X rays.

The American Cancer Society has developed a list of seven danger signals for cancer. These signs will in most cases be indicative of *other* malfunctions rather than the presence of cancer. However, they should be brought to the physician's attention for his investigation and diagnosis. The warning signals are:

1. **C**hange in bowel or bladder habits
2. **A** sore that does not heal
3. **U**nusual bleeding or discharge
4. **T**hickening or lump in breast or elsewhere
5. **I**ndigestion or difficulty in swallowing
6. **O**bvious change in wart or mole
7. **N**agging cough or hoarseness

TREATMENT FOR CANCER

With each cancer patient, the physician has the problem of deciding what treatment is best for that individual. In making this decision, he must take into account the type of cancer, the location, the patient's age, and general health. Consideration of these factors will lead him to recommend one of three basic forms of treatment or a combination of them.

Surgery is one of those basic forms of treatment. If the surgeon decides to perform the type of operation that is meant to cure the patient, then he will completely remove all of the cancerous tissue or organ, including surrounding tissues to which the cancer may have spread. Some scientists are wary of the term *cure* in dealing with cancers. They prefer instead the concept of *control of cancer,* where the cancer cells are held in check rather than allowed to grow to the point of destruction. Improvements developed in surgery have helped to make this form of treatment more effective. This has involved not only improvements in surgical techniques, but in the general care of the patient during and after operations.

Radiation is a second type of treatment for cancer. Two general types of radiation are used, namely, X rays and radio isotopes. From studies that have been done, man has learned that amounts of radiation that have relatively little effect on normal tissues can cause considerable damage to cancer tissue. The radiation may be beamed into the body from an outside source or placed directly on or in the body. Radio isotopes are used in the form of either solids or liquids. In either form they are placed as close as possible to the cancer. In recent years X-ray machines have been improved and made more efficient. Their rays are more penetrating than they have been in the past and there is less scattering of radiation throughout the body. The result is that a smaller zone of normal tissue is thus irradiated.

It is well known that radiation can cause cancer as well as cure it. For this reason the complex techniques involved in radiology must be performed with skill and caution. It has also been observed that different cancers react differently to various kinds of radiation. As is true of other diseases and treatments, patients react rather individually to them. Though there is a good deal to be learned about radiation treatment, it remains as one of the most effective procedures we have in combating cancer.

Chemotherapy is the most recently developed treatment for cancer. A great deal of research is going on in this area in attempts to find drugs that will effectively stop malignant growths. Drugs developed thus far have in some instances slowed cancerous growths or stopped them for periods of time. A wide range of drugs have been utilized in attempts to stop or retard tumor growths. They include such items as hormones, cell poisons (cytotoxic drugs), and metabolic antagonists. Even antibodies can now be counted among the new anticancer drugs.

Each year, thousands of drugs are screened and tested to determine their value as anticancer medications. For example, The National Cancer Institute scientists have reported successful drug treatment of a rare but highly malignant type of cancer (choriocarcinoma). The malignancy arises from the placenta during or after pregnancy. Methotrexate and the antibiotic actinomycin D resulted in a complete remission of the disease in 74 per cent of the study group used.

Drugs are sometimes helpful used singly, in combination with other drugs, or in addition to surgery and radiation. More and more there seems to be an attempt to combine the beneficial effects of various approaches to treatment.

THE OUTLOOK FOR CANCER

In the early 1900s, few cancer patients had any hope of cure. By the 1930s, some progress had been made, but still fewer than one in five could be saved. At the present time, of every six persons that develop cancer two are being saved and one could have been saved by early diagnosis and treatment. This represents, then, one of the immediate objectives in reducing the mortality rate from this condition.

The university of Minnesota Detection Center reports that those cancers diagnosed in routine checkups have a cure rate twice that of patients who see doctors after symptoms have appeared. The implications here for routine checkups and early detection are obvious. With regard to cancer, the unfortunate attitude still persists that what one does not know will not hurt him. The fact remains that of every twenty-four persons, six will develop cancer. In order to save three of these six, instead of the current two, we must make the most effective use of treatments, facilities, and medical personnel now available.

DISORDERS OF THE NERVOUS SYSTEM

Epilepsy

Epilepsy refers to repeated episodes of sudden overactivity of the nervous system. The episodes are associated with convulsions (or seizures) and lapses in consciousness. The EEG (electroencephalograph) is able to record the abnormal brain wave patterns developed in this disorder. Most causes of these convulsive disorders are unknown. In some known cases, it has been found that tumors or blood clots from accidents, infection of the meninges, or strokes are responsible. Faulty development of brain tissure during fetal life, birth injuries, deficient amounts of sugar and oxygen, high fever in young children, or defects in cerebral circulation are also possible causes. Though there may be a hereditary factor associated with some of the less understood forms of this disorder, it apparently is not associated with known causes of epilepsy, such as injury and disease.

Seizures occurring in epilepsy vary greatly. The *grand mal* type of seizure is often initiated by an aura, and the person sees flashing or colored lights and senses an unpleasant odor. The eyes and head turn to one side, and this is sometimes a warning of an oncoming attack. This is followed by convulsive movements. During the seizure, it might be helpful to remove furniture or any other objects against which the person might hurt himself during his thrashing moments. After the seizure, the person may have a headache or feel tired and sleepy.

In the *petit mal* type of seizure, the person may do nothing more than develop a blank stare for a short period of time. Sometimes the stare is as brief as the blinking of the eyes. This type of epilepsy is more prevalent in young girls, and its cause is unknown. The inattentive child or one who falls easily and drops things may in some instances prove to be suffering from petit mal convulsive episodes. Petit mal seizures can occur as often as two hundred times a day.

The *psychomotor* type of seizure usually results in purposeful motions that are not relevant to the situation, such as chewing or smacking of lips. Psychomotor episodes seem to be more prevalent among males. The incidence of the seizures is less frequent than in petit mal, but they may last from between three to five minutes. Sometimes disrobing becomes part of the actions taken during the seizure, with the result that the person is mistaken for a sexual deviate. In all three of the types of seizures described, total amnesia is part of the attack. In *focal or Jacksonian* seizures, involuntary actions may start in one part of the body, such as a foot or hand, and migrate upward to other parts. These attacks will often occur without loss of consciousness.

In the treatment of epileptics, drug therapy has been a very effective control. There are a number of anticonvulsant drugs used in varying combinations, dependent upon the symptoms and the reactions of the patient. It is felt that these types of drugs will ultimately be the answer to the complete control of this disorder. The difficulty, however, is that only one out of five epileptics at the present time is under a physician's care. Surgery is sometimes effective when the epilepsy cannot be controlled by drugs.

Maintaining emotional balance is important to the epileptic in that stress will often precipitate seizures. Some epileptics are sensitive to alcohol and therefore must restrict their use of it. Others have seizures triggered by flashing lights. Automobile driving for these people, then, can become dangerous. The biggest problem to the person suffering from a convulsive disorder is often the "normal" person, who does not understand his condition. He has to face the prejudicial actions and ignorance on the part of the society he lives in. Convulsive disorders are often not well understood, being erroneously confused with mental illness or feeblemindedness. This is one disorder in which some people feel that the sufferer is more handicapped by the regressive attitude of society than by his disability. While this attitude appears to be changing, many epileptics still face the possibility of chronic unemployment and poverty.

Cerebral Palsy

Cerebral palsy is a brain-centered disorder affecting the muscles. Because of damage to the motor area of the brain, cerebral palsied individuals are not able to control the voluntary muscles of the body. There are approximately 550,000 cerebral palsied persons in the United States. All the causes of cerebral palsy are not known; however, some causative factors have been identified. Rubella (German measles) contracted by the mother in the first trimester of pregnancy is one of them. Other causes include trauma, prematurity, Rh factors, anoxia (a lack of oxygen), and congenital malformations. The relationship of inheritance as a causative factor in cerebral palsy is receiving increasing attention.

There are several types of cerebral palsy, the most common being the *spastic* type. Spastics have a great deal of muscle tenseness and excessive contractions, making coordinated movements difficult. The *athetoid* type is characterized by slow, involuntary, and unorganized movements. The spastic and athetoid types represent 80 per cent of the cerebral palsy population. A mixed form of cerebral palsy occasionally occurs, severely incapacitating the individual. *Ataxia* is a third type of cerebral palsy in which a disturbed sense of balance is present. This usually will result in many falls. The fourth type is characterized by tremor, in which one or more limbs of the body may be affected. The shaking makes use of the hands and feet most difficult. A fifth type is characterized by rigidity of one or more limbs of the body. The rigid muscles resist movement and therefore make people so afflicted slow moving.

Many cerebral palsied individuals will have normal or above-normal intelligence. This is oftentimes masked by their inability to express themselves easily because of their muscular conditions. Preventive measures with regard to cerebral palsy center around good prenatal care, the reduction of premature deliveries, and the prevention of a lack of oxygen in the newborn baby. The control of Rh incompatibility and the prevention of accidents can also serve as preventive measures.

Multiple Sclerosis

Multiple sclerosis is a disease that affects the nervous system. It attacks the myelin sheath of the nerve and in doing so leaves scar tissue; hence the term sclerosis. The myelin sheath has the function of insulating the nerve fiber and preventing the overflow and loss of the nerve impulse. Since the disease can affect many parts of the nervous system, it is called *multiple.*

The onset of this condition is usually between the ages of 20 and 40 years. Symptoms that will appear when the myelin is destroyed in parts of the body will include partial or complete paralysis, numbness, double vision, slurring of speech, staggering, and general weakness. In the more advanced stages of the disease, problems in speech, swallowing, and loss of bladder or bowel control occur. The disease is not necessarily consistent in its progress. There will be periods of deterioration followed by temporary remissions. The prognosis for the disease varies, with most patients being ultimately disabled. In some people, the disturbance is relatively mild, permitting them to live long and productive lives. In the majority of cases; however, the life-span is shortened.

Muscular Dystrophy

Muscular dystrophy is a disease in which there is a degeneration of the striated or voluntary muscles of the body. In this condition the nerves are not affected. The number of persons afflicted with this disease is not known, but it is estimated that approximately 200,000 have the condition. More than one-half of these are children between the ages of 4 and 15. The cause or causes of muscular dystrophy are unknown, although there is general agreement that a hereditary basis exists in all types of the disease. Some research indicates a possibility that those so afflicted have the inability to utilize vitamin E. This and other theories with regard to causation are being investigated. The prognosis for the disease varies a great deal, dependent upon which of the four basic types of muscular dystrophy one is referring to.

While research holds the ultimate key to the prevention and treatment of this disease, we as a society have the responsibility to do everything possible for the present generation of patients now afflicted. There unfortunately seems to be at the present time the same kind of apathy about rehabilitation of the muscular dystrophy patient as there was approximately twenty years ago about those suffering from cerebral palsy. Rehabilitation programs for patients with dystrophy try to make the individual as self-sufficient as possible, physically, vocationally, and psychosocially. Successful rehabilitation programs keep dystrophy patients vocationally occupied longer and better adjusted for many years beyond the time that they could possibly be without this kind of help.

MENTAL RETARDATION

The term *mental retardation* describes an effect rather than a given condition. "The mentally retarded person is one who, from childhood, experiences unusual difficulty learning and is relatively ineffective in applying whatever he has learned to the problems of ordinary living; he needs special training and guidance to make the most of his capacities, whatever they may be."[8]

Some Causes of Retardation

There are many causes of mental retardation. Some may occur *before* birth, while others occur during birth or in early childhood. *Before* birth, brain development of a baby can be harmed by poor nutrition of the mother during pregnancy or by the presence of certain chemicals in her bloodstream. If the development of chromosomes is abnormal while the fetus is growing, the result may be a form of retardation known as Down's syndrome or mongolism.

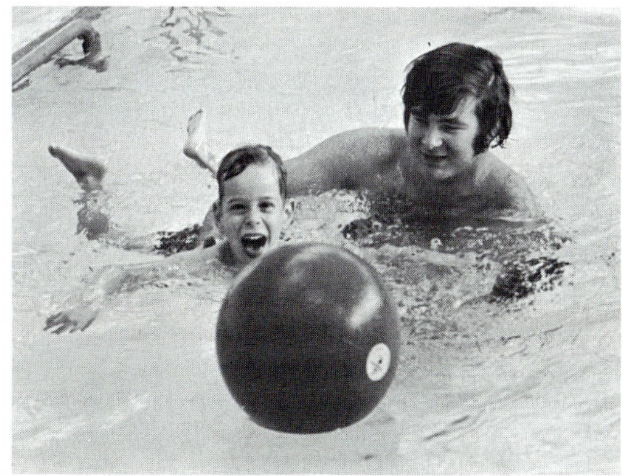

Figure 3–17

Making the most of his capacities.

(New York State Department of Mental Hygiene—Julian A. Belin)

[8] *Facts on Mental Retardation,* National Association for Retarded Children, Inc.

Sometimes if the mother gets German measles or takes unusually high amounts of vitamin D while she is pregnant, the baby will be harmed. An Rh incompatibility of the parents may also cause retardation. In these instances, the mental retardation exists at birth (congenital) and is considered a birth defect.

Mental retardation may occur *at* birth. During difficult deliveries there may be an injury or a reduction of oxygen supply to the infant's brain. Modern obstetrics have made significant contributions toward minimizing these as factors, particularly when prenatal care has been sought by the mother.

A "normal" child may become retarded as a result of such diseases as measles (rubeola), meningitis, encephalitis, whooping cough, scarlet fever, or other diseases causing high fever. Accidents such as a blow on the head or lead poisoning as a result of ingesting pieces of lead-based paints or window putty may cause retardation.

Attitudes Toward the Retarded

Societal attitudes toward the retarded have been undergoing considerable change. The era of hiding the retarded child in the home and having feelings of shame and guilt are rapidly disappearing. A more enlightened populace is recognizing that the many unknown causes of retardation make this a condition that could occur in any family. Where feelings of shame exist, it is often because the parent mistakenly feels responsible for the child's state. Thus it is that the parents' feelings of guilt are expressed in feelings of shame for

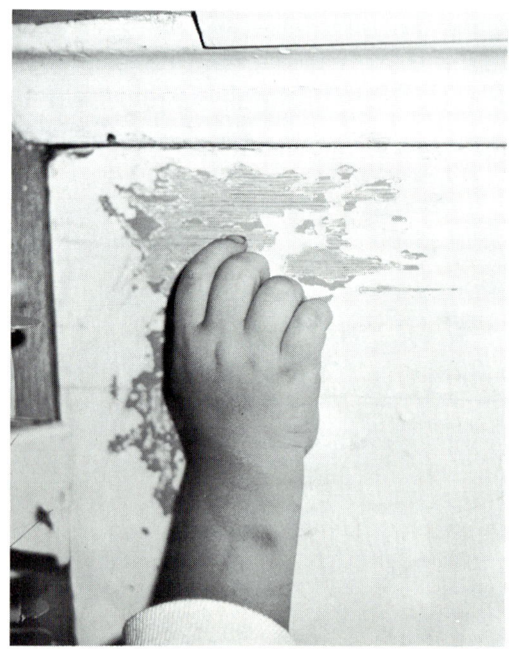

Figure 3–18

The presence of lead in paint poses a hazard when youngsters eat chips of paint. The accumulation of lead can result in mental retardation.

(*FDA Consumer,* October 1972)

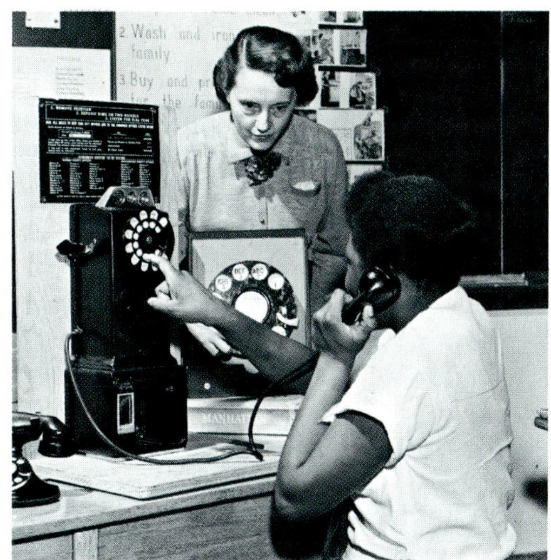

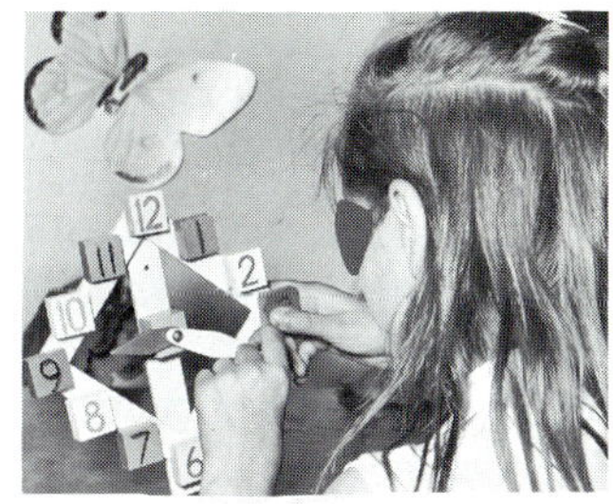

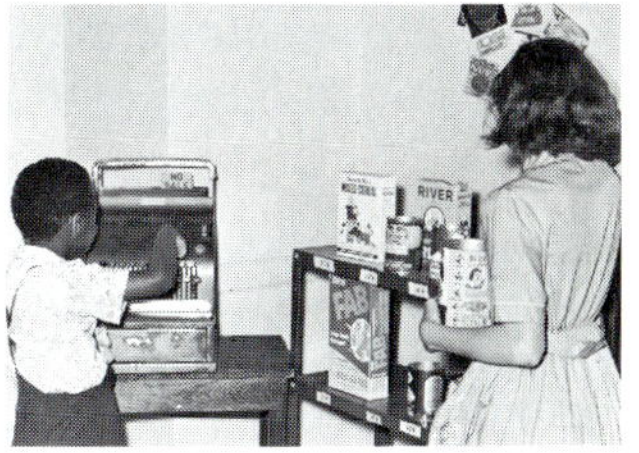

Figure 3–19

Retarded children learning some basic skills.

(New York State Department of Mental Hygiene and Capital Newspapers, Albany, N.Y.)

the child. In recent years, greater understanding of these conditions has resulted in more objective and positive responses to the problem. New and concerted efforts are being made to develop each retarded child to the maximum of his potential.

Comprehensive Programs for the Retarded

In order to diagnose mental retardation early, many communities have clinics where the type of retardation is diagnosed and proper treatment prescribed. Home visit programs are often provided so that parents may be counseled with regard to their child's condition and potentialities.

Special education classes in schools provide a curriculum for the "educable" children. The IQ's of these children range from 50 to 75, with most growing up to self-sufficient adults because of the education now provided them. This group makes up the bulk of the retarded. Special classes are provided for those children whose IQ's range from about 30 to 50. These children are referred to as "trainable." Their curriculum prepares them to care for themselves and to do less complicated kinds of work.

A third group of retardates consists of those that are severely or profoundly retarded. Their condition is complicated by a higher incidence of physical handicaps. The multiple-handicapped child is difficult to care for at home. For this reason these individuals are often institutionalized where they may be better cared for.

Except for the severely retarded or multiple-handicapped, most retarded children are reared at home. They do better in a home environment where enlightened parents and other family members as well as the community accept them. When one looks past the handicap to see the child beneath it, one realizes that the needs of these children are the same as those of any other. Love and acceptance are basic to their emotional development.

There are over 2 million retarded persons of work age in this country, and this figure is expected to grow. In the interests of the individuals involved as well as the national economy, it is important for retardates to be vocationally trained. Their contribution will be an increasingly significant one. It can only come about, however, with parental and community investment of time and effort in the training of the retarded leading to personal and vocational growth and worth.

Research

At the present time, research is our greatest hope for the prevention of the bulk of the cases of retardation. The research being conducted is as varied as the causes of this handicap. Some modest gains have already been made in the preventive area. We now have a vaccine for measles (rubeola), and German measles (rubella), childhood diseases that can cause not only mental retardation but hearing loss as well as a number of other afflictions. The development and mass distribution of these vaccines should eliminate these infections and their damaging effects.

Advances that have been made in modern obstetrical care are responsible for a similar contribution. Birth injury is not nearly as common as it used to be. Good prenatal care has also reduced the incidence of premature birth, which carried with it a higher incidence of retardation. There is now the awareness that malnutrition during pregnancy and infancy has a relationship to mental retardation. Where parents have an incompatible Rh blood factor, many a child's life and mental capacity have been saved by an amniocentesis (see Chapter 5), which alerts the physician to the problem before real damage occurs.

Research efforts will no doubt continue to make contributions to the prevention of retardation. These efforts deserve the enthusiastic support of the community they will serve. In the meantime, we have the obligation and need to utilize effectively that information we already possess in the area of prevention and rehabilitation of the retarded.

GENETIC DISEASES

At the present time it is known that more than 1,600 diseases are caused by defective genes that carry the inherited characteristics from parent to child. While many of the genetic diseases are rare, a number such as cystic fibrosis and sickle-cell anemia are rather common. It has been estimated that more than 25 per cent of children hospitalized are for genetic-related diseases.

New scientific discoveries are resulting in better control of these disorders. We are learning, for example, to better diagnose some of these diseases even before birth. The technique known as amniocentesis (see Chapter 5) results in the diagnosis of genetic diseases by examining the fluid surrounding the unborn child. Let us examine several genetic diseases.

Sickle-Cell Anemia

Sickle-cell anemia is an inherited disease affecting our black population almost exclusively, though it has been seen rarely in white families of Mediterranean origin (Italian, Greek). The abnormal structure of the hemoglobin causes red blood cells to pucker or assume a sickle shape. These twisted cells cannot pass through the capillary walls and often pile up eventually to block the flow of blood to body tissues. These red blood cells are also very fragile and are rapidly destroyed. "Their life span may be only 30–40 days instead of the normal 120 days. Although a person with Sickle Cell Anemia can produce new cells at a rapid rate, he becomes anemic because the rate of destruction of cells is greater than that of production."[9] When the flow of

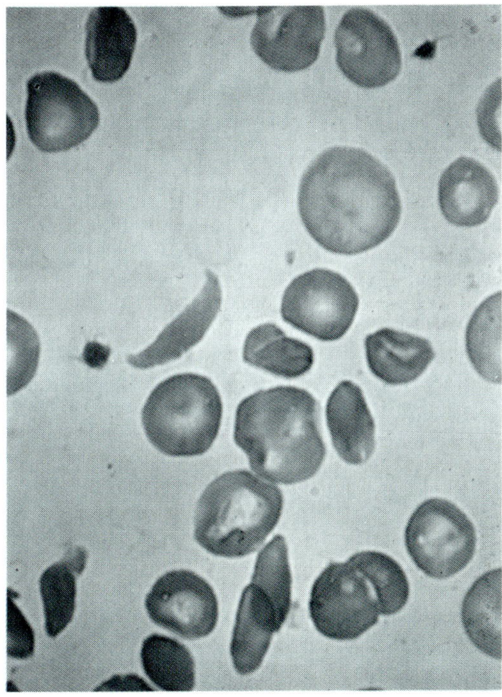

Figure 3–20

In sickle-cell anemia the abnormal structure of the hemoglobin causes the red blood cells to pucker or assume a sickle shape.

(Carl Pochedly, M.D., Director of Pediatric Hematology Dept., Nassau County Medical Center, East Meadow, N.Y.)

[9] Carl Pochedly, M.D., "Sickle Cell Anemia: Recognition and Management," *The American Journal of Nursing,* Vol. 71, No. 10 (October 1971).

blood to body tissues is hampered by the blockage of these sickled cells, the person is said to be suffering a sickle-cell crisis. These periodic attacks of acute pain, anemia with weakness, nausea, and jaundice are the plight of the person suffering this disease.

Many doctors feel all blacks should be screened for this inherited blood trait before undergoing basic training, surgery, or participation in strenuous athletics. Individuals with the disease and those merely carrying the genetic trait are advised against flying in unpressurized airplanes or engaging in any activity that might cause a moderate lack of oxygen, since a lowered amount of oxygen may lead to a sickling crisis.

It has been confirmed by studies conducted in Africa and the Mediterannean basin that sickle-cell hemoglobin makes the person more resistant to malaria. Throughout history those with sickle-cell hemoglobin thus had the advantage of surviving in malaria-infested areas and had the opportunity to pass on this characteristic to their offspring. It is estimated that 2 out of every 25 black Americans are carriers of the sickle-cell trait. Only 1 out of every 400 actually has the disease. When both the mother and father are carriers of the sickle-cell trait, out of every 4 children they have, chances are that 1 will have sickle-cell anemia; 2 will be carriers of the trait; and 1 will not have either the disease or the trait.

The Sickledex Test is used in mass screening for sickle-cell anemia. A positive reaction may mean the individual has either sickle-cell anemia or carries the trait. If a positive Sickledex is recorded, the person would then undergo additional tests which would determine whether the person had the disease.

Physicians now warn known carriers of the disease who are contemplating marriage what the disease risks are for any children born to them. This is one of the genetic diseases that *cannot* as yet be detected through amniocentesis. However, since the development of a simple blood test, the implications for *prevention* by genetic counseling are greatly increased. It has been noted in certain communities where massive screening has been conducted that there is a great need for mental health counseling in addition to the genetic counseling. The feelings of helplessness and hopelessness that result with the diagnosis of sickle-cell anemia are feelings that people must be helped to cope with. With improved treatment methods, hospitalization, and antibiotics to curb infections, the life-span of these patients has been increased, though it remains as a low 20 years of age. The disease is most severe in the young; once adolescence is reached, the sickling crises are not as severe and do not occur as frequently. Continued identification through routine testing, education, and follow-up programs remain essential.

Cystic Fibrosis

This is a disease that was not recognized until thirty years ago. At the present time, because of better knowledge and better diagnostic techniques, it is ranked as one of the leading causes of death among children. Cystic fibrosis is an inherited disease of children which affects the externally secreting glands of the body, including sweat and mucous glands. Instead of the mucous glands secreting the normally free-flowing fluid, they give off a mucus that it thick and sticky. Its effect is to clog and block the various ducts of the body. The thick mucus interferes with such bodily functions as breathing and digestion. In 80 per cent of the cases of cystic fibrosis the ducts of the pancreas become clogged with these secretions, inhibiting the flow of enzymes necessary for digestion. While the child's appetite may be enormous, his inability to digest some foods will result in early signs of malnutrition.

Chronic lung disease is a common complication of cystic fibrosis. The thickened mucus tends to block the passages of the lung, clogging air sacs and making breathing increasingly difficult. Bacterial infections occur repeatedly, leading to progressive, irreversible lung damage or pneumonia. It has also been noted that the cystic fibrosis patient has an excessive loss of salt. This may result in heat exhaustion during the summer months if extra salt is not taken.

Studies strongly suggest that cystic fibrosis is transmitted through a recessive gene. This means that both parents have to be carriers of the gene in order for one of their offspring to inherit the disease. When both parents are carriers of the recessive gene, there is a one-in-four chance that any child born to them will have cystic fibrosis. Tests have been devised for the early detection of the disease. The most common test is aimed at detecting the abnormally high salt content of the patient's perspiration. Early detection is necessary so that the condition may be treated before irreparable harm can be done to the child's organs. The test can be conducted while the baby is still in the newborn nursery, with the contents of the perspiration analyzed. Unfortunately cystic fibrosis cannot as yet be detected in the fetus by an amniocentesis. However, the presence of certain granules in the amniotic fluid of women who had previously given birth to children with cystic fibrosis has encouraged scientists to believe that prenatal detection is not far off.

Phenylketonuria (PKU)

Phenylketonuria is a congenital metabolic disease. It is caused by the absence of an enzyme required to convert an amino acid (phenylalanine) into a substance the body can use. Without this enzyme, phenylalanine is abnormally broken down into phenylketone bodies that cause damage to the brain in the young child, resulting in mental retardation. Phenylketonuria is transmitted through a recessive gene. The incidence of the disease was first estimated to be anywhere from one in 20,000–40,000 births. However, recent extensive screening programs have shown that the incidence is approximately one in every 10,000 births.

A test that has been developed for the detection of phenylketonuria is the Guthrie blood test. A drop of blood is taken from the child's heel shortly after birth and is tested for the presence of phenylketone bodies.

Because this disorder is detectable and the retardation often preventable, the Department of Health, Education and Welfare instituted in 1963 a nationwide screening program for the early detection of phenylketonuria by testing all newborn children.

Treatment of the disease thus far is through dietary management. Because phenylalanine is an essential amino acid, it cannot be excluded from the diet completely without ill effects. However, in the dietary management of phenylketonuria there is a drastic restriction of phenylalanine intake. With controlled amounts of the amino acid, the child will usually grow and develop without the expected retardation. The low phenylalanine diet is a pasty formulalike commercial preparation. As the child grows older, keeping him on this profoundly unattractive dietary regimen becomes most difficult. How long a child must be kept on this restricted diet will probably vary with individuals. Phenylalanine levels of the blood must be checked periodically to make sure that the diet is meeting the needs of the particular individual.

In addition to those characteristics related to mental retardation, phenylketonurics are often found to have schizoidlike personalities (withdrawn, with feelings of persecution and periods of incoherency). A patchy type eczema and/or convulsions may accompany the condition. Electroencephalograms are abnormal in 80 per cent of the cases tested. Phenylketonurics are usually blue-eyed and more blond than their parents.

It has also been found that there is such a thing as maternal phenylketonuria. In some cases, the mother is a phenylketonuric and has a high level of phenylalanine in her blood. When such a woman is pregnant, the high serum phenylalanine level will cause damage to the brain of the unborn child. This child will then, of course, be born mentally retarded. It has been suggested that perhaps all mothers of retarded children be tested for phenylketonuria as a means of preventing the birth of additional retarded children. These mothers are in many instances individuals who are not severely retarded but may have a mental capacity that is normal or just below normal. Where a mother is a phenylketonuric, physicians find that they can sometimes protect the unborn child by placing the mother on a low phenylalanine diet during her pregnancy.

Tay-Sachs Disease

Another genetic disorder associated with a specific enzyme deficiency is Tay-Sachs disease. Severe retardation, blindness, and early death, usually before 3 or 4 years of age, are the results of a massive accumulation of lipids in the brain. This occurs because an enzyme needed to break down fats properly was not developed in the child. One of the peculiarities of this disease is the fact that about 85 per cent of the children it affects are from Jewish families of Eastern European origin. An elaborate system of detection has been undertaken to detect and prevent new cases of this disease. Blood tests of both partners are performed prior to marriages among Jews. When both husband and wife are found to be carriers all their pregnancies are monitored by amniocentesis. The scientist who discovered the defective form of the enzyme followed twenty pregnancies in women known to be carriers. Seven of the twenty fetuses were affected with the disease, and in all seven cases the women chose to end the pregnancies through abortion.

Galactosemia

Galactosemia is an inherited disease caused by the absence of an enzyme required to convert galactose (a sugar substance found in milk) to glucose (a simple sugar the body can utilize). As a result, too much galactose accumulates in the body tissues, particularly the brain. Eventually the level becomes toxic and causes cataracts, liver damage, and brain damage resulting in mental retardation. With biochemical analyses of the amniotic fluid, the mother's diet can be modified prior to the birth of the baby. The diet of the newborn is also controlled and the disease arrested.

Down's Syndrome (Mongolism)

Mongolism is a common form of retardation that is genetically caused by abnormal chromosome formation. Where there should be only two of the 21st chromosome, there are three. Standard trisomy is the name used to describe this most common form of Down's syndrome that affects 1 out of every 600 births.

Down's disease appears more commonly in children born of older women. For example, in women 20 to 30 years of age, the risk of occurrence is 1 : 1500; in women 35 to 40, the risk is 1 : 600; and in women 45 or older, the risk of occurrence is 1 : 60. In mongolism the back and front of the head are flattened, making the forehead seem large. Oriental eyes are an added characteristic. The hands are often stubby, and the hand prints show definite characteristics different from normal prints. The child's degree of retardation may range from moderate to severe, and curiously enough genetically confirmed mongoloids are notoriously susceptible to leukemia.

A Chromosome Registry

The New York State Health Department's Birth Defects Institute has compiled via computer a Chromosome Registry that contains information on persons in New York State who have diseases caused by abnormal chromosomes. A physician concerned about a patient with a particular genetic disease can consult the Registry through one of its fifty member physicians and find out quickly if there are similar cases to compare notes with. This should permit physicians to provide better care to their patients and also prove a valuable aid in research. Ultimately it is hoped to have a nationwide Registry.

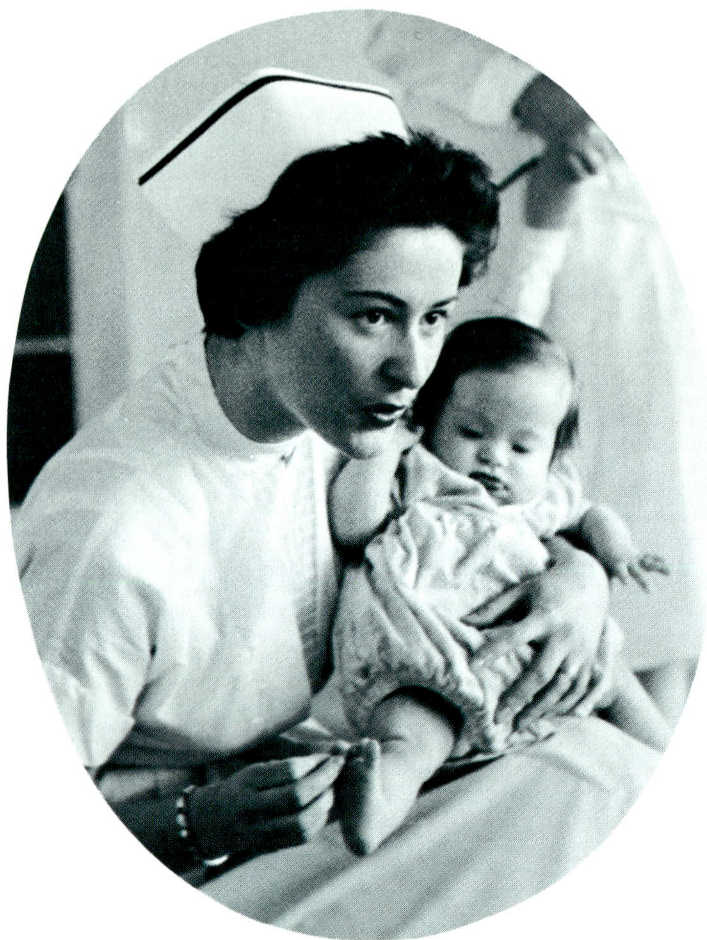

Figure 3–21

Love and understanding are basic needs of the retarded child as well as the normal child.

(New York State Department of Mental Hygiene—Julian A. Belin)

OTHER CONSTITUTIONAL DISEASES

Diabetes

Although significant progress has been made in the control of diabetes, it is still the eighth leading cause of death and the third leading cause of blindness. It is estimated that approximately 4 million Americans have diabetes. Half of these cases are undetected. There are two types of diabetes: diabetes mellitus and diabetes insipidus. Diabetes insipidus tends to occur in people over 40 who are overweight. The cause of this disease is not well understood, though it is believed to be caused by a dysfunction of the pituitary gland. Diabetes mellitus is caused by the insufficient production of insulin by the islets of Langerhans in the pancreas. This type of diabetes has its onset in childhood or adolescence and is sometimes referred to as the juvenile form of diabetes. The result of this insufficiency of insulin is the inability of the body to properly utilize carbohydrates as a source of fuel. The lack of insulin has a number of effects, such as raising the blood sugar level, inhibiting the conversion of sugar to glycogen, and accelerating the conversion of glycogen to sugar. The tissues of the body also find it more difficult to utilize sugar. As a result of all this, sugar is found in excessive amounts in the bloodstream and thereby excreted in the urine. This sometimes will result in an excessive loss of water and salt as well. Because sugar is not being utilized as a source of energy, the body will increasingly utilize proteins and fats for this purpose. The incomplete by-products of protein and fat combustion may also prove harmful. One of the harmful effects is to accelerate the hardening of arteries. An objective of early detection of diabetes, therefore, becomes the prevention of premature arteriosclerosis.

Symptoms in cases of diabetes may go unrecognized. Where they do appear, they generally consist of a constant hunger, thirst, and frequent urination. A tired feeling, loss of weight, itching, changes in vision, and slow healing of cuts may also be symptomatic of this disease. Tests for the detection of diabetes usually consist of urinalysis and blood analysis.

Heredity ranks as a primary contributing factor for this condition. The predisposition for the development of diabetes is apparently passed on through a recessive gene. Studies have also shown that where diabetes has appeared after 40 years of age, overweight appears to be associated with the condition. The sex of the individual may be another factor, in that women have one-third more chance of developing diabetes than men. It has also been noted that four-fifths of the diabetics are over 40 years of age. Diabetes that develops in later life is usually milder, whereas its incidence in children is usually more severe.

Many cases of diabetes can be controlled through diet alone. Where medications are necessary, it has been found that some cases respond to oral drugs such as diabanese or orinase. These are sulfonylureas. Their major function is to stimulate production of insulin in the still active parts of the pancreas. In the most severe cases insulin by injection is required. In these cases, the individual must develop a balance between the carbohydrates taken in the diet, the amount of insulin injected, and the amount of exercise participated in.

The failure to keep a balance between carbohydrates and insulin in the body can result in two dangerous diabetic reactions. The first of these is *diabetic coma*, or *acidosis*. In this condition, there is a lack of insulin present in the body, with the result that sugar and starches cannot be burned. Diabetic coma may be slow in onset. It is characterized by nausea, pain in the abdomen, thirst, deep breathing, and a pungent breath odor.

The second diabetic reaction is *insulin shock*, or *hypoglycemia*, which results from taking too large a dose of insulin, eating too little food, or exercising too much. Any of the preceding three factors will result in the presence of too much insulin in the body for the amount of carbohydrate. This can be remedied by the individual's taking a source of carbohydrate such as sugar or orange juice. The onset of insulin shock may be rather sudden, the symptoms being hunger, weakness, paleness, and drowsiness. The diabetic who can feel the reaction setting in can usually correct it by taking some carbohydrates. Diabetics who pass out from either reaction should receive medical help as soon as possible. Many diabetics carry identification cards indicating the need for medical help should they suffer from either diabetic coma or insulin shock. Too often, diabetics who are in difficulty are mistaken for people who are intoxicated and are in many instances ignored. A diabetic suffering from either reaction could be in very serious difficulty.

Allergies

An allergen is a chemical substance leading to an abnormal response called an allergic reaction. This reaction will often cause the release of histamine. Histamine, when released from the cells, may cause dilation and congestion of the blood vessels, forcing fluids from these blood vessels into the surrounding tissues of the body. This may result in a swelling of tissues (edema) or the development of hives on the skin. It may also cause a spasmodic contraction of some involuntary muscles of the body. If these muscles are in the bronchial tubes, asthma may be the result.

The causes of allergies are many and varied. There are airborne substances such as pollen, molds, insect fragments (hairs, stings, and scales of insects), dander or dandruff of dogs, cats, horses, or even mice. Ingested substances such as foods are possible causes, with milk, strawberries, and shellfish examples of more common allergens. Drugs of various types will also, at times, cause allergic reactions. The increasing sensitivity of many people to penicillin is characteristic of this. Injected materials such as a wasp or bee sting, insulin, and vaccines of various types may contain substances that become allergens for some people. The extent of this can be exemplified by the fact that more people die from allergic reactions to insect bites than from poison snake bites in this country. There are also contact substances that will cause allergic reactions, such as poison ivy, orange rind, and certain fabrics. Just about any substance has a potential for the development of an allergic reaction in a given individual.

Asthma is one of the more common allergic reactions that we see. Three million people in this country suffer from this condition. It results in general shortness or breath, coughing, wheezing, and even choking. Asthmatic attacks can be caused by a spasm of the bronchial muscles, the swelling of the bronchial mucous membrane, or the clinging of plugs of phlegm to the bronchial tubes. During an asthmatic attack, the individual, in essence, is attempting to breathe through a constricted opening. A complication of this condition can be emphysema, in which air is trapped in the lungs and cannot be properly exhaled. The child suffering from asthma will in most instances not outgrow the condition. Something should be done to attempt to correct the asthmatic reaction before the individual suffers physical, social, and economic difficulties which in turn may precipitate emotional problems.

The history and examination of the person are prerequisites to allergic management. Skin tests are often done to determine the varied substances to which a person may have a positive allergic reaction. Knowledge of the history of the patient's reactions of an allergic nature are most important at this stage. Controlling the allergy may mean doing such things as getting rid of the dog, cat, or certain types of clothing. It may also mean the installation of a filtering apparatus to filter out molds, pollens, or dust in the home that might be causes of the reaction. If certain kinds of foods are implicated, then substituting for these foods in the diet becomes necessary. This is sometimes difficult in infants who are allergic to milk.

Treatment for allergies may take various forms and should be administered by an allergist, the medical doctor best trained to treat these conditions.

Emphysema

Emphysema is a chronic lung disease more common than cancer and tuberculosis combined. Emphysema is the fastest-rising cause of death in the United States. In 1949 the death rate from this disease was 2.1/100,000 population; in 1960 it orse to 6.0/100,000 population; and in 1967 it reached 12.9 deaths/100,000 population. Alarming estimates indicate that over 10 per cent of our middle-aged and elderly Americans are afflicted with this disorder. The disease is more common among men than women.

In this disease the lungs are inflated with air that the victim cannot expel; hence the term "emphysema," which is a Greek word meaning inflating or puffing up. Chronic irritation of the bronchi often causes obstructions that trap air in the lungs behind them. The result is that less of the lung is working. The air sacs of the lungs may also be damaged by this trapped air and will lose their characteristic elasticity. This damage may be permanent in nature. While the normal person breathes fourteen times a minute, the emphysematous person may breathe anywhere from twenty to thirty times a minute and still not get enough exygen in the blood. The carbon dioxide level in the blood and tissues of these persons is high and it results in sluggishness and irritability. The person is constantly gasping for breath, wheezing, and coughing. The heart pumps harder in order to compensate for the lack of oxygen reaching the tissues, with heart failure becoming the ultimate hazard. Cigarette smoking increases the risk of dying from pulmonary emphysema and is a much greater hazard than atmospheric pollution.

Methods of treatment for this disease are currently under investigation. Cessation of smoking is essential if progress of the disease is to be stopped. Lung tissue that has already been destroyed cannot be replaced or repaired by current methods of treatment.

Rheumatic Diseases

Rheumatoid Arthritis is a severe type of rheumatic disorder that affects approximately 4½ million people in the country. This condition is recognized as being a generalized disorder and not one limited to the joints of the body. The disease, therefore, can affect the entire person. The cause of this affliction is still unknown. It is most commonly developed by young adults between the ages of 20 and 40, although cases of the disease may appear later in life. A form of the disease known as juvenile rheumatoid arthritis may even be found among the newborn. This type of arthritis can be most crippling, because it can do damage to the ligaments and coverings of joints and muscles as well as to some of the organs of the body. The joints of the hands, wrists, elbows, knees, ankles, and feet are often involved. These joints are weakened and distorted. The earliest symptoms very often are nothing more than fatigue, accompanied by a loss of appetite and weight and sometimes a numbness of the hands. It is oftentimes weeks and even months after the vague symptoms appear that the aching of the joints begins. These symptoms are most commonly experienced in the morning upon rising. A curious thing about rheumatoid arthritis is that although it may persist in the patient for weeks or months, it may at times suddenly go away. This sudden disappearance of the disease that occasionally takes place is responsible for so called "cures" that some quacks like to take advantage of. Spontaneous relapses of the disease may also occur. Treatment for the arthritic is aimed to prevent contraction and deformity of joints as well as to relieve discomfort.

Osteoarthritis is usually attributed to wear and tear, although it many times follows injuries and other diseases of the joints. This condition tends to occur in the weight-bearing joints of the body and occurs more frequently in those patients who are overweight or obese. Such patients are usually placed on a regimen that will result in weight reduction so as to take some of the strain off these joints and slow down the degeneration of the articular cartilage. A good deal of research with regard to osteoarthritis is aimed at uncovering the unknown factors related to the speeding up of the degenerative process in cartilage metabolism. Nutritional, genetic, and endocrine factors are being scrutinized to discover the role they play in determining the resistance of cartilage to wear and tear.

Gout is a rheumatic disease in which typically only one joint is affected, usually in the lower extremities. The condition is accompanied by severe pain and swelling, redness, and warmth about the joint affected. The sensitivity of the affected tissue is such that the mere vibration caused by someone walking in the room may cause unbearable pain. With treatment the pain can be terminated almost immediately, and in many instances the recurrence of an acute attack prevented. Without treatment, however, the acute phase of the illness may go on for days or weeks. The gout is caused by an excessive production of uric acid. For some reason, too little of it is eliminated through the kidneys. The tendency toward the development of an excessive amount of uric acid seems to run in families and is presumed to be an inherited factor. Because excessive amounts of uric acid precipitate gout conditions, physicians will restrict those foods that are rich in purines from which uric acid is derived. Examples of these foods are sweet-breads, anchovies, liver, and kidney. People trying to lose weight by adhering to diets high in proteins and fats (or ketogenic diets) tend to raise the levels of uric acid in their systems, sometimes bringing on a gout crisis. The prognosis for gout is quite favorable. The patient who seeks early medical help should be able to avoid the crippling effects of the disease and to enjoy considerable relief from medication during the acute phases.

Some types of arthritis have been found to be caused by specific types of bacteria. In these cases the disease is treated with an antibiotic and is cured. This brings up the possibility that there may be other infectious agents responsible for other forms of arthritis. Should this be the case, the identification of the specific agent or agents involved can lead ultimately to more effective treatment of the disease. Biochemical research is developing clues to other possible causes of arthritis. Researchers feel that they are not too far away from important breakthroughs in this area that could lead to more specific preventive and treatment measures.

REVIEW QUESTIONS

1. Describe the progress man has made in the control of communicable disease.
2. How can you distinguish between control of a disease and its eradication? What kind of effort would be necessary to eradicate a disease?
3. Define: (1) morbidity, (2) mortality, (3) immunity, (4) antigen, (5) antibody.
4. Distinguish between an active and a passive immunity.
5. What have been some of the difficulties in the development of preventive measures for influenza?
6. What is known about mononucleosis? Why is "kissing disease" possibly a misnomer for this condition?
7. How do infectious and serum hepatitis deffer? What have been some of the inhibiting factors in dealing effectively with the problem of infectious hepatitis?

8 Why is syphilis a difficult disease to detect and effectively treat? Why is it often referred to as the "great imitator?"

9 What can be the effects of advanced cases of syphilis?

10 Why is the detection of gonorrhea particularly difficult in the female? What can be the detrimental effects of this disease?

11 What are the implications of the increased resistance of gonorrheal infection to penicillin therapy?

12 What are some of the suggestions that have been made by public health leaders to bring our expanding venereal disease problem under control?

13 Describe arteriosclerosis. What are the factors related to the development of this condition?

14 What is a coronary thrombosis; angina pectoris? How are these conditions related to arteriosclerosis?

15 What are some of the varying causes of strokes? Describe some of the warning signals that may precede this condition.

16 How have advances in surgical procedures improved the outlook for individuals with rheumatic heart conditions?

17 What factors can contribute to the development of human cancer? With which forms of cancer has there been significant medical progress?

18 How has the public attitude toward cancer been changing? What is the outlook for cancer control in the future?

19 Distinguish between diabetic coma and insulin shock. Identify the two types of diabetes. What differences in these two disorders are now recognized?

20 What are some of the many causes of convulsive seizures? How are these reactions largely controlled?

21 What preventive measures can be taken to reduce the incidence of cerebral palsy? How do these types of conditions differ?

22 What is an allergy? What are the varied approaches used to alleviate or correct allergic reactions?

23 Describe the lung changes that take place in emphysema. What causative factors have been related to this condition?

24 What are the purposes of rehabilitation programs for people with muscular dystrophy?

25 How do rheumatic diseases differ? What is known about the causes of these conditions?

26 Mental retardation is an effect rather than a given condition. Explain.

27 How can genetic counseling control the incidence of genetic diseases?

4. Mental Health

THE PERSON who will probably be most comfortable, happy, and successful in life is the one who can accept himself. It is the person who can look in the mirror and say, "I'm OK!" The individual who is not accepting of himself will be preoccupied with making himself better. While self-improvement is a goal everyone has, the more secure personality spends more time being concerned for others and bettering the community in which he lives. It would seem that the development of persons who were self-accepting would be rather basic and easily accomplished. However, there are a variety of factors such as family, friends, teachers, heredity, societal values, and the environment that can detract from as well as contribute to a person's personality. Ultimately it is the person aided by self-understanding who must assert and accept himself as a worthwhile personality.

MENTAL HEALTH AND CIVILIZED MAN

Consider the simplicity of life for primitive man. He preoccupied himself with such basic matters as hunting, fighting, sleeping, and reproducing. It was an uncomplicated existence with a low incidence of "nervous breakdown." Civilization has made things much more complex and the satisfaction of needs more indirect. In order to obtain food, man does not hunt, but must train himself to acquire marketable skills that will earn the money to buy food. Man's instincts to fight have also been modified. When one becomes angry, he does not respond with a direct punch, but with due process of law, a carefully worded verbal response (lest he be sued for libel), or a nasty letter to the editor. The man who resorts to fisticuffs is behaving like the animal he *was* rather than the human being he is supposed to be.

The reproductive function has probably become the most complicated of all. This now requires marriage and the setting up of a home, which immediately embroils the individual in the most complex of legal and economic systems. Religious factors of even finite proportions related to the marriage become major considerations. Social customs surrounding the wedding further enmesh the original intent.

To the active primitive man, sleep was a simple reaction to fatigue. Now, however, loss of sleep due to tension is often dealt with by taking pills.

> Man's evolution is based on the fact that he has lost his original home, nature—and that he can never return to it, can never become an animal again. There is only one way he can take: to emerge fully from his natural home, to find a new home—one which he creates by making the world a human one and by becoming truly human himself.[1]

The maze that is civilization, then, requires a change of man's aggressive instincts and behaviors if constant frustration and unhappiness are to be avoided. Like the mouse in the maze, overly direct actions merely result in hitting one's head against a solid wall. The more indirect routes dictated by civilization can result in a life with greater meaning and abundance.

Civilized man is in a great period of change. He is in the process of adapting to a new self-created environment, an environment that has new elements related to both his physical and psychological self. That this adjustment should create some visible stresses and strains is to be expected. We are living in an era of such fundamental change that man's very soul seems to be the object of public discussion, if not criticism. Nothing is sacred. The very pillars of societal or individual strength appear to be crumbling.

> Faith has been replaced by a shallow rationalism, spiritual values by utilitarian ones, pride in one's work by interest in the profit it brings, tradition has been divested of its glory by historical criticism, and social conventions are for many no more than an object of ridicule.[2]

How does one play a game without rules? There will be those who will be intimidated by this lack of structure and be tempted to blame the previous generation for a chaotic state of affairs, as if a single generation could be

[1] Eric Fromm, *The Sane Society* (New York: Rinehart, 1955), p. 25.

[2] Oswald Schwarz, *The Psychology of Sex* (Pelican Books, 1962), p. 242.

responsible for man's current state—a development that has taken thousands of years.

Others will try to escape from it through the world provided by drugs. Some will try to return to the land, to live as their ancestors did, attempting to forget civilization and the technology it has wrought with its destruction of past values and social structures. It may be a futile attempt to escape the reality of things or merely a lull while one conducts an inner search for one's fundamental values. Basic in all this is that element of hope that marks the difference between animal and man. Life and living *happen* to an animal. He eats when he is hungry, he sleeps when he is tired, and mates during nature's predetermined time of year. With man, life is not so much a happening as it is something that he makes happen. *Man is the maker of his own destiny.* Those who are not faint of heart will come forward and build the new social structure based on greater human understanding resulting in a more humane world.

HUMAN NEEDS

Each human being has fundamental physical and psychological needs. These are fundamental to the survival and development of the individual as an organism and a personality. The child that does not receive love from its mother may become as emotionally deprived as one not receiving enough food is physically deprived.

Basic needs of a physical nature revolve around needs for air, sleep, food, and sex. We would not survive in an environment that lacked air for more than a few minutes. We spend approximately a third of our lives satisfying our need for sleep. The need for food serves as a prime motivator for a person developing marketable skills so that he can purchase this commodity. Sex needs are the ones most likely to be frustrated or sublimated because our culture has certain taboos with regard to sexual activity and because personal values of some people lead them to sublimate this drive until marriage.

Physiologists feel that the disruption of the functioning of any system of the body creates a basic physical need because the life of the organism can be endangered. A lack of oxygen or the inability of blood to clot could serve as two of many possible examples.

Emotional needs are based initially on receiving love, affection, and acceptance from parents in the early years of life. It has been dramatically demonstrated that infants who are separated from their mothers or a mother substitute for extended periods of time become extremely dispirited. They not only exhibit obviously poor mental health but can also become physically ill by this deprivation. Delinquency and varied emotional problems are related to the failure to receive normal love and affection at an early age. This emotional barrenness may cause the individual to grow up with a distrust for other people and the inability to give or receive love.

As the child grows older, added to the needs of love, affection, and acceptance by parents are needs for achievement and the development of status. The need to achieve is basic to our ego development. The means of satisfying these needs are of course many and varied. Some individuals have talent academically, others develop creative skills with paints, music, or dance, and some demonstrate multiple talents. Actually, the important thing is not so much the profoundness of the achievement as it is the satisfaction one derives from the experience. For instance, who is to say that the solving of a complex mathematical problem is a greater accomplishment than the successful growing of a beautiful rose?

Need for status is related to, and sometimes grows out of, the fulfillment of the psychological needs, namely love, affection, acceptance, and achievement. The person needs initially to have status in his family group; later in his development this need is extended to his peer group. As an adult, the person seeks added status in his or her field of endeavor. When a person's status is

Figure 4–1

Who is to say that the solving of a complex mathematical problem is a greater accomplishment than the successful growing of a beautiful rose?

(Betsy P. Thompson)

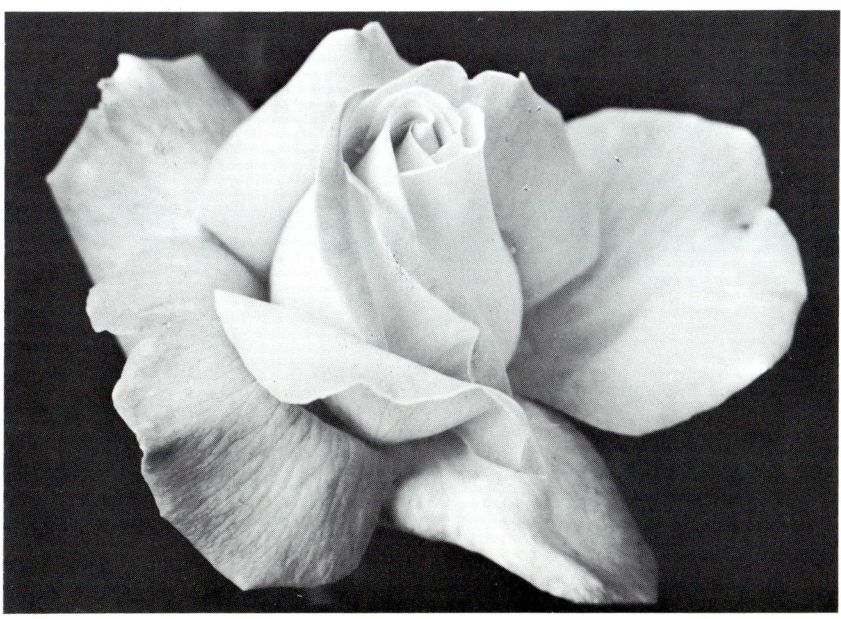

threatened, the assertive question, "Just whom do you think you are talking to?" may be heard or actions reflecting the question may be seen. This kind of response and its frequency reflect how important status needs are to the individual. Very often the desire for status will lead to the acquisition of material possessions that are not really needed but become psychological trophies for the individual (the expensive car, the mink coat, the bizarre wardrobe).

Maslow,[3] in his theory of hierarchy of human needs, states that people have physical needs that lead to personality growth and toward self-actualization. Maslow states that these needs must be successively satisfied. The organism seeks to satisfy the lower-level needs such as hunger before it becomes concerned with higher-level love needs. The epitome of personality development, according to Maslow, is the self-actualizing person. This person is dedicated to a profession, cause, or science. The self-actualizing person is dedicated not for the recognition or other rewards his work may bring him. He follows his dedication to wherever it may lead him, even though it may result in disapproval from others, or even persecution. Darwin, with his theory of evolution, and Pasteur, with his germ theory of disease, stirred up a great deal of controversy. These men did not, however, waver in their dedication and their work. This Maslow regards as self-actualization.

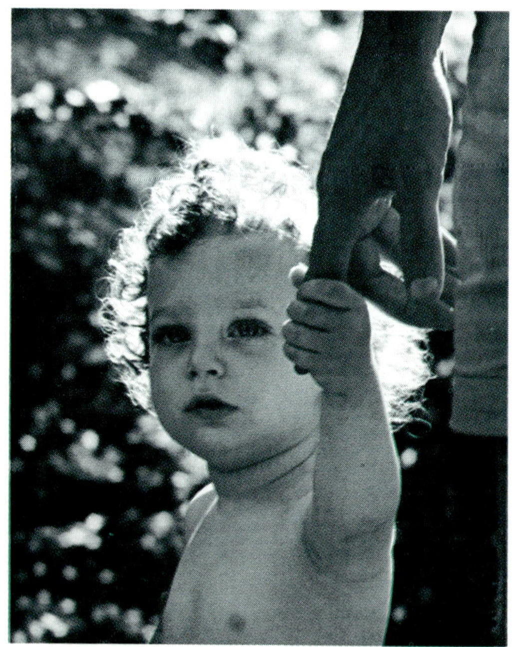

Figure 4–2

A person whose basic needs have been met early in life develops a strong personality structure.

(Susan Johns)

[3] Abraham H. Maslow, *Toward a Psychology of Being* (Princeton, N.J.: Van Nostrand, 1962).

PEANUTS
..SO THERE, SMARTY! NYAH! NYAH! NYAH!

8-30

THOSE "NYAHS" GET DOWN INTO YOUR STOMACH, AND THEN THEY JUST LAY THERE AND BURN
SCHULZ

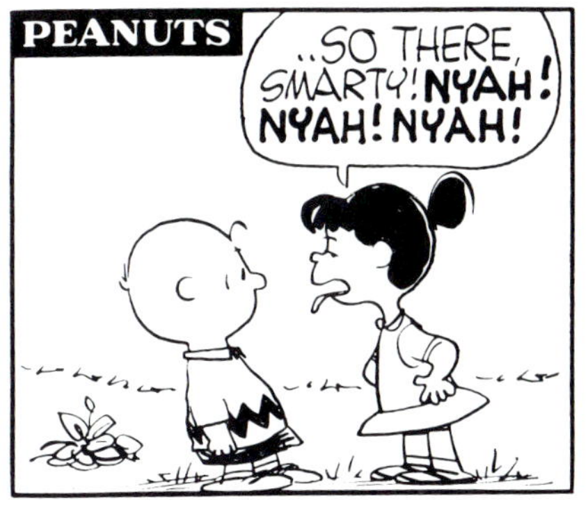

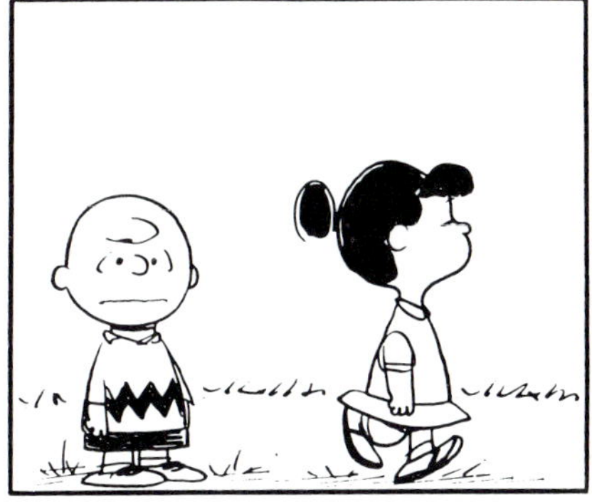

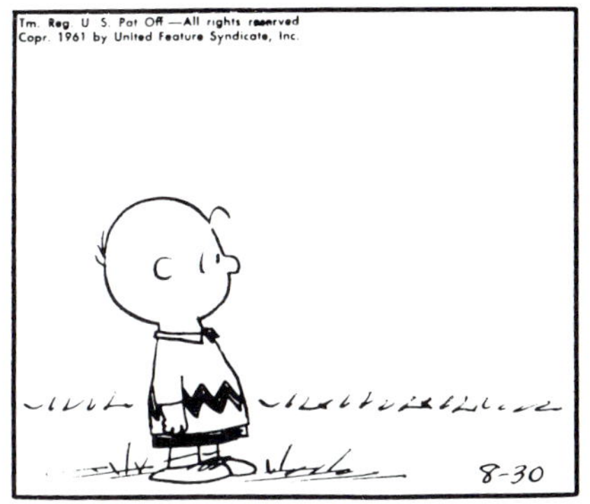

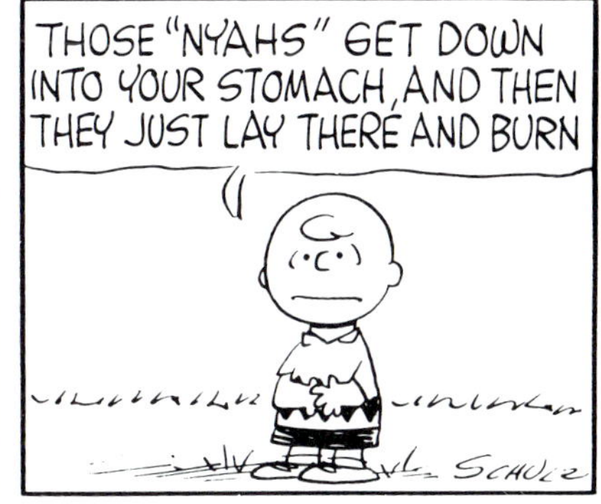

Figure 4–3

Peanuts cartoon by Charles M. Schulz.

Maslow also states that the person whose basic needs have been met early in life develops a strong personality structure. He is then capable to a much greater extent to weather opposition, rejection, and other negative conditions later in life. In planting a small tree one takes every precaution to protect it from the elements so that it will develop strong roots and have a good start in life. The transfer of this principle from trees to man on occasion falls short. This is exemplified by the father who feels he must subject his son to "rough" treatment in order for the boy to grow up to "be a man." The physical and emotional violence directed toward the youngster is comparable to stomping on the young tree and shaking it from its roots. Growth is not a response to overzealous, misconceived actions, but a reaction to nature's slow, positive, and constructive elements.

The ability to satisfy our psychological needs is reflected in our self-concept. How a person views himself is quite crucial to his mental health and to his effectiveness. Some people are so convinced of their inability to perform certain

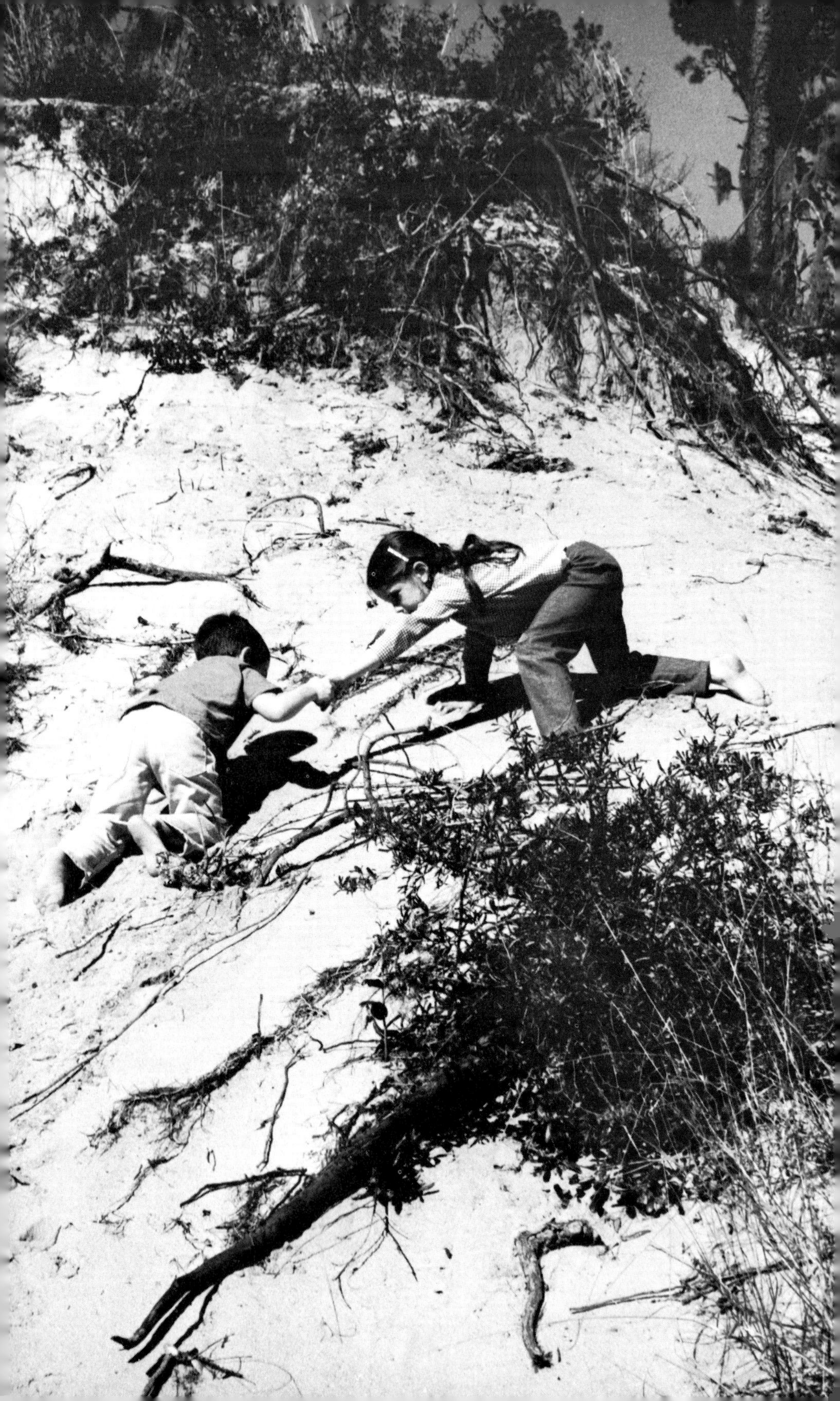

Figure 4–4

Opposite: It's always comforting to reach out and find a helping hand when needed.

(Susan Johns)

tasks that they inevitably fail. The coach's locker-room pep talk is often aimed at improving the self-concept of his team. As we know, this can at times prove an effective antidote to an uninspired group. However, we must also be realistic enough to realize that all cannot be accomplished by merely the will to do. A certain amount of talent is also necessary. A person whose self-concept is on a healthy level is one who is confident of his decisions, has set fairly specific goals, understands his values and ideals, and is comfortable with regard to opinions of others about him.

It is important to know that self-concept is learned. One's concept of self is strongly influenced by his childhood interrelationships with parents and siblings. The child becomes more and more aware of how he is being appraised by others. If these appraisals are positive, feelings of worth then develop. If the appraisals are derogatory, then the person is made to feel undesirable, worthless, and inferior. One's self-concept is always subject to change throughout life. Greater changes usually occur during childhood as compared with the adult years. One of the important responsibilities of parenthood is to help children to grow up feeling accepted in an environment reflecting warmth and affection. In addition, each of us has the opportunity to make a contribution in dignifying every human life we come in contact with. Self-concepts are made, not born.

WHAT, THEN, IS MENTAL HEALTH?

Mental health is sometimes mistakenly viewed as an absolute, something that a person either has or does not have. Actually it is more of an ideal that people strive for with varying degrees of success. It is reflected in our abilities to assume responsibility, to solve problems, to make decisions, to find satisfactions and happiness, and to live effectively with other people. To be sure, all people enjoy successes and experience failures in attempts to accomplish the difficult and to resolve conflicting drives and goals. Our level of mental health can be measured by our ability to take advantage of the buoyancy provided by success and to survive the depression of failure.

Many view the "well-adjusted" person as being mentally healthy. This is a person who has struck a suitable balance between himself, his needs, and his environment. Because there is a constant change taking place in our internal as well as external environment, adjustment is not a static condition but one that is in a constant state of flux. The only people who are permanently adjusted are those in cemeteries; the rest of us have to work at it constantly.

Leading psychologists and psychoanalysts have varying concepts with regard to what constitutes a well-adjusted or mentally healthy person. William Blatz, a well-known child psychologist from Canada, views self-reliance as the most important characteristic of the healthy personality. This means the ability to accept the consequences of one's decisions and actions. Alfred Adler. a psychologist who once worked with Freud, regarded social feeling or the ability to identify with mankind as a barometer of mental health. Otto Rank, an early psychoanalyst, viewed creativity as the important criterion in evaluating healthy mindedness. He felt the person who was not afraid to be different and to assert his individuality was self-assured. Sidney Jourard, a psychologist, views a healthy personality as one where the individual "has been able to gratify his basic needs through acceptable behavior such that his own personality is no longer a problem to him. He can take himself more or less for granted and devote his energies and thoughts to socially meaningful interests and problems beyond security, or lovability, or status."[4] Herbert Carroll feels that mental health depends upon the development of a mental hygiene point of view that would include:

1. Respect for one's own personality and for the personalities of others.
2. Recognition of limitations in the self and in others.
3. An appreciation of the importance of the causal sequence in behavior. (All behavior is caused; it does not just happen.)
4. A realization that behavior is a function of the whole individual.
5. An understanding of the basic needs that motivate behavior.[5]

Though there is not a universally accepted definition of what is mental health or a healthy personality, the foregoing provide us with some guidelines.

THE UNCONSCIOUS MIND

The unconscious mind serves to store the memory of past experiences. Electrically stimulating various parts of the brain with electrodes resulted in a conscious person's recalling periods of past experience. He relived the experience by hearing and seeing it with all the emotions initially related to it. The experience could be made to reappear with the reapplication of the electrodes.

There is evidence that unconscious thoughts influence our behavior, feelings,

[4] Sidney M. Jourard, *Personal Adjustment* (New York: Macmillan, Inc., 1967), p. 21.

[5] Herbert A. Carroll, *Mental Hygiene* (Englewood Cliffs, N.J.: Prentice-Hall, 1956), p. 13.

and decisions. These thoughts are sometimes "seen" in dreams or in purposeful forgetting. However, like the iceberg, most of it lies submerged and its great influence on us remains unrecognized. A student told this story when shown a picture of an old man stretching his hand toward the reclining figure of a younger man:

> This boy is having a nap. The old man, his father, is coming to get him out of bed so he'll get back to his studies. His father has been nagging him for ages about how lazy he is. The boy has been putting up with this for a long time. This is the last straw. When he wakes up, he'll be so mad he'll start beating on his father. He'll grab a chair and start mashing in his head. When he finishes, his old man will be a bloody pulp. The boy will get the electric chair, but he won't care, it was worth it.[6]

It is not too farfetched to infer there is at least some unconscious hostility toward authority figures in this young man.

The unconscious is often viewed in negative terms functioning to repress needs that the individual is afraid or ashamed of. In healthier personalities it can serve as a positive, creative source. When the unconscious is not preoccupied with the business of repression and inhibition, it is free to permit the surfacing into the conscious mind innovative ideas, solutions to problems, insights into oneself and others, and an otherwise surging forth of one's positive potentials.

Freud, basically responsible for the psychoanalytic theory with regard to the unconscious mind, felt that people tend to react in two ways, namely in relation to their environment and in relation to themselves. He therefore tended to categorize people's thinking into three component parts, which he called the id, superego, and ego. The "id" he described as that force of basic, primitive, uncivilized, and uninhibited drives related to man's nature, such as sex drives, infantile needs, and basic wants. As parts of the id these demand gratification without concern for the welfare of the individual or others.

Freud[7] regarded the superego as the conscience of the individual, acting to distinguish right from wrong. The superego has the function of making the individual conform with or uphold those values that he learned early in life from parents and other authoritative figures. The superego tends to make the individual conform to the cultural pattern of which he is a part.

The ego was conceived by Freud as being a mechanism that merges the id and the superego. It accepts the basic drives and instincts of the id and on the other hand accepts the regulations of the culture that the superego imposes. It functions as an intermediary, regulating the forces between the id and superego, particularly in reaction to the environment and reality.

[6] Jourard, *Personal Adjustment,* op. cit., p. 52.

[7] Sigmund Freud, *The Basic Writings of Sigmund Freud,* translated by A. A. Brill (New York: Modern Library, 1938).

The Endocrine System

How it influences mental health

The endocrine glands are ductless glands that secrete chemical substances called hormones. These substances are secreted directly into the bloodstream where they are carried to all parts of the body. The hormones of the endocrine glands can have profound effects on certain tissues. The tissue upon which a specific hormone acts is called a target tissue. Hormones also have an effect on other endocrine glands and can either stimulate or inhibit their actions. The hormones of the endocrine system have a strong influence upon both the physical and personality development of the individual, affecting growth, behavior, and varied body processes.

GLAND	FUNCTIONS
Pituitary (or master gland since it secretes hormones that influence other endocrine glands) Location: Brain	The pituitary secretes a number of hormones among which is one affecting growth. If there is an excessive secretion of this hormone during childhood, giantism results. Should the excessive secretion occur during the adult years, a disorder known as acromegaly develops. Although the person does not grow taller, he develops abnormally large hands and feet with a characteristic change in facial features. Should there be a deficiency of growth hormone of the pituitary in childhood, then the opposite condition, dwarfism, occurs. The mental ability of these persons will not be affected but will remain normal. The pituitary gland also secretes a hormone that has an influence on the gonads. The amount of this hormone produced can cause either early or late puberty. The pituitary also has an effect on the rate of metabolism in the body and together with the hormone thyroxin can affect the accumulation of fat. In animal experiments, the removal of the pituitary causes an aggressive animal to become a very docile one. Animals deprived of their pituitary glands are also unable to produce sperm or egg cells.
Gonads (**testes** and **ovaries**) Location: Testes are located in the scrotum. Ovaries are located on each side of the uterus.	The gonads' major function is the reproduction of sex cells. The testes produce sperm cells while the ovaries produce the egg cells. The gonads also secrete hormones that promote the development of secondary sexual characteristics such as the deeper voice and the beard. In the female the sex hormones result in the development of mammary glands and the feminine characteristics of the female body. They also serve to control menstruation, pregnancy, and lactation. The proper functioning of these glands has rather obvious implications for personality development. The person who feels inadequate sexually and unable to fulfill the role of "male" or "female" will no doubt face a number of emotional problems.

GLAND	FUNCTIONS
Thyroid Location: Base of the neck	The thyroid gland secretes the hormone thyroxin. The basic function of this hormone is to control the rate of metabolism in the body. The thyroid gland that is secreting an insufficient amount of the hormone tends to make the person sluggish, apathetic, and possibly emotionally depressed. Serious thyroid deficiencies in childhood result in a disorder known as cretinism. Retarded mental development and stunted growth are typical. When the thyroid deficiency occurs in the adult years, it causes a condition known as myxedema, which results from the atrophy of the thyroid gland. This disorder is characterized by a slowing down of both the mental and physical processes; the skin becomes dry and there is an accompanying loss of hair and teeth. Obesity is a common complication of myxedema, which can be corrected by the administration of thyroxin. The overactive thyroid gland secreting an excessive amount of the hormone thyroxin tends to have an accelerating affect on the person. Nervousness, excitability, and anxiousness are typical. Loss of weight, increased body temperature, and emotional instability may also occur. The condition is sometimes treated by the use of antithyroid drugs or by the surgical removal of part of the thyroid gland. Simple goiter is also a complication of the thyroid when there is a deficiency of iodine in the diet. This results in an enlargement of the gland in the neck. The prevention of the condition is through the administration of iodized salt.
Parathyroid Location: Usually 4 in number, located in the thyroid tissue	Their primary function appears to be that of maintaining the proper calcium and phosphorous ratio in the blood and tissues of the body. A decrease in the parathyroid hormone is most commonly caused by accidental removal or injury of the glands in an operation of the thyroid, causing irritability, muscle weakness, and spasms. Excessive secretion of the parathyroid results in the formation of kidney stones and the decalcification of bone.
Adrenal Location: On either side of the body above the kidneys	The inner portions of the adrenal glands secrete the hormone adrenalin that prepares the body for emergency action. The functions of the adrenal cortex are not well understood. Its absence is known to cause death; an oversecretion of its hormone causes a precocious sexual development in the boy prior to puberty and has a masculinizing affect on the female.

PSYCHOLOGICAL STRESS

A person's ability to function can be inhibited by physical stresses such as undue fatigue, nutritional deficiencies, illness, and injury. A person can be affected to a similar, if not a greater, extent by psychological stress. The origins of psychological stress are often not clear to the individual, and as a result it is difficult for him to take actions of a preventive or corrective nature. The sources of psychological stress are often quite varied and can arise from any part of the environment. There can be social or cultural stress as related to poverty or social status. There are many stresses that can be developed right in the home as a result of interactions between parents and children. Disciplinary actions reflecting disapproval or rejection can many times develop stressful situations. A source of stress may be the individual himself, who finds it difficult to make decisions and who does not adapt easily to change. Because stress tends to have a wearing effect on the personality, it becomes important that stressful situations be resolved within relatively short periods of time. While stress of a mild nature can act as a stimulant to help the person become more productive, in greater amounts it may cause a person to direct his attentions toward relieving the discomfort involved rather than solving the problems that are causing the stress in the first place. The person who has a "safety valve" for the accumulated tensions developed by psychological stress has a much better chance of surviving these kinds of conditions. The person with a recreational outlet or hobby has found a means of diverting the excess energies thus developed. Where these diversions do not exist, the "safety valve" then may consist of the improper use of alcohol, drugs, or other damaging substances.

It is difficult if not impossible to separate the physical from the psychological. What affects one invariably affects the other. When a child scrapes a knee, "treating" the child's emotional reaction to the injury may be as important as the care of the injury itself. This is not to imply that the child should be coddled. In fact, just the opposite type of reaction may be appropriate in some cases. It does mean that emotional feelings should be considered along with the physical.

It should also be recognized that real physical disorders and pain can be produced by psychological stress. Any person under tension is reacting not only mentally, but physically as well. In response to these situations there are secretions from the adrenal glands, the pituitary gland, and increased thyroid activity. There is oftentime involvement of the gastrointestinal tract, as indicated by the relationship of ulcers to long-term tensions. The acid production of the stomach is significantly increased during such periods of stress with resultant erosion of its lining. The physical reactions to stress are many and varied and could involve the cardiovascular system, with resultant cardiovascular disease, as well as the respiratory tract, with allergies and asthma being common reactions.

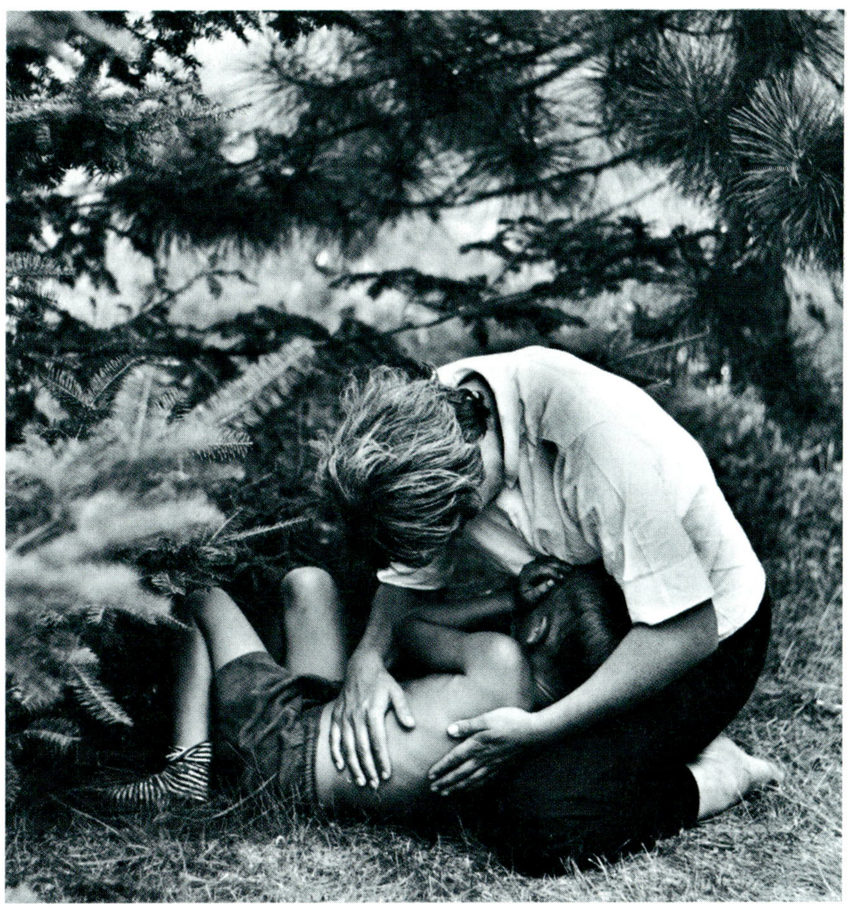

Figure 4–5

Emotional first aid.

(Ken Heyman)

HOW THE MENTAL AFFECTS THE PHYSICAL

The notion that the physical and the mental are two separate entities that have nothing to do with each other is poorly based. One need only watch a person cry. The tears are an obvious physical reaction to an emotion. There is not a gland or system of the body that cannot be influenced by emotion. This entity of mind and body is a human reality—we are made that way. It serves us well since it gives us a wholeness we would not otherwise enjoy. Because of this interrelationship, we are at times bothered by psychosomatic disorders; that is, physical disorders that are psychologically induced.

In reaction to anger, the body responds with the constriction of blood vessels, thus diverting blood to the skeletal muscles in preparation of the "fight" reaction and thereby raising the blood pressure. Where we have people who repress this emotion of anger, we find that the blood vessels remain constricted instead of returning to normal, resulting in chronic high blood pressure. Many people of this type give a rather calm outward appearance and are often referred to as "inside burners." There is evidence to indicate that when a person suffering from this condition is placed in a different psychological situation the condition is relieved. The modification of a chronic source or irritation and tension such as an unsuitable job or an incompatible marriage has a corrective reaction.

It is commonly thought that ulcers occur only in those personalities that are hard-driving go-getters. The easy-going and passive person, however, is also vulnerable to this disorder. In cases where an individual is overly dependent on another (such as a parent or spouse), if this relationship is threatened, enough anxiety is produced to cause physiological changes to take place in the digestive tract. Personality type is not so much a factor in ulcer development as is the excessive amount of anxiety that the person experiences.

Colitis is another malfunction of the digestive system sometimes related to emotional causes. The condition interferes with the digestion of food and disturbs the functioning of the bowels. Case histories of patients with colitis sometimes show that in childhood there was a mother whose domineering, antagonistic attitudes set up conflicts in the individual. The person therefore tended to grow up with a sensitivity to rejection or humiliation. Even minor failures resulted in emotional reactions that were out of proportion to the cause. The result is a sick colon.

It is thought that some cases of asthma are likewise psychologically induced. Attacks of asthma seem to be related to a child's fear of loss of mother love or psychological rejection. It is noted that many children and adults who suffer from asthma are overanxious and emotionally insecure. It must also be recognized, however, that many cases of asthma appear to be basically physical in cause.

THE EMOTIONS

The three basic emotions have been identified as anger, love, and fear. Our ability to control emotions has a great deal of bearing on how well we will be able to function. It has been found that moderate levels of emotion stimulate us to think more clearly, react faster, and achieve higher levels of accomplishment. Emotions also enrich our lives when we experience the warmth of love and affection which gives a crescendo to living that would not otherwise be there. Emotions also serve to unite people even when they are experiencing an emotion like fear. A group of people trapped in an elevator develop a feeling of comradeship as a result of experiencing fear together. Each section of the country has its small commercial airline with borderline efficacy that seems to inspire in their passengers a camaraderie not found in airlines with more sophisticated operations.

Intense emotion can have the effect of interfering with mental activity and break down our efficiency in various endeavors. For example, the lawyer who loses his temper in the courtroom is no longer capable of properly conducting his case. The adept fencer similarly swings wildly and ineffectively. Our ability to harness our emotions, therefore, is important to our effective functioning.

Emotions will often involve a number of physiological as well as psychological changes in the individual. The autonomic nervous system, for example, is concerned with the control of the parts of the body that function involuntarily. These include blood vessels, the heart, glands, and involuntary muscles. This system is made up of a series of nerve cell collections or ganglia. These ganglia lie along either side of the spinal cord and are connected to it by means of fibers. Some ganglia are located in the brain and control the tear glands and pupils of the eye. In an emotional state the autonomic nervous system prepares the body for a "fight" or "flight" reaction. It does this by diverting circulating blood to heart and skeletal muscles. Lung function is increased, the pupils of the eyes become dilated, and the skin becomes moistened with perspiration. The adrenal glands secrete adrenalin, which serves as a general body stimulant, and the liver releases sugar to serve as a source of additional energy. All systems are go!

A difficulty that can arise is that the emotional reaction may have been stimulated by a situation where a violent reaction is not appropriate. Many a person who is about to speak to a large group has experienced the increase in heartbeat and respiration as well as the clammy perspiration of nervousness. While the individual is geared for action, the situation calls for polite discussion. The emotional response then improperly prepares the person for the "emergency" situation. Some people have questioned whether fear and anger are emotions that serve an advantage or disadvantage to a person living in a highly technical society. The suppression of our emotions of fear and anger are in many respects related to headaches, backaches, tics of various types, and high levels of anxiety.

We also live in a competitive society where the fear of failure runs high. It is imperative that the individual become somewhat insulated against failure because he will experience a measure of this in the many highly competitive situations in which he will find himself. The real test of personality may not necessarily be measured in terms of degrees of success so much as it might be determined by the ability to deal realistically with failure. This ability might prove to be the ultimate success.

In a recent pole-vaulting event all contestants were eliminated save two. One of the men attempted to clear the new height the bar had been raised to and missed. His competitor noticed a flaw in his form that led to his missing his vault and informed him so. On the succeeding try he cleared the bar and won the event. By all standards in our competitive world the man who had placed second had failed. What would seem to be the greatest irony to many is that he contributed to his own "failure." "What is a man profited, if he shall gain the whole world, and lose his own soul?" Stated positively—if a man loses the world but gains his soul, has he really failed or has he in fact succeeded? It represents at the very least a selfless rather than a selfish act. It is also a religious concept too often forgotten in a self-centered, materialistic society.

THE MENTAL MECHANISMS

Mental mechanisms are means that we utilize to cope with anxiety. These mechanisms can be classified in three groups reflecting the kinds of actions that are taken in each, namely attack, flight, and compromise. The person in attack exhibits aggressive behavior that may be either physical or verbal in nature, directed at the source of frustration or a substitute for it. In flight, the person seeks to escape the situation or attempts to ignore it. In compromise, he decides to look at the problem once more and to live with it. These mechanisms tend to be generally used by people as a way of making life more comfortable by relieving anxiety. They can, of course, be symptomatic of personality difficulty when they are extensively used or when they are used rigidly and in fixed patterns. Usually mental mechanisms are unconscious in nature so that the person may be unaware he is employing them.

Daydreaming is a rather universal mechanism that is used by just about everyone from childhood on. It serves as a simple excape from situations that are unpleasant, boring, and perhaps even frustrating. It tends also to act as a bit of emotional relaxation. The boy pictures himself as the outstanding athlete or actor or whatever his unresolved dream might be. The girl might see herself in possession of great beauty, money, or fame. The opposite type of daydream might be the dreamer seeing himself as a victim of neglect, abuse, and mistreatment. This type of daydream might follow punishment that the individual feels is unjust. Daydreams that focus on success can many times have positive results. When they are not too unrealistic, they can often serve as goals and encourage constructive planning. The mechanism can serve useful purposes as long as it is not used to excess.

Regression is the return of the individual to a more infantile manner of behavior. The person who resorts to childish acts when he does not get his way or cannot face problems on the adult level is regressing. A temper tantrum is a common type of regressive action. If overused, regression may serve to make the person more dependent, indecisive, and overly cautious with regard to change.

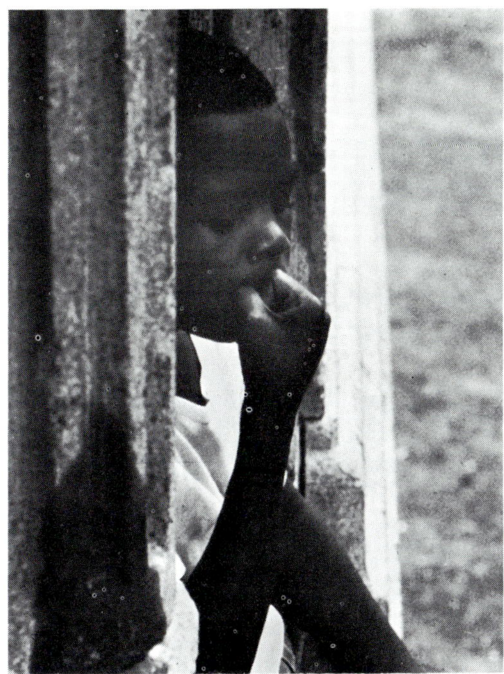

Figure 4–6

Daydreaming is a rather universal mechanism.

(Susan Johns)

Compensation is the mechanism whereby someone may offset his ability and success in one area against his failings in another. A person who feels he lacks status may seek to gain recognition through the purchase of an expensive item such as a car, suit, or dress as a means of compensating for his feelings of inadequacy. The person who tends to overcompensate for his feelings of inadequacy may become overly aggressive and domineering, and develop a fanatical need for power. On the other hand, compensation has its positive aspects as well. Some people who engage in community projects of various types are many times making a fine contribution, but are also compensating for unhappiness or boredom at work or at home. This kind of compensation might have a wholesome influence not only on the individual but on the community as well.

Substitution is a mechanism by which we tend to substitute one goal for another. A person may desire to own a very expensive car, but the reality of his bank balance motivates him to substitute the buying of a less expensive one. Where the person finds that he does not have the capability to perform well in a given activity or profession, he may decide to shift to one in which he can do better. This is a kind of substitute compensation. Substitution as a mechanism works out well only when the substitute goal is closely enough related to the desired one. Otherwise it is not really acceptable to the person.

An inadequate substitution gives relief that is only temporary in nature, and the anxiety that stimulated the mechanism in the first place will recur.

Suppression is the process of consciously hiding thoughts and feelings. Unexpressed fear, hostility, or even laughter, may interfere with the ability of the person to do routine things such as to read with comprehension, play the piano, repair machinery, and so forth. The ability to suppress thoughts and feelings and thereby to delay their expression can be a desirable thing. It may be inappropriate to laugh or express fear at a given moment. Delaying their expression could spare the feelings of others who might feel they were being laughed at, or whose levels of fear were already reaching unmanageable proportions.

Repression is similar to suppression except that it is unconscious in nature and the person does not have conscious control over this mechanism. It serves to push into the unconscious shameful or guilt-ridden thoughts, memories, or painful and distasteful experiences. A person who has witnessed a serious automobile accident or a soldier who has seen death will many times repress these painful, unpleasant thoughts. Repressed thoughts are often the bases of anxiety that we do not understand. A person may see an object or be in a situation that reminds him of an incident that has been repressed. This may cause a degree of anxiety that the person has difficulty understanding. The unconscious thought would have to be uncovered in order for the person to become consciously aware of the relationship.

Repression is generally regarded as an unhealthy mechanism because unconscious motives are sometimes unhealthy ones. When one permits himself to identify his needs accurately, then he can set about to deal with them. When for one reason or another a person is afraid, ashamed, or in conflict with regard to a basic need, he represses it. The need or what to do about it then remains chronically unfulfilled. Conscious reminders of the need develop in turn feelings of anxiety, fear, or guilt. Repression, then, is an attempt to hide a problem and therefore an unsuitable means of solving it.

Sublimation is the means by which instinctive and unacceptable impulses are transformed into socially useful goals. Primitive or aggressive impulses can be channeled into activities such as sports, art, literature, or religion. The mechanism of sublimation can serve an important function in the development of sound character and personality. Where sublimation is not possible, the personality finds itself in constant conflict.

Reaction-formation is exemplified by the submissive person who is actually covering up aggressive tendencies. Excessive amiability may be a façade for hostility. Reaction-formation, then, is a defense against the anxiety developed by disturbing and socially unacceptable feelings or impulses. The overly aggressive person may be covering up real feelings of insecurity. The overprotective mother who is obsessed with concern for her child's health and safety may actually be repressing hostility toward the child. This kind of false behavior usually becomes rather obvious. The mechanism does not reduce the tension caused by the conflict and somehow the underlying feelings seem to permeate the personality.

Fixation is the cessation of the development of the personality or a facet of it at an incomplete stage. There is normally a progressive development of the personality, not only in the psychosexual aspects, but in the ability to control emotion, to deal with frustration, and to assume responsibility. Why this process is arrested is not always understood. An example of this may be seen where child-parent ties persist for too long and the mother makes a son overly dependent upon her. His relationship to her remains childlike and he never reaches true adulthood.

Identification is a mechanism whereby the individual identifies with another. The girl may identify with a favorite actress, the small boy with a baseball player. The exaggeration of the abilities and attributes of these idealized figures usually occurs. The use of celebrities for commercials is based on their being viewed by many as being all-wise and near perfect. A second variety of this mechanism is in the association of one individual with another. On meeting a person, we may find we have a distinct impression of what the person is like and react accordingly. Because there has been no time to get to know the personality, we have actually identified him with someone we knew previously and attributed to him the characteristics of the other personality for better or for worse.

Rationalization is one of the most commonly used mechanisms. This is a means whereby a person gives a plausible reason for his behavior rather than the actual reason. The person who rationalizes is unconscious of his motives, and is not making a deliberate attempt to distort the truth. Rationalization makes the person feel better about playing golf instead of mowing the lawn, or helps the person feel guiltless about going to a dance instead of studying. He might rationalize these situations by indicating that he has been working too hard and is in need of a recreational outlet. If rationalization is used beyond the degree of moderation, the individual may rationalize his way out of many of his basic responsibilities.

Projection is a means of shifting blame and responsibility for an act or a thought to someone else. The person who fails the course blames the instructor, or the salesman having difficulty selling blames the product. Another form of projection is scapegoating, whereby the blame for situations may be focused or projected on to other groups in the community. A weak minority tends to serve this negative purpose well. Even though projection may many times relieve anxiety, it often carries with it a sense of guilt that can lead to a need for self-punishment.

These internal mechanisms which are used universally are generally unconsciously selected and used automatically by the personality. Because they help to manage anxiety, aggressive impulses, and frustration, they make life a good deal more bearable during difficult times. The manner and extent to which they are used can serve as barometers of a healthy personality.

NEUROTIC ADJUSTMENTS

Neuroses are undesirable means whereby the individual deals with anxiety that has been produced by frustrations and conflicts. Many psychologists feel that the bases for neurotic reactions are developed in childhood and that they are particularly related to parent-child relationships. As stated by Kaplan:

> The typical family patterns encountered are those in which protective anxious parents prevent the child from growing up. Perfectionistic parents make the child feel that he can do nothing right. Overly strict parents make him feel mistrusted or ashamed of his natural impulses, and rejecting parents make the child feel worthless and unloved.[8]

Because neurotic reactions are motivated by unconscious thoughts, the individual is perplexed by them and will many times take inappropriate actions in dealing with them. The person who goes from one doctor to another hoping to find a cure for his physical ailments (that are psychologically caused) usually will not cooperate with the doctor because the physical symptoms he is exhibiting hide his real emotional problem. Because he is not conscious of all the factors involved in his condition, the neurotic is in a sense on a merry-go-round. He consciously seeks to relieve the symptoms of his neurosis while unconsciously he wants those symptoms to persist because they hide the real problem that he feels incapable of facing.

Types of Neurotic Adjustments

Anxiety Reaction. Anxiety is a feeling of apprehension or dread that something unpleasant is going to happen. Under normal circumstances, the person realizes why he is experiencing the feeling of anxiety. A person may have anxious moments about losing his job if he hears that his company has to cut back on employees. A mother may become concerned about her child who she knows has been exposed to a serious disease. Anxiety, however, is neurotic when there is no apparent cause for its occurrence or where a very slight cause results in a highly exaggerated response. The latter is exemplified by a person who has a pain in his chest and imagines that he is having a heart attack, or the person with a slight cold who is sure that it is pneumonia. When the reason for anxiety is not apparent, it is usually because it is due to a repressed and usually unacceptable emotion. The closer the repressed emotion comes to making its way into the consciousness the greater is the anxiety developed. Anxiety can cause a number of physical symptoms and reactions such as headaches, indigestion, chronic fatigue, dizziness, constipation, and loss of appetite. The anxious person usually has difficulty sleeping and when he does get to sleep he is many times bothered by fearful dreams. This

[8] Louis Kaplan, *Foundations of Human Behavior* (New York: Harper & Row, 1965), p. 270.

person usually seeks a physical explanation for his distressing mental state. The person generally reflects feelings of apprehension and helplessness and is quite indecisive. He also lacks confidence, feels chronically fatigued, and will often complain about the inability to concentrate.

Dissociative Reaction. In this reaction the person disassociates or separates himself from his personality. One of the most common of these reactions is amnesia. When a person faces a problem that overwhelms him, forgetting his identity and therefore his problem becomes one means of escape. How well amnesia serves the person is indicated by how unperturbed the individual is in regard to his loss of memory. In this condition, the person will forget who he is or even assume a different identity and will not recall people or factual events related to his past. It must be remembered that amnesia is not purposeful forgetting. The reaction is quite unconscious and beyond the conscious control of the individual. While most dissociative amnesias last a relatively short time, some can blot out a person's entire previous life. The fictional story of *Dr. Jekyl and Mr. Hyde* exemplifies this mental condition. Another example is *The Three Faces of Eve,* which is an actual case of multiple personality where three quite different personalities occupy the same body and predominate it at different times. Most cases of amnesia, however, are not as dramatic as *Dr. Jekyl and Mr. Hyde* nor as involved as *The Three Faces of Eve.* Quiet, neurotic forgetfulness better describes most cases of this type.

Conversion Reactions. A conversion reaction or conversion hysteria, as it is sometimes referred to, can oftentimes be quite dramatic. A sudden loss of vision or hearing, paralysis of an arm or leg, or the loss of sensation in the skin can be typical types of reactions. After a thorough physical examination, it is found that the person has nothing organically (physically) wrong with him. The basic difference between this type of disorder (psychogenic) and a psychosomatic one is that in the latter the psychological stress results in the development of a physical disorder. The symptoms that develop in a conversion reaction provide to some extent the solution to a problem facing the person. The soldier who is the army is trained to kill may find himself unable to pull the trigger as a result of a paralysis of his arm. This occurs because of the conflict created with his early upbringing that indicated "Thou Shalt Not Kill." The girl who is about to marry someone that she does not really love may suddenly find her legs paralyzed and unable to walk down the church aisle. Lesser kinds of conversion reaction involve twitches and spasms of the muscles of both the face and limbs. It can also include the experience of imaginary symptoms of illness to the point where the person actually feels pain. The solution to these problems of course does not lie with aspirin or other such medication but with psychotherapy and with the person's understanding of his problems. Where unconscious motivation is a factor, the person cannot be in a position to diagnose the nature of his difficulty objectively.

Obsessive Compulsive Reaction. If a person has a repressed thought or emotion, he may occupy himself with an obsessive thought or a compulsive act which takes the form of a ritual. When the mind occupies itself with these obsessive or compulsive functions, it does not have the opportunity then to think of the distasteful thought that it is trying to keep repressed. Obsessive compulsive acts have a wide range in terms of activity, thoughts, and significance. Just about all people have found themselves experiencing the compulsion to double-check the front door that they know is locked and the alarm clock that has obviously been set. Likewise, we have all experienced obsessive thoughts like the inability to get a certain jingle or tune out of our minds. While these obsessive thoughts or compulsive acts have, at worst, nuisance value, more intense forms of these behaviors can prove to be real handicaps. In some instances, people develop rather elaborate rituals or ceremonies. There is a case of one woman who when retiring to bed would fold her clothes very meticulously and in a complicated manner. Her preparations to retire usually took two hours. People most prone to the development of these types of reactions are those who would be described as hair splitting and stubborn, submissive and yet in need of asserting their importance. They are usually overconscientious in tasks that they perform and are intolerant and highly critical of others. Kleptomania, the compulsive urge to steal, pyromania, the compulsion to set fires, are more serious forms of obsessive compulsive reactions.

Phobic Reaction. A phobia is an intense fear of a specific thing or situation that is of no real danger to the individual. While all people have fears, generally these fears are based on a real threat or at least a potential threat. Phobic fear is based on a fear reaction when no real cause for it is observable. The principal causes of phobias are traumatic experiences that a person may have had and forgotten. Anything that reminds the individual unconsciously of that experience would stimulate a phobic reaction. A person may also be conditioned as a child to fear certain situations or things. The mother, for instance, who has a phobic fear of mice could very well condition her daughter to react likewise. In many instances, the real cause of a phobia is repressed so that it is unknown to the sufferer.

Phobias are many in number and examples of a few follow:

Acrophobia, fear of high places.

Agoraphobia, fear of open places.

Algophobia, fear of pain.

Hematophobia, fear of the sight of blood.

Hydrophobia, fear of water.

Mysophobia, fear of contamination.

Nyctophobia, fear of darkness.

Photophobia, fear of strong light.

Toxophobia, fear of being poisoned.

Zoophobia, fear of animals.

PEANUTS
Tm. Reg U. S. Pat Off —All rights reserved
Copr. 1961 by United Feature Syndicate, Inc.
AND SOME PEOPLE HAVE WHAT IS CALLED "HAPHEPHOBIA"
WHAT IN THE WORLD IS "HAPHEPHOBIA"?
6-28
AUGH!
A FEAR OF BEING TOUCHED!
SCHULZ

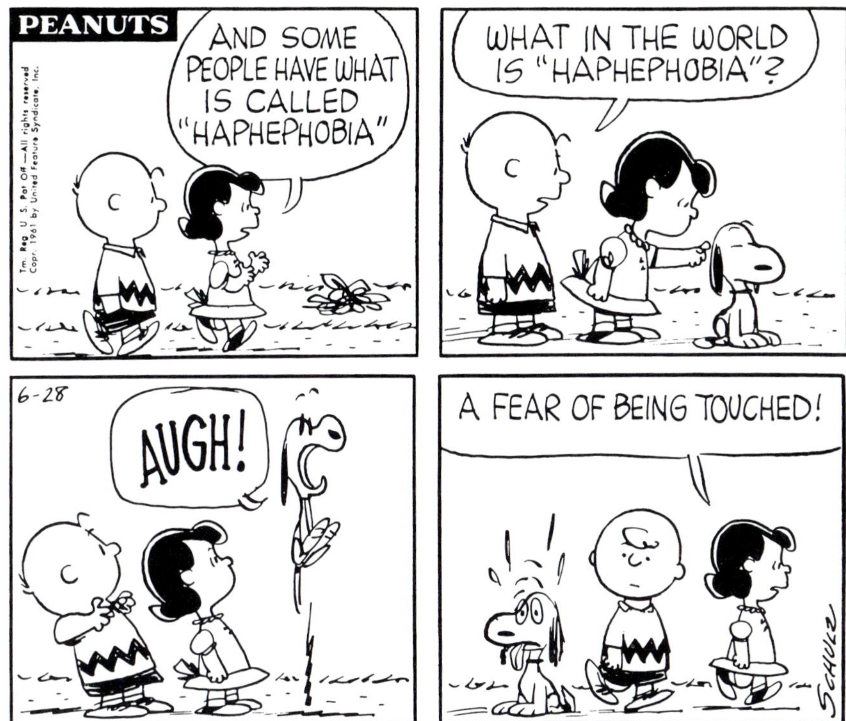

Figure 4–7

Peanuts cartoon by Charles M. Schulz.

Phobias are of varying intensities and quite common. When they begin to interfere with one's work and activities, then it is time to seek professional help to correct them. Because phobic reactions are often unconsciously stimulated, individuals should not attempt to correct them themselves. One college student suffering from claustrophobia asked his classmates to put him in a dumbwaiter, lock the door, and not open it regardless of his reactions. This was his erroneously conceived approach to solving the problem by fighting it directly. Upon placement in the dumbwaiter, he panicked and fortunately his screams did induce his colleagues to open the door, although by the time they did he had already fainted. The experience did nothing more than aggravate the condition for the individual. The treatment of a phobia lies within the realm of the professional and not the amateur. People who like to play pranks with the phobic fears of others are in essence playing with fire. The hysteria that may be triggered by aggravating a phobic reaction can lead to even more intense psychological problems.

Depressive Reactions. Neurotic depression lies somewhere between normal discouragement or grief and the intense psychotic depression that is accompanied by suicidal desires. We are all familiar with the reactions that take place when the individual experiences a deep personal loss. However, after a period of time the depression following this kind of event is lessened as the individual gets back to the routine of living. In neurotic depression, the feelings that develop occur without any apparent cause. In other instances, a minor disappointment triggers a reaction that is completely out of proportion to the event. In neurotic depression, the person has the feeling of being unloved and a failure. The depression will usually be of long duration basically because it is fulfilling a neurotic need. The depression in this instance is a symptom and is in essence an indirect expression of a repressed feeling of guilt or hostility. Depression is considered a most common mental disorder.

There are a number of basic differences between a neurotic adjustment and a psychotic one. Neurotic adjustments are not only less serious than psychotic ones but are always functional (psychological) in nature, whereas psychotic reactions may sometimes be organically caused. In a number of psychotic reactions there is actual physical damage to the brain that precipitates the reaction. In the neurotic there also does not occur the kind of personality disorganization that takes place in the psychotic. While the neurotic may misinterpret reality, he does not replace it as the psychotic does. The neurotic person has an awareness that something is wrong, whereas the psychotic individual has replaced reality with fantasy. Freud described neurosis as a situation in which we are dealing with scars, whereas the psychosis is one where we are dealing with bleeding wounds. One description distinguishing between the two is illustrated by the statement that the psychotic believes two plus two equals five, whereas the neurotic knows that two plus two equals four, but it bothers him.

THE PSYCHOSES

The psychoses refer to a broad range of mental illnesses that have wide variations in terms of their severity, duration, and nature. As mentioned earlier, they are basically characterized by personality disintegration and loss of contact with reality.

The following discussion of mental disorders we hope will lend some understanding of the breadth and nature of mental illness. The broadly based classifications of mental illness referred to are intended to serve as a guideline to understanding. They are not intended for the overzealous, amateur diagnostician who is invariably found in every group and who enthusiastically categorizes friend and foe alike as having one type of mental illness or another . . . like a hypochondriac turned outward.

Schizophrenia is the most common of the mental illnesses. It is sometimes erroneously referred to as split personality, when it really is a disintegrated personality. Although schizophrenia is referred to as a single disorder, psychiatrists feel that it is actually a grouping of disorders. Most cases of schizophrenia have their onset during the adolescent or early adult years. A rather small percentage occur between the thirties and middle age. The early signs of schizophrenia are evident many years before the person undergoes the actual breakdown and often these signs go unnoticed. In these people there develops a general tendency toward greater withdrawal, feelings of unworthiness, and increased sensitivity to being rejected and unloved. There is a continual development toward a lack of response to people and activities about them. There appears to be a kind of drifting into an unresponsive state. Oftentimes there is a great and abnormal preoccupation with such abstract things as life, good, evil, and God. In some cases, the schizophrenic loses his identity, sometimes thinking that his body no longer belongs to him and that he is literally beside himself. The reactions that are stimulated by the hallucinogenic drugs are considered to be very much like those experienced by the schizophrenic. Recent experimentation has shown that a substance very similar to mescaline, a hallucinogenic drug, was isolated from the urine of most schizophrenics. This has led to the conjecture that possibly schizophrenics form hallucinogens because of defective body chemistry and are in effect on a permanent hallucinogenic kick. Statistics show that the incidence of schizophrenia is 1 per cent (1 in 100) in our population. However, where there has been some schizophrenia in the immediate family, the incidence is 14 per cent (1 in 7). This does not mean that the condition is inherited; it does imply that the person may inherit a weakness which if abused could result in the greater tendency to develop the illness. It has also been noted that in the use of LSD, those individuals who experienced permanent mental illness were usually those who had genetic inclinations along these lines. Individuals with such a genetic weakness can with the use of a hallucinogenic drug create enough stress to "tear the fabric" and cause mental illness.

For the purposes of diagnosis, greater understanding, and treatment, schizophrenic reactions have been subdivided into four major groups:

SIMPLE TYPE. Simple schizophrenia is characterized by indifference and apathy. The person develops the attitude that it is much more comfortable *not* to try and lives essentially through his daydreaming. Vagrancy, prostitution, and delinquency are frequently "occupations" of the simple schizophrenic.

Case Study—Kevin M.

This third admission to the hospital at thirty-three, was the final one for Kevin, and he was to remain until he died of natural causes at seventy. During his first few years on the ward he was dull, uncommunicative, and evasive. There was a marked lack of emotional tone, with the same apathetic affect accompanying his every behavior. He was slovenly in attire,

> and seemed utterly indifferent to any question of personal appearance. He was listless on the ward, and although he worked on various jobs as assigned, did so very slowly and apathetically. He had no plans for the future and was quite satisfied to remain in the hospital.[9]

HEBEPHRENIC TYPE. Hebephrenic schizophrenia is probably most closely related to the layman's conception of insanity. The behavior is characterized by inappropriate laughter, smiling, and smatterings of hallucinations and delusions. The person's speech is quite incoherent and illogical. The person's personal habits with regard to cleanliness and sanitation tend to deteriorate. The auditory hallucinations of hebephrenics are often related to God and religion. When the patient hears the voice of God, psychiatrists feel that this is in essence the voice of conscience reflecting feelings of guilt. In many instances, the patient will regress to an infantile level which he creates and in which he seeks protection.

An example of an interview with Robert follows:

Case Study—Robert A.

DOCTOR: What are you talking about?

ROBERT: I've been lured, I've been lured time and time again. I've been lured by mobs and lured by money to build space. They talk about pleasure principle, pleasure purpose, it's merely false sex.

DOCTOR: What do you mean?

ROBERT: I know what I'm doing. I'm living out my grandfather's life. They had to tell me, my mother went. America sees its own heirs.

DOCTOR: Does God talk to you?

ROBERT: No, I don't get voices. I just used that for a sex point.

DOCTOR: Do you see some particular pattern for the world?

ROBERT: It's immaterial. I don't day I can't use the moon. God made the moon so let it have it. I'm like a psychiatrist and I'm trying to help my mother.

DOCTOR: What's wrong with her?

ROBERT: I've got intuition. She doesn't seem to want to be a father. If she'd show me a written statement I'll be a priest.

DOCTOR: Have you ever seen any visions?

ROBERT: I don't see visions. I see God in word and deed. My mother couldn't stand any such program.

DOCTOR: What does that chair look like to you?

ROBERT: Sex. It's immaterial. The legs are like the moon, sexy to a point. They tell me that the clothes were divided. I want to see who's lying. They've got the greater part of the money. They live out lies. When I meet God I can live out a clean conscience.[10]

[9] Melvin Zax and George Stricker, *Patterns of Psychopathology* (New York: Macmillan, Inc., 1969), p. 61.

[10] Ibid., p. 65.

CATATONIC TYPE. The behavior of the catatonic schizophrenic varies from one extreme to the other. In some instances, the patient may remain in a fixed position without movement for days and even weeks on end. During these periods of catatonic stupor, the patient is conscious and though he shows no reaction to activities around him, he is aware of their presence. The waxy and statuelike positions assumed by these patients is typical of the catatonic condition. On the other hand, the catatonic also experiences periods of wild excitement. He becomes very aggressive, hostile, and destructive. He may attack people, smash objects, and tear clothing. Speech during these wild periods of time is meaningless. The catatonic reflects a negativism and an antagonism that result in his not eating or sleeping, to the point of physical exhaustion. Developing catatonia is sometimes seen in introvertive individuals who will sit quietly, sullenly, and motionless in a room for long periods of time. These persons usually show unstable temperaments and a characteristic exhibition of fits of anger.

Case Study—Henry E.

During the year previous to his current hospitalization, Henry did not walk, talk, or eat unless he felt he was specifically instructed by God to do so. Occasionally he would become excited and violent, and when these episodes occurred he was indiscriminately destructive. The chaos this caused in the family home led his brother to seek his rehospitalization. When admitted, Henry was in an emaciated state, and refused to eat or talk. He would only lie passively in bed, staring fixedly at the ceiling. His occasional changes of expression suggested the possibility that he might have been actively hallucinating. Henry did not seem to be distressed by holding himself in uncomfortable positions for long periods of time.[11]

PARANOID TYPE. The paranoic schizophrenic is characterized by delusions of persecution and grandeur. It seems that the disorder develops slowly and appears somewhat later in life than other schizophrenic reactions. The paranoid appears frustrated with regard to his abnormal need for achievement or status. He concludes that others have schemed and are scheming to keep him from success. He will trust no one, particularly those he is most closely associated with, such as members of his family. In some cases, he develops the feeling that people want to destroy him and he may in "self-defense" kill them first. Not all paranoic patients, however, are dangerous. The feelings of inferiority that these people experience are usually compensated for by the psychotic belief that they are God, Napoleon, or some other omnipotent figure.

Case Study—Olive W.

She began to express the idea that someone was following her with the intention of doing her harm. She noted that people passed her house

[11] Ibid., p. 77.

> in groups of threes and felt that this had special significance for her. Finally, she began to experience auditory hallucinations and lost interest in caring for herself or her home. When she became very disturbed and assaultive toward members of her family and accused them of plotting her demise, it was necessary that she be hospitalized.
>
> She was also grossly delusional. Olive insisted that the electric meter on her house was her own broadcasting station which was registered by President Truman and in Atlanta. This station was thought to cover the entire world. Its workings were vaguely described and she termed it a Westinghouse Triple No. 99. It was said to have been installed by former President Roosevelt, since he intended to live in her home, and she insisted she had a chair belonging to him which was left when he spent a night there. She indicated that because of Roosevelt's intention to move to her house, General MacArthur visited there several times.[12]

Schizophrenia has the highest frequency rate accounting for approximately one-fifth of all admissions to mental hospitals in the United States. Because it is a chronic kind of mental illness that psychiatrists have had the most difficulty in treating, approximately one-half of all patients in mental hospitals today suffer from this ailment. Research that will identify more specifically the nature of the illness is needed before we can significantly reduce its incidence and duration.

Manic Depression Psychosis. It is quite normal for people to experience changes in mood. We tend to be in a pleasant mood when things are going well and become rather unhappy when we fail in one task or another. However, when a person's moods are extreme, ranging from very high elation and hyperactivity to severe depression, particularly without apparent cause, then something is wrong. Manic depressive reactions do not have the effect of causing personality deterioration or disintegration, as occurs in schizophrenia. Rather they seem to be an exaggeration of normal behavior. In the manic stage of this condition, the person becomes quite elated and talks very rapidly, sometimes so rapidly that he becomes incoherent. The person in this stage has all kinds of energy and everything seems completely simple. He feels he has little time for sleep, and in spite of great activity shows little sign of fatigue. He resembles a car that has been thrown out of gear with the motor racing. While it is making a lot of noise, it is not really going anywhere. The manic who begins to express his antagonism for others may lose what little control he has over himself and do others bodily harm.

In the depressive stage of the condition, the depression may range from a mild state to a very severe one. Rather intense feelings of guilt are usually present during the depressed state, along with feelings of hopelessness, confusion, and dejection. In the depressive stage, people sometimes express feelings of being in need of punishment and think about, or even attempt, suicide. In manic depression, the patient may alternate between manic and depressive

[12] Ibid., p. 86.

phases. In other instances, the person may experience just the manic or just the depressive phase. The incidence of recovery from this condition is quite high. It does not appear to be as serious an illness as schizophrenia. In schizophrenia, the patient gradually withdraws from reality, whereas in manic depression there seems to be an accumulation of frustration which suddenly bursts forth and may prove to have catharsis value. It is felt that manic depression generally results from too much stress for too long a period of time. Some authorities feel that gifted people with a certain amount of mania have an increased drive that makes it essential that they work long hours and therefore accomplish many and great things during their lifetime.

Other authorities feel that there may be a genetic factor associated with manic depression. Dr. Franz Kallman, of Columbia University found in his study of identical twins, that if one twin suffered the disorder, the chances were 85 to 90 per cent that the other twin also suffered from manic depression. Dr. Kallman has concluded that at least one type of manic depressive psychosis has all the markings of a hereditary disease. Scientists are now attempting to find biochemical causes of the illness and ultimately its correction.

Organic Psychosis. Mental illness can be caused by a number of physical factors. The most common is probably that caused by cerebral arteriosclerosis. The narrowing down of the arteries by deposits that accumulate along their walls reduces the amount of blood carrying food and oxygen to brain tissues. The result is that many older people suffering from this condition show signs of confusion, incoherency, forgetfulness, and bewilderment. There are fairly large numbers of older people in mental hospitals because of cerebral arteriosclerosis. Paresis is another example of organically caused mental illness. The spirochete that causes syphilis attacks nerve tissue and ultimately migrates to the brain. In spite of an increased incidence of syphilis, fewer new cases of paresis (brain damage due to syphilis) now occur, because of effective treatment with penicillin.

Large amounts of bromides act as toxins in the body and can cause psychotic conditions. People who douse themselves with some of the patent medicines containing bromides can run this risk. Discontinuance of intake of the substance will return the person to normality.

Alcohol intake by the chronic alcoholic will cause Korsakoff's Psychosis, which is a reaction to a toxic level of alcohol in the body over a prolonged period of time.

SUICIDE

Approximately 25,000 suicides occur in the country each year. An additional 175,000 to 200,000 make unsuccessful attempts to kill themselves. About 2 million people in the country have made at least one attempt at suicide. These statistics with regard to suicide attempts and incidence are probably conservative estimates. Suicides are often disguised and certified as accidents because of the stigma associated with it or because insurance policies do not cover suicide. The circumstances of death are many times unclear so as to make it difficult to determine if death was caused by an accident or suicide. It is estimated that the underreporting of suicide may be as high as 200 per cent.

Historically some societies responded to suicide with crude vengefulness. The bodies of suicides were dragged through the streets or impaled on stakes for public view. His property was confiscated and burial denied in church and city cemeteries. In the last century or so the suicide was viewed not as a criminal but a lunatic, which represented but a slight improvement, in view of the maniacal attitudes toward the mentally ill. In recent years these attitudes are changing in more positive directions with the suicide being recognized as a person in difficulty and if the person were helped the suicide would be prevented.

Emil Durkheim, a French sociologist and suicidologist, describes three basic types of suicide, each being the result of man's relationship to his society. "Altruistic" suicide is the first type he describes where there are social pressures to commit suicide under certain circumstances. The Japanese who committed hara-kiri serve as examples of altruistic suicide as do Hindu women who were expected to cremate themselves on the funeral pyres of their husbands.

"Anomic" suicides are described by Durkheim as those occurring when the relationship between an individual and his society is suddenly destroyed. The shocking and unexpected loss of a close friend, or fortune, or position might precipitate suicidal actions. Surprisingly, sudden wealth can also cause the suicide of some people. Serious social readjustment either in the form of sudden growth or unexpected catastrophe can apparently set off self-destructive inclinations in some people.

"Egoistic" suicide, a third kind described by Durkheim, is the form most commonly seen in the United States. The individual in egoistic suicide has few ties with his community and tends to have no strong attachments to church, home, or the political life in society. In essence he is uninvolved.

Youthful suicide is causing increasing concern in the United States. It has risen in prominence as a cause of youthful death in recent years. Research at the University of Southern California School of Medicine[13] reveals the profile of the suicidal adolescent often involves problems relating to family. A large percentage of these adolescents had one or both parents missing from the home because of death, divorce, or separation. Many had parents who were married more than once. Those with stepparents were not adjusting well to the newcomer. Many had both parents working or in one-parent families, the one parent worked. A large percentage lived with persons other than their parents.

[13] Joseph D. Teicher, M.D., "Children and Adolescents Who Attempt Suicide," *Pediatric Clinics of North America,* Vol 17, No. 3 (August 1970).

Poverty also seemed to be a significant factor with regard to suicide. A young person who is suicide-prone is attempting to cope with the stresses and strains of growing up without the support of important family relationships.

As a society we have attempted to sweep suicide under the rug and pretend that it does not exist—then alternately express surprise and shock when it does occur. The lack of discussion of this topic has made it possible for a number of misconceptions about suicide to establish themselves in the public thinking. Some of the more common ones follow:

1. *People who talk about suicide won't commit suicide.* It is estimated that up to 80 per cent of people who commit suicide have communicated their intention to do so. Persons who hint or threaten suicide should be taken seriously and help sought for them.
2. *Suicide happens without warning.* In addition to verbal warnings persons may communicate suicidal intent by writing a will, leaving a note, or giving expensive gifts without apparent reason. It must also be added that most suicides are not impulsive acts but are planned.
3. *Suicide and attempted suicide are the same class of behavior.* While 5 to 10 per cent of those who attempt suicide unsuccessfully will later succeed, most people attempting really want to live. They use this desperate means of drawing attention to themselves and their problems, hoping someone will come forth to prevent the suicide and help them to correct their problems.
4. *Suicide involves only a specific class of people.* Suicide is neither "the curse of the poor" nor "the disease of the rich." All levels of society are rather equally represented in its statistics.
5. *All suicidal individuals are mentally ill, with suicide always the act of the psychotic person.* Studies of suicide notes indicate that many are logical and rational and not psychotic. So, while some suicides may be psychotic, others are just extremely unhappy people.
6. *Suicide is inherited.* In studies reported on twins there is not a single case where both twins committed suicide, although there are a number where one twin has committed suicide and the other has not. There is no evidence that suicidal behavior is inherited as the color of one's hair or eyes.
7. *Once a person is suicidal he is suicidal forever.* A person's desire to kill himself may last for only a short period of time or until he is helped to face and overcome his problems.
8. *Improvement in a suicidal patient means the danger is over.* It has been noted that with depressed patients the greatest risk of suicide is during the period of improvement. The patient may regain sufficient drive and energy to take his life at this time.

9. *Only a psychiatrist or mental hospital can prevent suicide.* While psychiatrists and mental hospitals can be most helpful, there are a variety of religious, lay, and community groups making up the developing suicide-prevention movement.

Is it possible to identify the potential suicide? Almost everyone seriously considering suicide gives indications of his interest. Some indications are rather obvious; in other instances they may be subtle. The suicide decision is usually not an impulsive one, but a planned one. The person is disturbed and very often depressed. He (she) feels hopeless about the direction of his life is taking and feels helpless to do anything about it. This pessimism in combination with depression can serve as initiators of the act.

There are often verbal threats and cries for help such as "You won't have to put up with me much longer." "They'll miss me when I'm gone." "This is the last straw—I wish I were dead." "I'm good for nothing." "I'll show them!"

Other common signs include withdrawal, loss of initiative and motivation, loneliness, disturbed sleep, loss of appetite, inactivity, a drop in academic performance. More subtle signs might include boredom, antisocial behavior, restlessness, defiance.

Obviously any *one* of the above signs by itself is not an indication of suicidal intent. A changed pattern of behavior including a number of the above *is* cause for concern.

> No one knows what it is like to be dead. At best, one can only imagine what it would be like if one were alive to watch—an invisible personality—at one's own funeral. Often such an attractive fantasy intoxicates the suicidal mind, and tips the scale to death. But until the very moment that the bullet or barbiturate finally snuffs out life's last breath—while the ground is rushing up—the suicidal person terribly wants to live. No doubt, he also wants to die. But it is an ambivalent wish—to die and to live. Until he dies, a suicide is begging to be saved. Before his death, the suicidal person leaves a trail of subtle and obvious hints of his intentions. *Every suicide* attempt is a serious cry for help. This cry can be heard, and suicide can be prevented.[14]

An increasing number of suicide prevention centers are being established in communities and college campuses across the country. They are manned by mental health professionals as well as carefully selected lay personnel. Such centers are usually available for services twenty-four hours a day. Such a center in the city of Los Angeles averages 500 persons contacting it each month. Their help is as close as the nearest telephone, since they have "hot lines" manned twenty-four hours a day by lay personnel who can be of immediate help to a person calling for help.

[14] Edwin S. Schneidman and Philip Mandelkorn, *How to Prevent Suicide,* Public Affairs Pamphlet #406, p. 6.

DEATH—A PART OF EVERY LIFE

Death is an inevitable part of every life. It is a normality of life, just as a sunset must follow every sunrise. It has often been stated that "nothing is more certain than death and taxes," yet there are in our society many inappropriate responses to death. Death is often denied or repressed, resulting in an inability to cope with it when it occurs. The hysterical reactions of friends and relatives as well as the frantic, fruitless efforts of health professionals do not enrich one's last moments. When the death of an individual is expected *and* inevitable, it is time for solace and compassion.

In years gone by, the family would be called together when "grandfather" lay on his deathbed. It was a time to tidy up one's affairs, a time for sorrow and final goodbyes. When the man died it was in the company and comfort of family and friends. With the advent of "civilization," grandfather dies in the sterile environment of the hospital under the glaring lights of the intensive care unit surrounded, punctured, and manipulated by gadgetry designed to save life rather than to delay death long after the individual is prepared to

Figure 4–8

Death is an inevitable part of every life, just as a sunset must follow every sunrise.

(New York State Department of Mental Hygiene—Julian A. Belin)

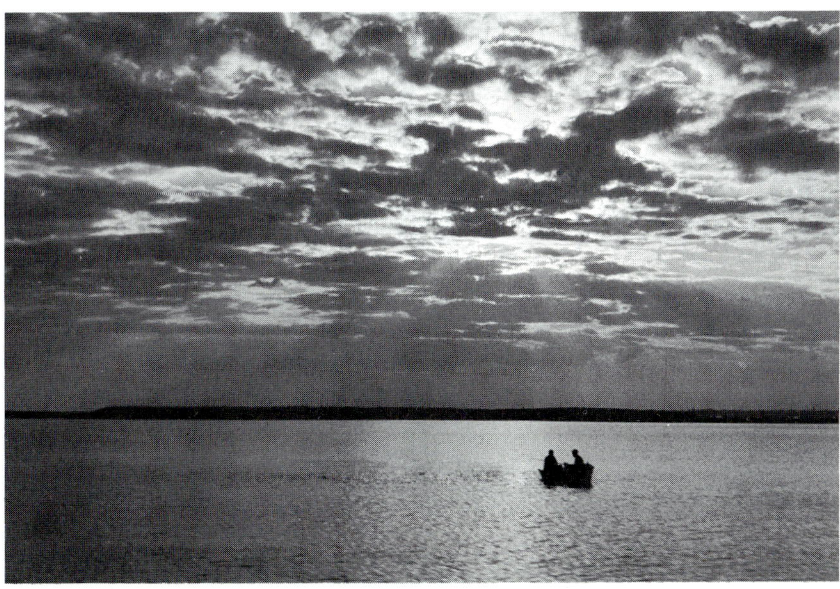

accept it. The family is herded oftentimes in a waiting place down the hall so that they may not interfere with hospital procedure. Dying with dignity should be the last humane act permitted and should not be lost to the superfluous efforts of technology.

As stated by Reverend Carl Nighswonger, "In 12 years of hospital chaplaincy, I have yet to find a family that could cycle their grief according to the hospital schedule. . . . How much better it would be when the doctors give up, if the patient could be moved to a dimly lit, quiet room where the family could sit at his bedside and hold his hand."[15]

The physician and health professionals are trained to sustain life. It is understandable that to them death is viewed as being synonomous with failure. The technology now available to the physician is no doubt in many instances life saving. The decisions become more difficult when it becomes questionable whether "the machinery" is sustaining life or delaying death. To sustain a vestigial fragment of life obviously misses the point.

Some people have developed and signed documents called *living wills* in which they state that should they reach a time when their lives are being sustained artificially, without hope of recovery, that they be permitted to die naturally. Legislative bills have been introduced in several state legislatures to make living wills legal documents rather than just the written expressed wish of the individual.

In an effort to remove the dying process from its depersonalizing, technological context and to give it back to humanity, a new medical subspecialty has evolved called thanatology (The Study of Death). At the Billings Memorial Hospital in Chicago, health professionals are offered a course on The Dynamics of Death and Dying. The objectives of the course are to make the health professional more aware of the psychological adjustments a person makes to his impending death. The health professional is thus trained to help the patient during this difficult period. Physicians who undergo this training seem more capable of handling their own emotional reactions to their patients with regard to their life expectancy and to help prepare them psychologically for life's final act.

MENTAL HEALTH SPECIALISTS

The Psychiatrist is a medical doctor who specializes in the treatment of mental and emotional disorders. In addition to the M.D. degree, three additional years as a resident physician in an institution where mental illness is being treated is required. After two additional years of experience in the area of specialization, the physician must pass an examination by the Board of

[15] "Death: Making It Easier for Patient and Family," *New York Times,* May 9, 1971.

Psychiatry and Neurology of the American Medical Association, The American Psychiatric Association, and the American Neurological Association.

The Psychologist is an individual without a medical background who concerns himself with applying scientific methods to the study of human behavior. If he is a *clinical psychologist,* he has earned a Ph.D. and has completed a supervised internship at a psychiatric clinic. If the clinical psychologist meets the standards set by the American Psychological Association, he is then qualified to diagnose and treat behavior disorders, usually through testing and other psychological diagnostic devices.

The Psychoanalyst can be either a psychiatrist or a psychologist who devotes his time primarily to psychoanalysis, which is a method of studying the emotional problems of a patient with the purpose of alleviating them.

The Psychiatric Social Worker usually has a master's degree in social work and then concentrates on psychiatric case work. Field work in a mental hospital, clinic, or family service agency is part of the training of the psychiatric social worker. After graduation, this professional will work in one of those three settings. The National Association of Social Workers sets accreditation standards for its members.

The Psychiatric Nurse is a graduate nurse with additional training in the care of the mentally ill.

TREATING MENTAL AND EMOTIONAL PROBLEMS

Psychotherapy is the treatment of mental and emotional problems by psychological means. The therapist meets with the patient and through verbal exchange determines the nature, cause, and possible solution of the patient's problem. Psychotherapy is often of a supportive variety, where the patient is given reassurance and emotional support in facing his problems.

When the therapist deduces that repressed thoughts and emotions are underlying factors in the person's problems, he attempts to bring these factors to the surface or to the conscious level. He may do this through dream analysis and free association. In free association the person responds to a stimulus, such as a word or picture, with the first thing that comes to his mind. These responses give clues as to the nature of the repressed thoughts. Dreams often reflect unconscious thoughts and their analyses sometimes prove helpful in the better understanding of the patient. Hypnosis may also be used as a means of overcoming patient inhibitions and amnesia with regard to his past. Under hypnosis, the patient is very suggestible and responds more easily to the questions and suggestions of the therapist. It helps the therapist to discover the causes of the person's difficulty and to give guidance for the reeducation of the personality. Often, the closer the therapist gets to uncovering the repressed thoughts or feelings, the more uncomfortable the patient becomes.

As some people proceed through the therapy, they may decide to stop seeing the therapist because they are being "upset." This is often an indication that the therapy is proving successful and moving toward the root of the problem. Psychotherapy is in many ways a learning process. The person is learning about himself and how to react more appropriately to life situations.

Group Therapy. The therapist will often bring a number of people together for group therapy. Here patients have an opportunity to react to each other as well as to the therapist. The situation itself is helpful to the patient as well as the therapist, for it gives the therapist the opportunity of seeing the patient in a different setting which invariably reveals other facets of the personality he is dealing with.

Sensitivity Training. There is a wide range of activity that may be classified as "sensitivity training." Encounter groups represents one of these. These are often candid confrontations with the person made to acknowledge his rationalizations. Drug and alcoholic patients are often involved in such encounter groups to assist them in acknowledging the real reasons they use drugs. Various forms of nonverbal communication may also be used as part of this approach. Care needs to be taken in the use of this approach lest the abrasive confrontation prove to be psychologically destructive rather than constructive. It is a technique best left to the highly qualified and experienced rather than to amateur psychiatry.

T-Groups represent another form of sensitivity training. It tends to focus on how people feel rather than on how they think. It encourages people to be open and candid about how they feel about others. The theory is that criticism will develop honesty, self-understanding, and trust in others. Because it can also result in conflict expert leadership is necessary for such groups. A person lacking ego-strength could find such a group session to be threatening and emotionally destructive. Widespread use of these techniques has caused some concern where groups are led by people not prepared to cope with the emotional responses they may turn loose in the group.

Psychodrama or Role Playing is a technique whereby patients act out their problems. As a result they often gain some insights with regard to their solution. Closed circuit television is sometimes used to play back the psychodrama to the persons involved. A person watching himself on television often "sees" himself for the first time. It has often resulted in the development of a more positive self-concept.

Play Therapy is another form of psychotherapy, one that is used with children. How a child feels about various members of its family, for example, may be revealed by its play reactions to dolls that represent mother, father, brother, or sister. Repressed thoughts are often communicated via this approach.

Drug Therapy. The two basic types of drugs used in drug therapy are tranquilizers and psychic energizers (stimulants). Tranquilizers such as chlorpromazine and reserpine (there are many brand names for them) are used mostly

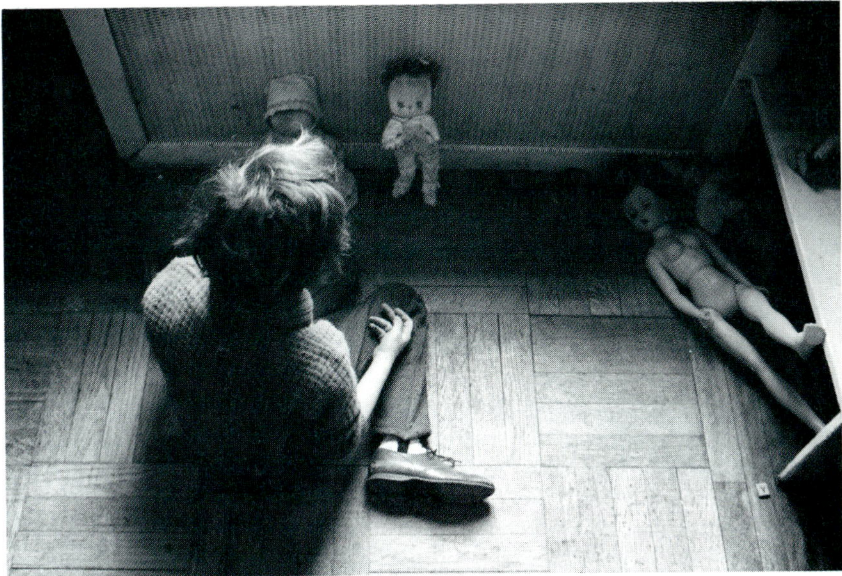

Figure 4–9

Play therapy often reveals how a child feels about himself and members of his family.

(Susan Johns)

for psychotic patients with schizophrenia and manic-depression as well as for acute alcoholics. These drugs have a quieting effect, blunting the exaggerated threats commonly experienced with psychotic patients. The stimulants or antidepressants are used for depressed patients and alcoholics with success in counteracting these depressed conditions. Drug therapy is used in conjunction with psychotherapy, and in many instances, even when drugs are used alone, they provc helpful to the patient and his management.

Shock Therapy was much more widely used before the introduction of drugs. In one form of this therapy, insulin is administered to reduce the blood level of sugar and cause the patient to go into a coma. In another form of this therapy, a small electrical current is passed through the patient's brain for several seconds causing a convulsive reaction. The use of shock therapy has declined since the 1950s when antidepressant drugs such as thorazine and marplan came into expanded use. Shock therapy to treat depression gets faster results than psychiatric counseling and drug therapy. When carefully administered, it is reported to be effective in a vast majority of the depression cases within days and surely within a month. Shock therapy is very often used in conjunction with psychotherapy and/or drug therapy.

MENTAL HEALTH TREATMENT FACILITIES

Until the early nineteen fifties, the only places of treatment available for people with serious mental illness were the state mental hospitals, Veterans Administration hospitals, and small private hospitals for those who could afford them. In recent years, general hospitals have increasingly developed psychiatric wards. The development of drug therapy for the mentally ill person has helped to make this possible because it affords greater control of the patient. Patients who stay at general hospitals are usually those requiring short-term care.

The Community Mental Health Center

In 1963 the Community Mental Health Centers Act was passed. This legislation was introduced at the request of the late President John F. Kennedy. The legislation authorized federal funds to states for the construction of community mental health centers. These centers are designed to provide a wide range of services for the mentally ill and to keep them in the communities where they live. Too often sending a person to a mental hospital a distance away from home cuts him adrift from family, friends, and job, thus superimposing an additional problem on the one the patient already has. President Kennedy believed that community mental health centers would reduce the number of mental patients by at least half by providing services that would focus on diagnosis, care, rehabilitation, and emergency service that would be available both day and night. It is felt that the cost of per patient care would also be reduced by such a center. At the present time the cost of patient care per day in a psychiatric ward would be six times that in a public mental hospital. Psychiatric care at a local general hospital averages a period of two or four weeks, whereas in a public mental hospital the stay averages six months. The nature of a community mental health center will vary from community to community. The functions of the center could include prevention as well as treatment.

In the early 1970s the concept of community mental health centers received some setbacks as the federal government cut back on funds for this purpose. Economy-minded governors of some states have added to the problems of the mentally ill by closing down state mental hospitals. The patients discharged from the state hospitals returned to their local communities to find that mental health facilities for their continued care was nonexistant. The program for community mental health centers had as its initial objective the establishment of 2,000 such facilities around the country. At this writing, less than 400 are still functioning.

HOSPITAL MANAGEMENT OF THE MENTALLY ILL

In the past, mental "hospitals" were such in name only. They were essentially institutions where the mentally ill were locked up and detained. Within recent years, mental hospitals have been developing a more liberal policy with regard to patients, and more and more of these institutions have been adopting an open-door policy. At the present time, at least two-thirds of the mental hospital population enjoys the freedom, as well as the dignity, of the open ward. The time that was spent by nurses locking and unlocking doors is now directed toward more positive measures. Hospitals have recorded rather dramatic changes in the attitudes of their patients when the bars came off the windows and the doors were unlocked. This approach in itself has created a better therapeutic atmosphere. It is recognized, of course, that patients in some of the acute phases of illness need to be secluded for their protection as well as that of others. This open-door policy has also made it more possible for patients to leave the hospital and continue treatment in outpatient clinics. The patients have

Figure 4–10

Treating the mentally ill takes many forms.

(New York State Department of Mental Hygiene—Julian A. Belin)

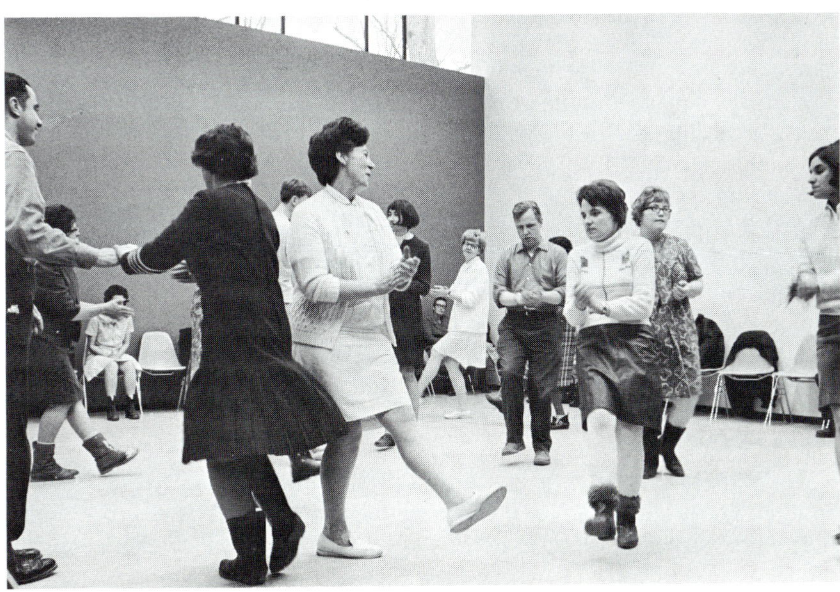

also been encouraged to go home for visits during weekends to help maintain family ties and relationships. It is felt that this greater flexibility in hospital management has helped to decrease the average length of hospitalization of the mental patient.

On being admitted to a state mental hospital, the patient is generally given a course in intensive treatment which could include drug therapy, psychotherapy, and possible shock therapy. How long this intensive care lasts depends on how well staffed the hospital is. Because of the shortage of personnel in this area, some mental hospitals will have a doctor-patient ratio of 1 to 100 or worse. This ratio needs to be reduced if intensive care is to be given over longer periods of time to ensure a greater percentage of successful therapy. Many state mental hospitals that are properly staffed can discharge up to 75 per cent of their patients within three months after admission and 85 per cent within a year. Some of these patients will not require any further treatment. Others will need to follow a prescription of psychiatric drugs for several months or several years. In other instances, psychiatric clinics in the community will provide follow-up services to support the patient through further rehabilitation.

The community psychiatric clinic is staffed by a team consisting of a psychiatrist, a clinical psychologist, and a psychiatric social worker. In addition to follow-up treatment given to a patient from a hospital, many of these clinics will provide treatment for individuals not requiring hospitalization. These clinics often serve a preventive function by giving early assistance to those with emotional problems. Where emotional problems are not permitted to fester, they do not develop to the point where hospitalization becomes necessary. Persons may be referred to an out-patient clinic of this type by a physician or another community agency such as the school. In other instances, a person may initiate treatment by merely walking in and asking for it. The treatment cost for the patient at most of these clinics is usually nominal, with payments scaled according to the patient's ability to pay. In a number of states the community psychiatric clinic is liberally subsidized by the state government.

Veterans Administration hospitals treat veterans with service-connected mental disorders. Where a veteran is mentally ill with a disorder that is not service-connected, he can be admitted to these hospitals if he cannot afford to pay for needed mental health services. There are approximately sixty Veterans Administration hospitals in the United States. These hospitals are usually more completely staffed and better equipped than state mental hospitals and as a result can often provide more thorough treatment.

Types of Admission

There are four basic ways in which a patient may be admitted to a mental hospital. The first is the *informal admission:* the patient merely enters the hospital and indicates that he feels he needs help. Under this type of admission, the patient is free to leave at will. At the present time, there are comparatively few states that permit this type of admission. In *voluntary admission,* the patient again approaches the hospital, indicating that he is in need of help, signing a paper asking for treatment as well as hospitalization. He can leave the hospital whenever he chooses, provided he gives the hospital notice of intent to leave several days before. An increasing number of states have developed a voluntary admissions policy. Many, however, still do not have such a policy and require commitment of the patient. *Commitment by medical certification* occurs, in the usual case, when a relative approaches a doctor, indicating that he believes a member of the family to be mentally ill and in need of treatment. After examination of the patient, if the physician feels that the person should be hospitalized he will sign a certificate to that effect. In some cases the medical certificate for admittance can be given by the admitting physician at a mental hospital. In *legal commitment,* the patient is brought before a judge for a sanity hearing. The judge will often ask a medical doctor to act as his adviser, to hear testimony, and to help him come to a decision with regard to hospital treatment. The physician, unfortunately, is not always a psychiatrist; in fact, in most cases he is *not.*

OUR CHANGING ATTITUDES TOWARD MENTAL ILLNESS

There was a time when the mentally ill person was locked in a cell and was the recipient of much physical abuse. He was the object of ridicule and was regarded as something to be ashamed of. Ignorance invariably stimulates fear of the unknown. Clifford Beers' manuscript, *A Mind That Found Itself,*[16] described his own experiences as a mental patient and drew early attention to the need for the better understanding of mental illness and the mentally ill person. His writing set off the Mental Hygiene Movement, which stressed prevention of mental illness as its goal. It also sought to correct the distorted idea that it was a disgrace to be or to have been mentally ill. In his writings, Beers indicated that mad men were too often man-made. He felt that mental "hospitals" that deprived the person of his dignity and rights were just as disturbing to the mentally ill person as they would be to a well person. Although many of our mental institutions may now be called hospitals, there are a number, even today, that are in need of great improvement.

Present-day attitudes toward the person with an emotional problem are improved, but by no means perfect. There persist fallacious ideas with regard to mental illness that distort reactions to it. Many unfortunately still believe that a mentally ill person is usually a wild, dangerous lunatic. It is undoubtedly safer to be on the ward in a mental hospital than in a room where two "normal" people have lost their tempers. Mental illness is still not a completely socially acceptable disease, although giant strides have been taken in this

[16] Clifford Beers, *A Mind That Found Itself* (New York: Doubleday, 1948).

direction through public education. A reason for the inability to accept the mentally ill person as sick is that he does not behave the way "sick" people do. The sick person usually expresses some feelings of helplessness, and in response is helped and cared for. The mentally ill person often does not realize that he is ill and therefore does not ask for help and does not expect any. If help is forced on him, he begins to feel abused, which is a reaction that any one of us would have.

A further complicating factor in dealing with the mentally ill is that families cling to the irrationality that mental illness constitutes a shameful disease. This attitude not only inhibits the seeking out of treatment but blunts its effectiveness as well. The patient, after receiving treatment, returns to family, friends, and job, and acceptance of the former mental patient by those closest to him becomes important if he is to be helped to continue his recovery and make a good readjustment to normality. In response to negative attitudes toward mental illness, Dr. Karl Menninger once stated that many patients recovered from their mental illness, but not from their diagnosis.

Mental illness has become a highly treatable disorder. When mental hospitals are fairly well staffed, 75 per cent of the patients admitted are discharged within a three-month period. While we certainly do not know all the answers as far as mental illness is concerned, current treatment can prove to be quite helpful. The difficulty at the present time is that there is a lack of mental health facilities as well as personnel. The shortage of psychiatrists and other mental health professionals is critical. As a society we are just beginning to come to grips with one of our major health problems—mental illness. We need to develop more realistic, less prejudicial attitudes toward these disorders. We must be willing (we are certainly able) to invest in the facilities and in the training of the professional personnel so urgently needed. Research in this area also needs to be significantly increased if newer and more effective preventive and treatment procedures are to be developed.

REVIEW QUESTIONS

1. Describe what you would consider to be the "mentally healthy person."
2. What are man's basic physical and emotional needs? How are these best fulfilled?
3. What does Maslow regard as self-actualization?
4. "Self-concept is learned." Describe those influences that contribute to the development of one's self-concept.
5. Distinguish between the conscious and the unconscious mind. How does Freud describe the unconscious mind?
6. Why are man's emotional responses sometimes inappropriate in our current level of civilization?

7 The test of personality is often measured by its ability to deal with failure. Explain.

8 Describe how anxiety can be helpful to the individual.

9 Describe the nature of the mental mechanisms and the purposes they serve.

10 Give examples of mental mechanisms that you have observed others using.

11 What are some of the relationships between the proper functioning of the endocrine system and mental health?

12 How has civilization affected man's behavior? What kinds of changes does it demand of him?

13 What are the objectives of the new medical subspecialty called thanatology?

14 What are the reasons for neurotic adjustments? How can unconscious thought complicate the understanding of neurotic reactions?

15 What is a phobia? Describe the dangers inherent in playing pranks with the phobic fears of others. Why do phobic reactions often require professional help to overcome?

16 Though schizophrenia and manic-depression are both psychotic conditions, there are marked differences between them with regard to their nature. Explain.

17 Distinguish between the functional and organic psychoses. Give some examples of the latter.

18 Suicides are not as spontaneous and as singularly caused as they are often considered to be. How would you support the aforementioned thesis?

19 Define: (1) psychiatrist, (2) psychologist, (3) psychoanalyst, (4) psychiatric social worker, (5) psychiatric nurse.

20 Describe the types of therapy currently used with the mentally ill.

21 Mental illness is a highly treatable disorder. Explain.

22 The mentally ill are people! How does the open-door mental hospital contribute to the dignity as well as the recovery of the person with a mental disorder?

23 Describe the various types of admission to a mental hospital: (1) informal, (2) voluntary, (3) commitment by medical certificate, (4) legal commitment.

24 Describe the changes in attitude taking place in our society toward the person with an emotional problem.

25 What are three basic types of suicide and their sociological rationale?

26 Why are there so many misconceptions about suicide even as late as the twentieth century?

5. Human Relationships & Family Life

Love probably starts when the I becomes WE. It does not happen so much as it develops, and it is not as exciting as it is comforting. Love is like an oasis; it serves as a kind of solid spot—a piece of rationality in an irrational world. It is a constant in an era of rapid change. It gives a person purpose and direction as the North Pole does a compass. Fickleness and self-centeredness are immiscible with it. Love is tough, durable, and unshakable because it is a kind of personality fusion, welded by time and understanding.

LOVE HAS BEEN DESCRIBED as both a human emotion and an accomplishment. It is the outcome of successful human interaction. Certainly good lifelong relationships cannot be without it. An ingredient it requires is the ability of the individual to invest of himself in another; the willingness to care for another with the hope that the concern will be returned. "Whatsoever a man soweth, that shall he also reap." Those who invest wisely, will know human contentment; those who do not, can know the depths of despair. Love then can serve as a measurement of the richness of one's life and how well one has learned to live.

CONCEPTS OF MASCULINITY AND FEMININITY

Determining what represents maleness and femaleness by physical standards is quite simple. Femininity and masculinity, on the other hand, are learned and psychological in context. Cultural influences play significant roles in the determination of standards here. In our society, emotional and intuitive qualities and sensitivity for the arts would be classified as feminine in nature. There are societies, however, where these would be masculine qualities, where unemotional, calculating, reasoned reactions would be considered feminine qualities. Cultural standards in this area can exhibit wide differences substantiating the thesis that behavior is learned.

Though the foregoing may sound confusing, it is not particularly disturbing to the individual who never or rarely leaves his environs. He or she can reject the standards of another society as being wrong, undesirable, or placed in the "that's interesting, but . . ." category. When the individual is in a society such as our own, where the standards for feminity and masculinity are undergoing change, the bases for some adjustments present themselves.

In the past in our society, the epitome of femininity was exemplified by the woman who was coy and demure and cultivated ineffectualness and inferiority to man. A woman who dared challenge a man intellectually or professionally during that era was at the very least "no lady!" These concepts of femininity have been rapidly undergoing change. In order to achieve this end a whole new concept in elementary school textbooks is evolving where little girls' mothers are not always in the kitchen. A woman may be portrayed as a professional, i.e., doctor, lawyer, architect. Physical Education classes and competitive sports are becoming increasingly coeducational. Now over 50 per cent of the women who are college graduates are working professionally and quite successfully. Women are seeking equality in their interactions with the opposite sex, professionally, socially, and in marriage.

Outcomes of this reevaluation of our standards of femininity appear to be greater companionship in marriage and greater socialization of the sexes. The woman sees in the newer developing concepts of femininity greater intellectual and social freedom and the opportunity of being, to a much greater extent, herself.

Definitions for masculinity are also undergoing change in our culture. Historically, masculinity referred to muscular strength and the ability to protect. The "Prince Valiant" swinging his singing sword could serve as the model of manhood defending spouse and country. Wars are no longer fought with swords, and rifles are already obsolete. The scientist, the engineer, and the technician prepared to push "the button" are the present-day Prince Valiants. They do not swagger, and they may have trouble picking up, much less swinging, a heavy sword. Although muscular strength and skills are still admirable qualities, their identification with masculinity is waning.

The male clinging to the more traditional concepts of masculinity and femininity may feel threatened by the changes taking place. The more aggressive female who does not recognize his concepts of masculinity can emasculate him. He can retreat to the coy, demure, "old fashioned" girl, or to the solace of equally bewildered, sympathetic males.

The male who will not have difficulty in this era of change is he who can develop his masculinity around other kinds of strengths. These are inner strengths that give him the courage to admit his mistakes and not be shattered by them; that render him unafraid to make himself be heard; that make him dedicated to his work and help him influence the course of events around him. This self-actualizing male is one who is not a "yes man" at work or a nonentity at home, but one whose moral strengths and values make him a masculine model for a son to identify with and for a woman to love.

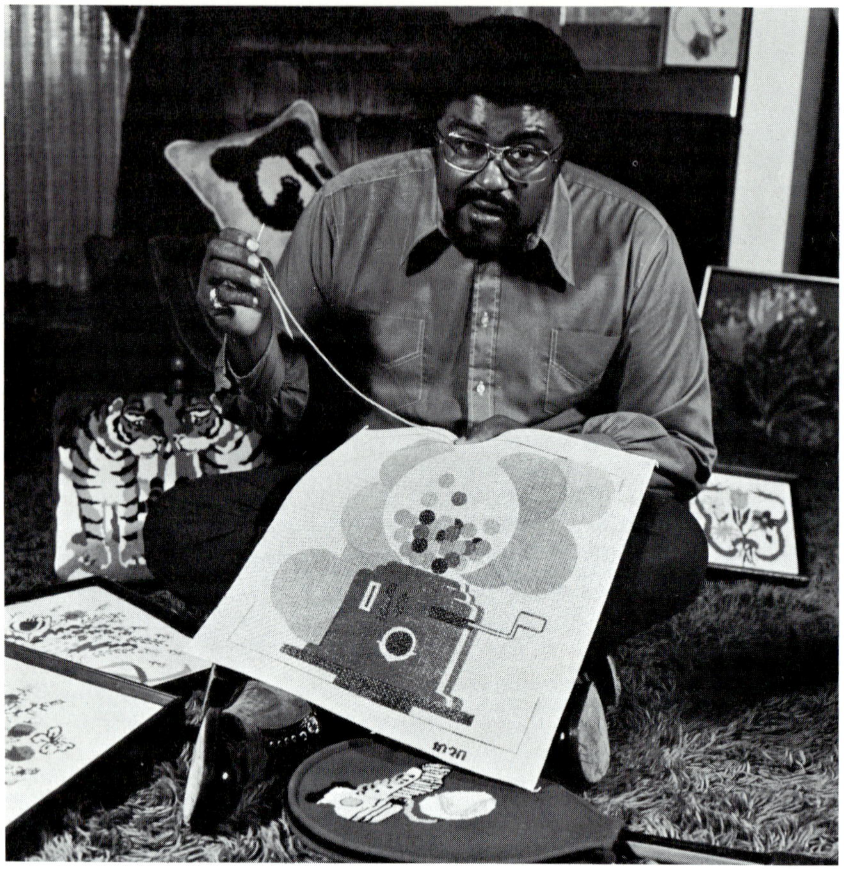

Figure 5–1

Rosey Grier is best known for his awesome bone-crushing tackles as a professional football player. Anyone who would like to tell this gentle giant that needle point is for sissies can do so at his own risk.

(From the book Rosey Grier's *Needlepoint for Men,* by Rosey Grier. Published by Walker and Company, 720 Fifth Avenue, New York, N.Y. 10019. © 1973 by Walker and Company, Inc.)

THE FEMINIST MOVEMENT

"We hold these truths to be self-evident; that all men *and women* are created equal."[1]

"Women are helpless . . . because men control the basic mechanisms of society."[2]

[1] The Declaration of Sentiments—The first Women's Rights Convention held in 1848 at Seneca Falls, New York. Leaders were Lucretia Mott and Elizabeth Cady Stanton.

[2] *Time Magazine,* August 31, 1970, p. 14.

"The average man, including the average student male radical wants a passive sex object cum domestic, cum baby nurse, to clean up after him while he does all the fun things and bosses her around—while he plays either big-shot executive or Che Guevara and he is my oppressor and my enemy."[3]

"There is no way out of such a dilemma but to rebel and be broken, stigmatized and cured. Until the radical spirit revives to free us, we remain imprisoned in the vast gray stockades of sexual reaction."[4]

"Heaven has no rage like love to hatred turned, Nor hell a fury like a woman scorned."[5]

The message coming through is quite clear: women do not want to be regarded as second-class citizens. At the present time women make up about 9 per cent of all professional groups. Women constitute 9 per cent of the doctors, 5 per cent of the lawyers, and 1 per cent of the engineers. Starting salaries for women in these fields are lower than for the men. The average full-time salary of a woman is about half that of a man. Financial independence is thus a primary goal of the women's liberation movement and lack of it a primary gripe.

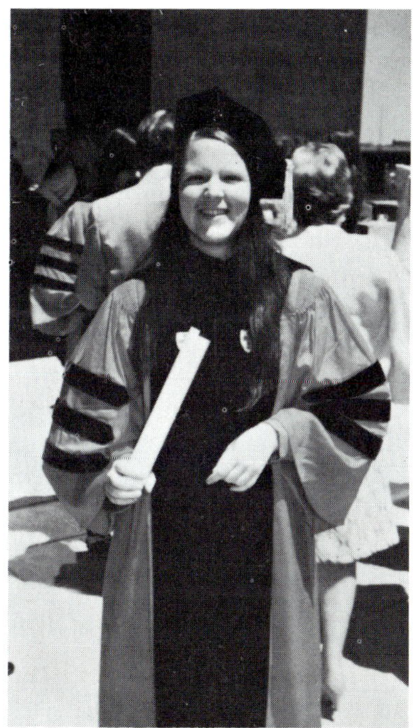

Figure 5–2

A law student graduates to increase the ranks of women lawyers. However, women still make up only 5 percent of the profession.

---

[3] Ibid., p. 14.

[4] Kate Millett, *Sexual Politics* (Garden City, N.Y.: Doubleday, 1970), p. 233.

[5] William Congreve, *The Way of the World,* Act III, Scene 8.

The fury that has been generated around the issue goes beyond pure economics. A great deal of resentment revolves around the woman being regarded as a thing, a sex object, a housekeeper, an intellectual inferior, and generally a subsidiary to that of the man. The term "male chauvinist" became not only a common expression, but a battlecry for women and a thrust at any male who exhibited any signs or symptoms of male supremacy.

Practically all women liberationists are agreed on such issues as equal pay for equal work, an opportunity to fill jobs traditionally reserved for men only, abortion reform, child-care centers to free mothers for work, more equitable income tax laws, and male respect. The more radical feminist groups see their mission as one of destroying the patriarchal system (male dominated), to be replaced presumably by the only other alternative, an equally unequal matriarchal system (female dominated). This represents not so much a change in the system, but rather *who* is in charge of it. A basic difference one sees therefore in the feminist movement is that while most are calling for equality, some are seeking to shift the power from others to themselves. The latter is hardly a quality found in just some women; some men have also sought power for the same self-centered reasons. Suffice it to say that acquiring and abusing power is unfortunately a human quality—but not a humane one.

Should the women's liberation movement succeed, the following would be some of the outcomes. The woman would assume many more positions in the ranks of the professions, in administration, and in the political arena. She will therefore become more independent financially, have a greater range of choices as to what she may choose to do with her life and have greater impact on influencing the course of events around her. She may choose not to marry, preferring a career. Fear of being called an "old maid" will become a thing of the past. She may choose to be a wife, mother, or professional or she may choose a combination of all three.

The man on the other hand may also benefit from the change. He may not have the pressures of being the sole or even the major source of income for the family. He may therefore have greater choice in the kind of work he selects, which may pay less, but is more satisfying to him. He may be free to spend more time with his children and thereby truly share the responsibility of raising them as is done in Sweden. Gloria Steinem, editor of the feminist magazine entitled *MS,* is credited with saying that ideally men and women should not reverse roles, but they should be free to choose their roles according to their individual talents and preferences. It is felt that role reforms will change the sexual hypocrisy we have now.

Studies have shown that societies that were most peaceful were those where sex roles were not polarized—a society where men were not expected to be the aggressive warriors and women the subservient peons. Rather, differences in dress and occupation were minimal, with men and women as true partners. The feminist movement, which started out with a warlike attitude, may have as its outcome a more peaceful society, where men and women will have freedom of choice as the kind of life they see for themselves.

SOME WRONG REASONS FOR SEXUAL INVOLVEMENT

It is important to note that a sexual relationship is a kind of social interaction. The motivations of the person in this type of relationship will not vary to any extent from those carried into other social situations. The level of maturity and healthymindedness are also reflected in sex as well as other social relationships. The heart of the matter is in one's personality and not in one's physiology! Let us first consider some of the negative bases for this kind of involvement.

SEX—A THING. A person may view sex as a kind of thing that is bought, sold, and paid for. The man with this point of view spends money on the girl he dates and regards it as an investment. He expects repayment in the form of physical pleasures that the female can provide. A girl who understands the rules of this game complies. The focus in this case is not on persons relating to each other, but on services bought and paid for. Whenever people are regarded as things and the ability to purchase is valued above the ability to relate, then there is indeed confusion with regard to one's values and behavior. It must be added that if a young person is confused with regard to sex values here, it is not the young person who introduced either the confusion or the value—but a society that views commercialism as the ultimate objective.

EXPLOITATION. While the previously mentioned situation involved a type of reciprocal trade agreement, exploitation is based on the principle of getting something for nothing. The Don Juan needs to exploit others as a means of alleviating his fears with regard to his masculinity. Some people contend that we encourage an exploitative male attitude in our society. They cite as evidence our concern with the problem of the unwed mother and the all-but-oblivious attitude toward the unwed father. A recent study of unwed fathers indicates that perhaps there is cause for concern here. It presents evidence that the experience is also damaging to the unwed father. He is first of all denied identification with his own creation and is further emasculated by his inability to see, much less take pride in, his offspring. Feelings of guilt that he may have are often heightened by the lack of punishment. The girl in the case usually is unwilling to identify him and in essence protects him. This serves to have a further distressing effect on the male who has been reared in a society where it is the masculine role to protect, rather than to be protected by, the female. The idea is fostered that pregnancy is the girl's responsibility. Any girl that engages in sexual activity is no good, but—boys will be boys! It is contended that we equate male sexual irresponsibility with masculinity rather than with immaturity. The male who accepts the exploitative attitude, it is charged, betrays the "wholesomeness" of his activities when he reacts with all kinds of indignation if the girl in a like situation is his sister or later on his daughter.

FEELINGS OF INSECURITY. The woman who places undue importance on her physical attractiveness needs constant assurance of its presence. She often becomes involved in a "Mirror, mirror on the wall" kind of game, seeking assurance from every male of the species that she is still "the fairest in the land." While it is quite natural and normal for a woman to want to be attractive to the opposite sex, preoccupation with the thought reflects a neurotic rather than a healthy need. When promiscuity is a result, the activity has hardly anything to do with sex, even though sex may be the distorted basis for attempting to satisfy security needs.

THAT BIOLOGICAL URGE. Satisfying the biological nature of the sex urge may be the sole motivation in some sexual involvements. Some find difficulty in acknowledging the existence of this aspect of their nature. Self-deluding attempts are made to believe that love was a motivating part of the experience. Marriages that result from a lustful relationship cannot be well based. A common cause of failure of early marriages is that they are often predominantly based on a sexual relationship. The young couple never learn to communicate on a higher level, preventing the fulfillment of each other's personality needs and the development of a more mature personal relationship. An erroneous conclusion that is drawn when such a marriage goes sour (as it inevitably must) is that each made a poor choice of a marital partner.

There is an erotic element in man-woman relationships—even in one as casual as a verbal exchange. Those who recognize the potential of this powerful erotic force deal with it appropriately so they can control it rather than have it control them. They seek to avoid situations and behavior that would stimulate and unleash these forces with inappropriate partners. *There is nothing quite so ashen as meeting the gray light of dawn with the throbbing realization of overinvolvement with a person one cannot love.*

THE RELATIONSHIP OF SEX AND LOVE

Much has been written and said about the relationship of sex and love. It is rather basically agreed that they mutually benefit each other. Some feel strongly that sex without love is a barren experience, being equated to speech without thought. It lacks meaning. As expressed by Schwarz in referring to sexual activity, ". . . if we meekly submit to the physical impulse, we incur guilt. Because it fails the essentially spiritual nature of man, a purely physical intercourse is essentially immoral."[6]

The relationship of sex and love is often more casually viewed by the male as compared with the female. The male is more erotic in nature and his sex

[6]Oswald Schwarz, *The Psychology of Sex* (Baltimore: Penguin, 1962), p. 22.

drive is more physiologically based. His sex drive can serve as the motivating factor leading to intimacy, even with women he would otherwise have no regard for. Love, then, does not always fit into the sexual pattern of things, particularly for the immature or exploitative male. Most girls are more prone to view sex as part of a long-term relationship. Premarital sex is therefore stimulated in the female more commonly by the idea of not losing someone than by sexual urges. Where a girl's romantic notions are mixed with some naïveté, she may be coerced by the exploitative male to "prove her love." In recent years, however, with the biological protection of the contraceptive pill there has been a greater tendency for young women to accept sex activity on a more casual basis paralleling those of men. Each period of liberation accompanied by the new-found freedoms requires careful preparation of the individual to make those most important decisions, lest we unshackle ourselves from the rigidities of the past to fall precipitously off the nearest cliff of licentiousness.

If love is viewed as the indispensable aspect of an ideal interpersonal relationship, one's interpretation of what is love becomes basic. Dr. Popenoe has reacted to the false values spewed out via the mass media by stating:

> The mass media picture love as a mysterious visitation that comes out of the nowhere and grabs hold of you like measles. Once it has you, the rest of your life should be an effortless ecstasy. If it turns out later that some effort is involved, it proves that you were mistaken in thinking this was your predestined soul-mate and there is nothing to do but throw him or her out and try again. . . . The net result has been to produce a culture that is based far more than is tolerable, on sex without love and marriage without responsibility.[7]

The nature of love is often overidealized with the emphasis on a sacrificial and an unrealistic selflessness. This interpretation gives it a saccharine flavor that could in time nauseate even the most romantic. The ability to give love is unquestionably an essential quality for the lover. The person's ability to receive love is equally important. It should be recognized that some of the person's own needs are being met by the relationship. The love relationship is characterized by a couple's feeling of warmth, pride, and identity with each other. There is also the mutual satisfaction of security needs. A oneness emerges from the interaction of the two people involved. There develops a related emotional dependence and an ability to communicate, not only in terms of words, but in attitudes, feelings, and thoughts. In a new or developing relationship each person tries to put his best foot forward as a means of impressing the partner. In a mature love relationship, this kind of thought and action is not necessary. A man and woman can stand before each other and bare their complete psychological and physical selves with all inherent

[7] Paul Popenoe, "Sex Education," *Family Life,* Vol. XXII, No. 8 (Los Angeles: The American Institute of Family Relations, August 1962). Used by permission of the author.

strengths and weaknesses. The commitment is complete. Sexual expression in this context then becomes a physical enactment of an existing mental, emotional, and social state of unity. In a love relationship, sex plays the secondary role of expressing and complementing the emotion. A mature love relationship is not one that all people are capable of attaining. Nor is it a state that once reached is forever propelled under its own power. It is a relationship that requires consistent attention or it dies of neglect like the unwatered plant.

SEXUAL OUTLETS

Masturbation is the self-stimulation of the genitals to effect sexual arousal and often orgasm. For the young male, masturbation is the most common sexual outlet until marriage. Over 90 per cent of the males have masturbated by the time they reach their sixteenth birthday. It is estimated that over half of the females have also masturbated. The frequency of the practice is usually much lower in the girl.

There were at one time many misconceived ideas about masturbation. It was erroneously related to just about everything from club feet to poor vision. Because uninhibited mental patients were observed to masturbate openly, it was even considered a cause of mental illness. Concern with regard to masturbation revolves around its use as a source of comfort and an escape from problems. Those who have been taught that masturbation is evil or sinful will often develop guilt feelings when they participate in this activity. Views with regard to masturbation in our society are becoming more objective. It is no longer regarded as often with alarm, but increasingly with the knowledge that it is a part of psychosexual development.

Nocturnal Emissions occur as a result of dreams of a sexual nature. An orgasm occurs during sleep and in the male semen is ejaculated, hence the term "wet dream." Females may have similar dreams, but of course ejaculation is not associated with them. The individual has no control over these experiences; they just happen.

Athletes are sometimes troubled by nocturnal emissions because they feel that they are weakened by them. It is believed that a decline in performance following a "wet dream" is psychologically induced by the thought that it may have this effect rather than by any actual physical changes that have occurred.

Occasionally, sexual dreams may involve a person the individual would not consciously consider as a sex partner. This could result in the development of guilt feelings. These feelings will be reduced if the person does not attach too much importance to the dream and places it in proper perspective. To attach moral meanings to nocturnal emissions is inappropriate because they are beyond the control of the individual.

Petting can include a wide range of activity from kissing to the stimulation of the partner's genitals to orgasm. There are varied motivations for petting. It may serve as a means of expressing love and affection or it may be stimulated by a curiosity with regard to the opposite sex. In other instances, the person may be seeking to establish that he or she is attractive to the opposite sex. It becomes important to give definition to a petting situation. Does one indulge for the pleasure of the moment, or does it mean the development of a more serious relationship between two people? If one person gives the activity one meaning while the partner gives it another definition, difficulty will inevitably be an outcome. Petting tends to be progressive, with greater intimacies developing on a given occasion or with succeeding dates. Understanding one's motivations and those of the partner becomes increasingly important. It is also important to understand one's physiological reactions as well as those of the partner. A girl's slower sexual response may lead her into underestimating the male's level of excitation. The young man, conversely, may misjudge the girl's response by his more rapid reactions. Petting leads so naturally to sexual intercourse that a couple may reach the point of no return before they realize it. When intimacy goes beyond the level desired by those involved, strong feelings of guilt and degradation may follow. If the intent is to keep petting under control, its limits should be decided beforehand as a guard against impulsive behavior that one will later deeply regret.

Studies show that petting to orgasm is becoming more common as a solution to sexual tensions short of intercourse. As stated by Hettlinger:

> It is of course, possible to be a "promiscuous virgin" and to engage in petting to orgasm with a variety of casual partners and without any serious commitment. In such cases, the technical preservation of virginity is purely superficial, and the level of sexual maturity is less than that of the person who has intercourse with one partner in the context of a loving relationship.[8]

Sexual Intercourse can serve to enhance a love relationship, particularly when the relationship is protected by the sanctity of marriage. Whether to participate in premarital intercourse is often a difficult question for a couple to resolve. "Premarital" would in this case be defined to mean that the couple have made commitments for marriage to each other. Intercourse without such commitments would be considered "nonmarital" in nature. Some couples have reported that as a result of premarital sex activity they felt they had developed a closer relationship. Others report negative reactions. Where sex activity is undertaken accompanied with fear of discovery, pregnancy, and guilt, more may be done to tarnish the feelings the couple have for one another, than to strengthen their relationship. Good sexual adjustment after marriage may

[8] Richard F. Hettlinger, *Sexual Maturity,* Basic Concepts in Health Science Series (Belmont, Calif.: Wadsworth, 1970), p. 47.

also be negatively affected by hurried, fearful, and guilt-tinged premarital attempts. Because it may take a period of time for a couple to adjust to each other sexually, early premarital relations often give false indices as to the kind of sexual adjustment they will ultimately be capable of. Careful consideration must be given to the decision of premarital sex to determine if the couple will be helped or hurt by the experience, particularly in view of the circumstances and attitudes that often surround such practices. What effect an unexpected pregnancy will have on the relationship must also be taken into account. It has also been noted that when a couple engages in premarital relations, feelings of jealousy and greater possessiveness often develop. The result is that the couple limit their social life making it impossible for them to meet others who might make more suitable marriage partners. Sex before marriage can thus "cement" couples into unsuitable marriages. Where premarital sex is practiced, should one of the partners decide to break off the relationship, it becomes more difficult to do so. A more unstable personality in this circumstance may threaten to expose the couple's premarital relationship. In a few cases, one of the partners may even threaten suicide. These latter actions usually do no more than demonstrate instability and confirm the individual's unsuitability for marriage.

The question of nonmarital sexual relations has also been raised. There are those who advocate complete sexual freedom in reaction to past sexual repression. Most people see both these points of view as creating their own sets of problems, with neither being a solution for the other. Reducing sex to the fun-and-games level with indiscriminate premarital intimacy appears to bear the same seeds of destruction as would the indiscriminate use of just about anything else. The difference, if any, is that here we are dealing with a sensitive part of life, requiring sensitive considerations. Equating sex that is based on sadism, masochism, exploitation, or self-indulgence with sex based on sincerity, love, and understanding cannot be justified by stating that sexual activity is "natural." There are mushrooms and there are mushrooms; there are berries and berries. Some will sustain the person; others will poison him. The skill comes in distinguishing between the two.

HOMOSEXUALITY

Homosexuality and heterosexuality are often viewed in terms of absolutes. Actually, there are various degrees of sexuality from one extreme to the other. Many psychiatrists view homosexuality as those persons who seek sexual gratification primarily with members of their own sex. There is apparently a rather large percentage of the population who may be erotically aroused by members of both sexes. Research shows that approximately 37 per cent of all males have had some overt homosexual experience to the point of orgasm. However, studies show that only 4 per cent of males are exclusively homosexual all their lives.

There are various theories to explain the possible causation of homosexuality. Increasingly, researchers in this field are finding agreement that psychological, social, and cultural factors are more important than genetic or glandular ones. A number of studies indicate that identification with the parent of the opposite sex can be a strong contributing factor.

There is general agreement that multiple factors probably play a part in the development of the homosexual state. Some of these include disturbed parent-child relationships, arrested psychosexual development at an immature stage, and cultural overemphasis on "masculinity" resulting in feelings of inadequacy in males.

In 1969 the Gay Liberation movement had its birth in the form of a riot at a gay bar in Greenwich Village, New York. The movement represents a revolt against social persecution and seeks to assist the rights of the homosexual. The North American Conference of Homophile Organizations put forth the following formal statement.

> In our pluralistic society the homosexual has a moral right to be a homosexual, and being a homosexual, has a moral right to live his homosexuality fully, freely and openly, free of arrogant and insolent pressures to convert to the prevailing heterosexuality, and free of penalties, disabilities or disadvantages of any kind, public or private, official or unofficial, for his nonconformity.[9]

The Gay Liberation movement has also taken the stand that homosexuality is not pathological and does not belong in the realm of the psychiatrist and psychologist but view it instead as a sociological problem in which prejudice and discrimination are directed against a minority in much the same way that other minorities are recipients of such treatment. "It is society that is defective and at fault and needs our attention, not the homosexual."[10] In 1973 The American Psychiatric Association changed its position on homosexuality, no longer classifying it as a "mental illness" but rather as a "sexual orientation disturbance." The emotionalized attitudes toward homosexuality in our culture are found to inhibit research in this area and add the problem of social rejection and persecution to the difficulties of the homosexual.

PREPARATION FOR MARRIAGE

Preparation for marriage does not start at the time that one begins to give consideration to marital possibilities. To be quite precise about it, since one's genetic makeup represents an initial contribution in this area, preparation for

[9] Joseph A. McCaffrey, ed., *The Homosexual Dialectic* (Englewood Cliffs, N.J.: Prentice-Hall, 1972).

[10] Ibid., p. 188.

marriage starts at the time of conception. Because the individual has no control over his inherited characteristics, he must accept it all gleefully or philosophically, as the case may be. Regardless of genetic endowments, the kind of marital partner a person *will be* is determined to a greater extent by the kind of person he *has become.* Marriage is essentially a close, intimate, social relationship between two people. The most important thing a person brings to this union is himself.

The prerequisite to a successful marriage is maturity. The complexities and responsibilities of marriage are not for the immature. Because the term "maturity" is subject to interpretation, it would seem appropriate to give some indices of its presence.

The mature person can accept responsibility for his own acts. This means that he is not trying to blame others for his failures or to exaggerate his accomplishments. He also does not take offense easily in reaction to what others may say or do. The immature often feel that people are picking on them. This kind of oversensitivity will hardly prove to be an asset in marriage, or in any interpersonal relationship, for that matter.

Maturity also means the ability to endure present deprivation in order to effect more meaningful future gain. A young couple may decide to rent an inexpensive apartment and furnish it with inexpensive, used furniture so they can save enough money to ultimately buy a house of their own and furnish it to their liking. Their present sacrifice will eventually pay off.

The person whose wants and urges need immediate gratification has not outgrown a childlike mode of behavior. This also implies a nonexploitative attitude toward others. The immature regard other people as things to manipulate and use for their own purposes.

The mature person is also socially responsible. His natural regard for others and his sense of responsibility make him one who has a concern for other individuals as well as for his community. He participates in community activity without the expectation of personal reward other than the satisfaction of contributing to a better-functioning society.

The selflessness characteristic of the mature makes them better prepared to live in close association with others and to contribute positively to their lives. The close interpersonal relationships that exist in successful marriage require acceptable levels of maturity as prerequisites.

WHY PEOPLE MARRY

The reasons why people marry are many and varied. The wholesomeness and unwholesomeness of the reasons may run an equally wide range. Positive motivations for marriage revolve about the desire to develop a close interpersonal relationship with another. This is usually described as a love relationship. The marriage serves to give this union religious sanction and legal protection. Thus protected by marriage, the relationship is provided an environment in which it can best grow. It is thus also regarded as a favorable environment in which to bring the products of this relationship—namely children. Many people see in marriage a stable structure within which love relationships and families are best developed.

There are also some negative motivations for marriage. Many times a girl has been indoctrinated with the unfortunate notion that her major function in life is to "get her man." In this case, the focus is not the development of a meaningful relationship with someone, but how to get him to the marriage ceremony. The wedding then becomes a day of triumph and a celebration of accomplishment. The groom in such an unfortunate circumstance is not loved, but is a piece of property that represents some temporary social status.

An individual may use marriage as a way of removing himself from an unhappy home situation. Where the predominant motive to marry is one of escape, the basis for another unhappy marriage may be in the making.

People who have been thwarted in a love relationship may decide to salve their bruised egos by impulsively marrying "on the rebound." The business of marrying the next eligible person to come along is an emotional reaction aimed to prove that the person *can* find someone to marry him or her. It also is designed to show that the rejecting party was not really needed, anyhow. Generally, such marriages are as likely to be successful as a series of shots in the dark.

Sometimes wealth may serve as a prime motivator for marriage. People who would use marriage for this purpose usually feel unloved and unsuccessful and strive to marry profitably as a means of compensating for both. The most that can be hoped for under the circumstances is misery in comfort. The close personal relationship necessary to a marriage cannot be based on a bank account. The price for fraud in marriage can be brutally high for both the victim and the perpetrator.

The unexpected pregnancy sometimes serves to initiate marriage. However, the biological father may not be emotionally mature enough to be a husband, much less a meaningful father—to say nothing of the readiness of the girl for motherhood and marriage. The compatibility of the couple may in other instances leave much to be desired. When all these things are considered, perhaps other means should be sought to resolve a difficult situation, rather than to aggravate it further by forcing an unsuitable marriage.

Social pressure cannot be overlooked as a motivating factor in marriage. The person who does not succeed in marrying is often viewed with a degree of suspicion or regarded as a kind of failure. Mothers often develop a good deal of the social pressure when they act as "coaches" and regard their daughters as "players." According to the rules of the game, the idea is to see how soon and how well the daughters can marry. How well the daughters can marry is usually measured in terms of nabbing someone's son a little higher on the social ladder.

In recent years some young people have been appalled at some of the poor marriages they have observed or have been the products of. They have seen people with the poorest of relationships who have entombed themselves in the concrete of marriage, thereby sentencing themselves to a lifetime of incompatability and unhappiness. Their reaction has been to reject marriage and indict *it* as the perpetrator of the crime. Others see those who inappropriately enter marriage as the precipitators of their own misfortunes. Relationships that are ill founded should not seek the religious sanction and legal protection of marriage. Perhaps it is time to stop viewing marriage as an end in itself and to recognize that not all people are suited for lifelong relationships. Despite the contrivances that may exist, our society generally expects people to marry, and many of our laws and customs are based on this expectation.

LOVE

Most people, when asked why they married, will aver that they were in love. The meanings given to the word "love" are many. The word is used in innumerable contexts such as love of country, parents, siblings, animals, clothes, fishing, and so forth. However, its meaning even in regard to one's intended spouse varies widely. Some people feel that they "fell in love" or that they experienced "love at first sight." Both of these experiences imply a sudden happening, something on the order of a chemical reaction. It could easily be rationalized that one no longer has control over a situation where "love has taken over." ("It's bigger than both of us!"). All that is left to say where such thinking prevails is "lover—beware!"

Closely akin to this kind of thinking is the concept of the "one and only." The thought is that there is only one person in the whole wide world with whom one could possibly fall in love. The fact that a large percentage of people marry individuals who live but a few miles from their homes represents a rather extraordinary level of coincidence that is blithely overlooked.

"Love conquers all" is a concept that leads a person to believe that love is an impenetrable shield against all problems. Such thinking is either a rationalization devised to ignore problems or potential problems a person does not choose to own up to, or an unfortunate naïveté. The thought that love will solve problems related to finances, education, children, parents, and religion by a magical waving of its wand cannot be equated with a realistic approach to life and living.

The decision of whether one is in love is an obviously important one. The rest of one's lifetime will be affected by it. A person about to abandon himself to love, needs as criteria for judgment more than wishful thinking or a hunch. As indicated, love is based on rather complete understanding, communication, and commitment between two people. The bases of understanding, communication, and commitment are not established by a sly glance across the room.

The criteria listed here for the evolution of love probably do not rate very high with the romantic. However, without these basics the most violent of infatuations is nothing more than a blazing star. Physical attraction and infatuation are usually pleasant, exhilarating factors in the initial stages of many love relationships as stated earlier. Love, however, probably starts when the *I* becomes *We.* It does not *happen* so much as it *develops,* and it is not as exciting as it is comforting. Love is like an oasis; it serves as a kind of solid spot—a piece of rationality in an irrational world. It is a constant in an era of kaleidoscopic change. It gives a person purpose and direction as the North Pole does a compass. Fickleness and self-centeredness are immiscible with it. Love is tough, durable, and unshakable because it is a kind of personality fusion, welded by time and understanding.

THE ENGAGEMENT

The engagement period affords the couple a period of time for the development of a closer relationship prior to marriage. This period of belonging to each other tests the relationship of the two people in a manner that casual dating cannot. It is assumed that engagement follows a period during which the couple have had the opportunity to become well acquainted. Some people establish an informal or preengagement period before making the more formal and public commitment of marriage. The informal engagement period gives the couple the opportunity to get to know each other better without the public commitment to marry. If the relationship does not work out, it is socially more comfortable to ease out of the situation.

The engagement period serves as a last trial run to test compatibility before marriage. There may occasionally be a gnawing doubt about the whole thing, but this is not unusual. There are, however, a number of engagements which for one reason or another do not make it to the wedding ceremony. Studies show that anywhere from one-fourth to one-third of engagements are broken. A number of relationships run into difficulty because they were not well founded in the first place. When it is apparent that an engagement should be terminated, it is best to face this reality squarely. There are some who have managed to avoid the issue until after marriage, with resultant divorce. It is better to break an engagement than become involved in the more complex business of disassembling a marriage. The philosophic thought, that an engagement broken is a divorce prevented, helps.

Engagement should be synonymous with a deepened relationship and a comfortable feeling of belonging to each other. There is a security that is not found in other kinds of relationships in being able to share life's experiences with another. The feelings of elation at having "found" each other is generally present in engaged couples. In good relationships, this feeling remains as the couple continue to complement each other throughout life.

THE PREMARITAL CHECKUP

A complete physical examination is appropriate before marriage. Those defects that may be found are in the vast majority of instances remediable. In some few cases, the examination may reveal that a partner is sterile and that the couple would be incapable of having children. This kind of information could at times alter the marriage plans. Genetic counseling has created the possibility of avoiding or preventing birth defects. It is the couple's responsibility to seek out such advice, to determine the prospects of their possibly producing children with avoidable genetic diseases.

The premarital physical examination will occasionally reveal minor infections in the genital area that are common in women. In a pelvic examination the physician can also detect whether the hymen will prove to be a problem after marriage. The opportunity to receive from a physician information about contraception and sexual intercourse also presents itself during the premarital examination. The couple may want to discuss these matters jointly with the doctor.

Increasingly, physicians are using the premarital examination as an opportunity to give the Papanicolaou (Pap) test, a means of detecting cervical cancer. The greatest value from this procedure does not come from the comparatively rare incidence of cervical cancer in the young age group tested. Rather it can serve as a means of initiating a routine yearly "Pap test" habit. Most states in the United States require that a blood test be performed on prospective marital partners as a precautionary measure against syphilis.

Physical examinations should be routine procedures in preparation for marriage as well as throughout life. The person owes it to himself, to the prospective marital partner, and to the marriage they are establishing to assure as completely as possible full preparation for a lifelong partnership.

ON HAVING CHILDREN

In his earlier days, man viewed his ability to reproduce with a certain amount of anxiety as he struggled against the elements to assure the survival of the human species. He suffered, at that time, losses from high rates of maternal mortality and even higher rates of infant mortality. If a child survived his first year of life, he was then challenged to weather a variety of childhood infections. As child and adult he was exposed to the plague and other epidemic diseases.

With the advent of modern medicine, there has been a significant recession of the epidemic diseases, with their virtual disappearance in more highly developed communities of the world. It is now possible to immunize against many of the childhood diseases. The advances in pediatrics and obstetrics have reduced to all-time lows the infant and maternal mortality rates. Gradually man is becoming preoccupied with problems related to overpopulation. In this context, the tendency to view the creation of life with a disdainful casualness becomes possible. An appreciation of this phenomenon may be enhanced by the realization that man can initiate life, but he cannot create it. Man's role in this process is really no different from that of lower animals.

The motivations of people who desire or do not desire children can be more involved than at first appears. In primitive societies, a great premium was placed on having children to perpetuate the race, and establish a large work force. It was also recognized that the children would later care for the parents in their declining years. The child became an almost necessary form of old age insurance. In our more sophisticated society, which boasts medicare and varied retirement income plans, the child no longer serves this function. The decision therefore to have children can to a greater extent be based on a couple's desire to have them or not.

The bases of such a decision could include religious beliefs and whether or not the parents feel physically, psychologically, and financially capable of taking care of a child. They should have enough love and energy to share not only with each other but with a new baby as well. An interesting point was made in a study done at the University of Pennsylvania, where sociologists found that children raised in large families very rarely followed that pattern. In fact they tended to have small families—smaller than average. Therefore the size of the family from which the individual comes may be the determining factor in the projected size of his family.

A complicating factor in deciding to have children is that many people grow up with the idea that they *must* have children, or that they are not very wholesome people if they avoid parenthood. The influence of religion can be felt on this issue. Some religious organizations strongly encourage parenthood. In those cases where religious belief delimits birth control methods, choice as to parenthood is also delimited, as well as the size of one's family. How effectively *any* birth control measure is used is another factor. When people genuinely do not desire to have children and are forced by a vague sense of morality or obligation into a childbearing situation, we have the basis for a problem. While babies coo and are cute, they are also demanding. They want to be fed, changed, and loved. When these needs are not fulfilled, they cry at all hours of the day or night. The parent who does not really want the child in the first place feels put upon and becomes indignant. The end result is not only a disturbed parent but also an inevitably emotionally disturbed child. The high incidence of child abuse appears to reflect the frustration that a number of parents experience in child caring.

In recent years an organization has evolved that proclaims "None is Fun." The organization seeks to promote child-free marriages and nonparenthood

So You Want to Get Married...

Have you considered:

Values and background

If you are a city girl or boy, could you live in the country or vice versa?

Would you be able to move away from your family?

Is your level of education much higher or lower than your future spouse's?

Do you feel comfortable when you are out with his or her friends or family?

Are your parents and prospective in-laws happily married?

Finances

Are you a pinch-penny or do you like to throw your money around?

Do you think two can live as cheaply as one?

How dependable is your income?

Are you expecting financial help from parents? Do they know it?

If you are both working now, could you make it on only one salary in the future?

Do you think your parents have spent too much time and energy acquiring the material things in life?

Roles in marriage

Do you feel fixing beds, washing dishes and vacuuming is the woman's job?

Who should be the *head of the household?*

Is it worng for the wife to make more money than her husband?

Should the father share in the caring of the baby, i.e., bathing, feeding and changing?

Who should fix the screen door, dig up the garden, paint the kitchen?

Who should attend the Community College's class on income tax preparation?

Personality

Can you make decisions on your own?

Do you seek advice from parents or people in authority?

Are you subject to fits of anger and do you stay moody and sullen for days after an argument?

Can you express affection easily?

When things get rough do you panic or keep you cool?

Are you basically optimistic and feel that things will get better?

Are you considerate in dealing with other people's shortcomings?

Religion

Do you view yourself as ''religious'' as your partner?

If this is to be an interfaith marriage, have you made an effort to understand the differences in religious philosophy?

Do you think your religion is the only *true* religion?

Do you feel you will iron out the religious differences after the wedding?

If this is to be an interfaith marriage, which religious affiliation will the children follow?

Could you change your religious affiliation without alienating your family?

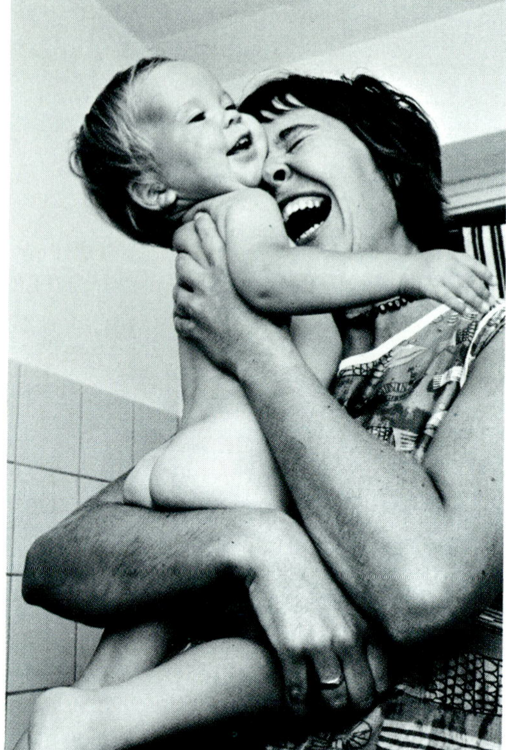

Figure 5–3

While some believe that "none is fun," others obviously disagree.

(Ken Heyman)

for those so inclined. They are rejecting the cultural bias that has made parenthood a requirement of marriage and seek to dispel the idea that non-parents are selfish, shallow, and neurotic. This group parts company with the women liberationists who say: "Yes, have children." "Yes, be a professional." "We must set up day care centers which will care for your children while you are working." The organization for nonparenthood is saying: "No, if I had children *I* would want to provide the environment in which they grow, but since I cannot or will not do that, I choose *not* to have children."

The question of whether a mother should work while her children are quite young or living at home is a common issue. Ideally, children should have a great deal of contact with *both* parents. In a farming economy this was easily accomplished with both parents working at home. As our economy became industrialized, it was the father who went off to work leaving the child-rearing responsibilities largely to the mother. The family role of the father has hereto-fore been minimized. Studies are beginning to show, however, that the absence of the father contributes in his children (particularly sons) a low motivation for achievement, the need for immediate gratification of needs at the expense of long-range benefits, low self-esteem, and an unusual susceptibility to peer group influence. It is being realized that prolonged absence of either parent can be potentially damaging to the child. The issue of how children will fare with one or both parents working will largely depend on how much time the parents spend with their children daily and the *quality* of these parent-child relationships. An interesting comment was made by a working mother to the editor of a magazine expressing her views on liberated women. She said that she was a female who had been liberated all her married life. She had worked through six pregnancies, received a high salary and had always had help to take care of housework and babysitting. She closed with, "What has been the result of all this? My children are grown, and I never really knew them."

The many social changes that have taken place in this country during the last twenty years warrants our reevaluating the role of the family as it concerns bringing up one's children. A number of factors have diminished the opportunities for adults to come in contact with children. The nuclear family no longer has access to grandparents, aunts, and uncles. The working mother rationalizes that a child is better off in a "professional" child care situation. Gone is the apprentice system where a father taught a son his trade. We have followed this up within the home by relegating the children to the "playroom" and leaving them with babysitters while parents "get away from it all." As described by Dr. Urie Bronfenbrenner we are experiencing an age of segregation and

Figure 5–4

The *quality* of parent-child relationships are all-important.

(Susan Johns)

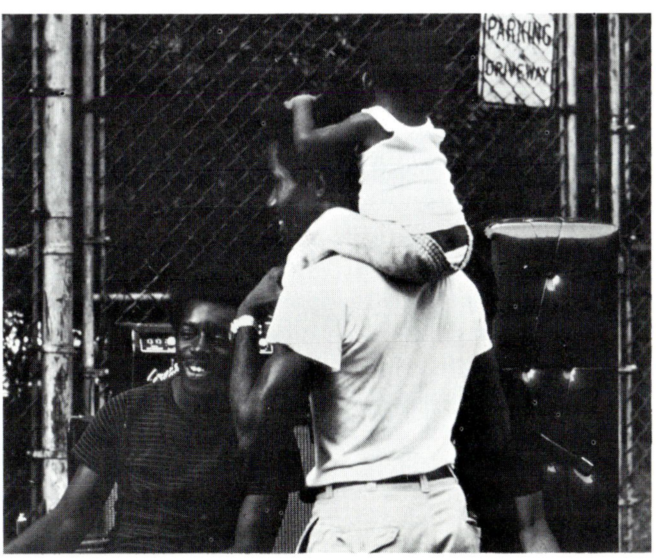

"PEANUTS"
CHARLIE BROWN WILL BE THE DADDY, I'LL BE THE MOMMY AND YOU'LL BE OUR LITTLE GIRL...
NOW, DON'T BOTHER ME! I'M WASHING DISHES!
AND DON'T BOTHER ME! I'M READING THE PAPER!
I QUIT!!
WHY SHOULD I PLAY SOMETHING I HAVE TO GO THROUGH EVERYDAY?!!
7-18
SCHULZ

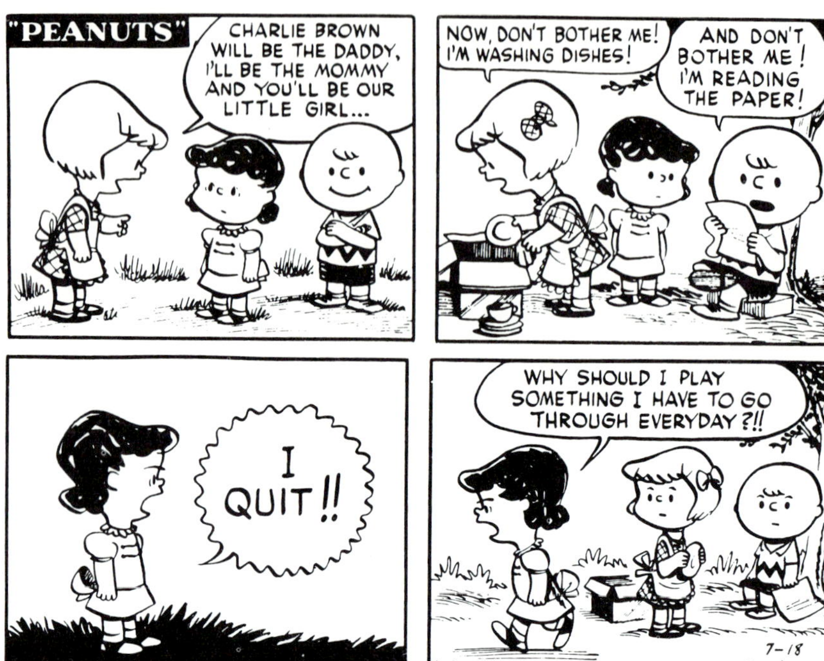

Figure 5–5

Peanuts cartoon by Charles M. Schulz.

must make every effort to "bring adults back into the lives of children and children back into the lives of adults lest we complete the breakdown in the process of making human beings human."[11]

At the risk of sounding ambivalent, we must also emphasize that determining whether one genuinely *desires* children is a difficult assessment to make. In essence, the person is asked to make a judgment in an area where he has no experience. Many a couple initially cool to the idea of parenthood become ecstatic over their firstborn. The creation of another human being in one's own image can obviously have profound effects on the individual. The miracle of birth can bring with it an unmatched humility and a sense of awe that accompanies only human creation.

How completely a person can understand all his motivations in any area is open to question. Unconscious motivations cannot be accounted for by the individual. The unconscious desire to prove manhood or womanhood may, for instance, be the prime mover in parenthood. Although self-understanding

[11] *Today's Health,* June 1972, p. 37.

is never complete, discussion can lead to greater insight into one's own motivations and those of one's partner.

The concept of family planning and contraception too often is interpreted solely as a means of keeping families small or childless. There are many other indications for use of contraception within marriage. These include some medical reasons such as advanced diabetes or cancer. Kidney disease, neurological diseases, and some inherited conditions might require strict use of contraception or even sterilization. For many, the basic purpose *is* to regulate family size and to effect a more judicious spacing of children, particularly since it has been shown that repeated closely spaced pregnancies have a higher incidence of stillbirths and premature births.

Contraception outside of marriage has become a current issue which is being dealt with in several ways. Social agencies concerned with birth control and illegitimacy will advise and prescribe contraceptives to anyone seeking them. Their theme is if you are going to be sexually active, then you must be responsible for the prevention of any births outside of marriage.

There are various devices and methods related to contraception. They can take the form of mechanical devices, chemical substances, or natural methods. No contraceptive method is foolproof, but each helps in producing the desired results. Ideally a contraceptive should be harmless, reliable, free of objectionable side effects, inexpensive, readily reversible, simple to use, and should not interfere with the sexual satisfaction of either partner.

PRENATAL CARE

Modern medicine has made childbirth much safer for both mother and child. A major contribution to this accomplishment has been better prenatal care. While pegnancy is a natural process, hazards related to it are minimized when this period is supervised by the obstetrician. The expectant mother will usually see the physician once a month during the early months of pregnancy. The visits are increased to every two weeks in the latter stages. The physician will take a medical history to evaluate the woman's capability to handle the stresses and strains of pregnancy. He will also give a complete physical examination including the pelvic region. He checks the size of the pelvis to make sure it will permit the passage of a normal-sized child at birth. The physician will routinely check the weight of the expectant mother as well as chart the rate of growth of the unborn child. Weight control during pregnancy is desirable. The common old wives' tale that a pregnant woman needs to eat for two can serve as a bit of misleading information resulting in undesirable, if not dangerous, weight gain.

The need for a well-balanced, nutritious diet is important to the expectant mother. The child will draw from the tissues of the mother for its growth.

Where inadequate diets are followed, it is the mother who will suffer the deficiency, not the unborn child.

Urinalyses serve to check that the pregnancy is progressing routinely. During this period, the kidneys are under the double strain of excreting wastes for both the mother and child.

There are few organisms that can pass from the mother's body through the placenta to the child. However, a few disease-producing bacteria and a number of viruses can. Rubella (German measles, or three-day measles), while not dangerous to the adult, can cause harmful effects to the fetus in its first trimester. Fetal death, mental retardation, cataracts, and deafness are among its varied effects. Since a vaccine for rubella has been developed (see Chapter 3), it is hoped that routine vaccination of children will eradicate this disease and thus avoid a variety of serious defects. The mumps and other viral diseases can also affect the fetus. When expectant mothers are exposed to viral diseases to which they may not be immune the physician may recommend injections of gamma globulin. Gamma globulin is a derivative of human blood that contains antibodies and will give the person a temporary immunity that serves to protect the fetus. It is wise for the expectant mother to avoid people with various infections as a precautionary measure. We cannot discount the fact that our information in this area is incomplete. The number of diseases that can affect the early pregnancy is not known at this time.

Part of the prenatal care involves informing the mother about the various changes that will take place during the pregnancy. This is particularly important for those who have not had children before.

The use of drugs needs to be handled more cautiously at this time. The thalidomide* drug disaster resulted in the birth of thousands of deformed babies in Europe. This demonstrated with resounding impact that a normally harmless drug can be dangerous during pregnancy. Even the use of nonprescription drugs should be checked with the physician. The current inappropriate use of sleeping pills, pep pills, alkalines, tonics, and alcohol singly or, worse yet, in combination, can be threats to the unborn child as well as the prospective mother.

It has also been noted that those children who are X-rayed in utero have a higher incidence of leukemia later in life. For this reason it is wise for a woman to inform a physician other than her obstetrician of her pregnancy.

Tooth decay is another possible source of difficulty that should be corrected preferably before pregnancy. Tooth decay is in essence an infection and its elimination deletes any possible toxic effects on the child from this source.

The maintenance of good muscle tone is always desirable, but it becomes particularly important during childbirth. Strong abdominal and back muscles will not only make a pregnancy more comfortable for the expectant mother

* Thalidomide was a drug prescribed for women to curb their nausea during early pregnancy. The drug was used primarily in Europe. The FDA had not approved the use of the drug in the United States.

but will also play a significant role in the birth process itself. The woman who has always exercised regularly is better prepared for the function of childbirth.

BREAST FEEDING

The question of whether or not to breast-feed the newborn is a decision each mother must make. Attitudes toward breast feeding are often consciously or unconsciously developed fairly early in life. The woman is often faced with the decision without having given it much prior thought. Some advantages of breast feeding are found in the development of a closer child-parent relationship. Mother's milk is also rarely one that does not agree with the baby. Allergy and other feeding problems have greater incidence with formula-fed babies. Some women prefer this method of feeding because it does away with nipples, bottles, sterilizers, and so forth. It is also cheaper, which is a factor in some families. Several studies have also shown that the incidence of breast cancer is lower among women who breast-feed their young. There has, however, been a growing tendency away from the breast-fed child in our society. Some mothers are repelled by the whole idea and see only animal-like qualities in the process. There is also the fact that where babies are bottle-fed the father can give the 2 A.M. feeding as well as the mother. The decision as to how to feed the newborn is dependent to a great extent on the psychological preparation of the mother for this function and what are perceived to be the advantages and disadvantages of either method.

THE RH FACTOR

This factor is an inherited protein substance found in the red blood cells. Approximately 85 per cent of white people have this protein material and are therefore designated as being Rh+. The other 15 per cent are described as being Rh−. Approximately 93 per cent of blacks are Rh+, and the factor is even higher among Asians. The Rh symbol was given to this blood protein because it was first detected in the rhesus monkey.

The Rh factor has caused some concern because under certain circumstances it can be responsible for such conditions as mental retardation, cerebral palsy, and spontaneous abortion. These developments are possible only when the mother is Rh− and the father is Rh+, and the fetus is Rh+. Not every pregnancy of this type is necessarily affected. In order for there to be a reaction, some of the Rh+ blood of the fetus must leak through the placenta to the mother's bloodstream. The mother's blood in reaction to the blood of the

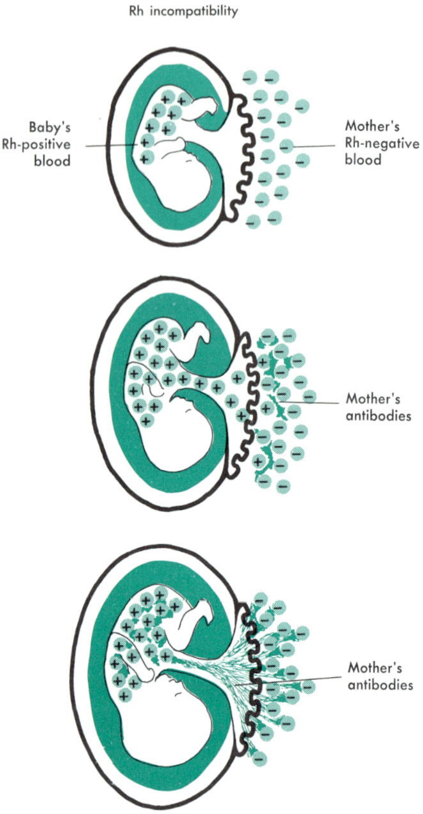

Figure 5–6

As diagrammed, some of the RH+ blood of the child leaks through the placenta to the RH− blood of the mother. The mother's blood reacts by developing antibodies that return to the baby's bloodstream and destroy some of his red blood cells. If enough antibodies reach the child, anemia of varying severity will result.

(Adapted from René Dubos, Health and Disease, *Life Science Library*, 1965)

fetus will develop antibodies. The quantity of antibodies developed is in proportion to the amount of fetus blood that leaks into the mother's bloodstream. In large enough quantities, these antibodies could begin to destroy the red blood cells of the fetus, resulting in anemia, a jaundiced condition, or even death. The first such pregnancy will probably produce no reactions. It may take several pregnancies before the mother's blood has been sensitized enough to produce sufficient antibodies to affect the child. Up until now, when the obstetrician had a case with an Rh− mother and an Rh+ father, he would periodically check the mother's blood for antibody level. If necessary, the child's blood was replaced by an exchange transfusion immediately after birth, or the child was delivered prematurely in order to save its life. Newer medical techniques now enable the physician to give the baby a blood transfusion while it is still in the womb.

Early in 1968 a new *preventive* treatment was developed. A vaccine, called anti-Rh immune globulin, is administered to an Rh− mother within three days after the delivery of an Rh+ baby. In the mother, this blocks the development of a sensitization against the baby's Rh+ red blood cells that entered her circulation. This protection lasts long enough for the baby's blood cells circulating in her body to wear out and disappear. The mother whose blood has already been sensitized against the Rh factor by previous pregnancies or blood transfusions may not benefit from this new preventive measure. It is therefore important for the girl with Rh− blood never to receive blood transfusions with Rh+ blood and for her to receive anti-Rh immune globulin within the first three days following the delivery of an Rh+ baby, miscarriage, or abortion. This process will be repeated after each pregnancy involving an Rh+ baby. Since the use of the vaccine has been so nearly 100 per cent effective, parents with an Rh incompatability can look forward to having additional children safely.

CHILDBIRTH

Childbirth starts with the onset of labor, the somewhat rhythmic contractions of the uterus. During the pregnancy, the muscle cells of the uterus increase in number and size in preparation for the birth process. Labor can be subdivided into three stages. The first and longest stage starts with the first uterine contraction and ends with the complete dilation of the cervix of the uterus. The second stage starts at this point and terminates with the birth of the child. The third stage extends from the birth of the child to the expulsion of the afterbirth (placenta) and the final contraction of the uterus.

The amniotic sac ("bag of waters") which surrounds the child in the uterus and is filled with fluid will often break during the first or second stage of labor. This occurs in response to the increased pressures created by the contracting uterus. The breaking of this sac is usually a signal for the expectant mother to get to the hospital if she is not already there. The amount of fluid released is anywhere from a cupful to a quart. Increased uterine contractions usually follow the "breaking of the water." Obstetricians will sometimes break the amniotic sac in order to induce greater uterine activity.

When an expectant mother arrives at the hospital during this first stage of labor, a number of routine procedures are performed. Her contractions are timed, the baby's heartbeat is recorded, and body temperature is taken. Preparation is then made for delivery. For hygienic reasons, the pubic hair is shaved and an enema containing antiseptic fluid is given to clean out the lower bowel.

The obstetrician can then check the progress by a vaginal examination to determine the extent of dilation of the cervix. When the cervix is completely dilated, the second stage has begun. Contractions become quite strong and are assisted by abdominal muscles when the mother bears down with each contraction. She is guided in this process by nurses encouraging her to bear down at the proper times. It is particularly important that the mother be prepared for this part of the birth process so that she knows what to expect and what is expected of her. The most difficult time comes when the baby's head reaches the muscles surrounding the vaginal opening. If the physician deems it necessary, in order to prevent the tearing of these tissues, he may perform an episiotomy. This is a small incision made at the bottom of the vaginal wall, usually at an angle to the side rather than straight down. This type of incision heals fairly quickly and functions to facilitate the birth. Once the head of the child is cleared, the body follows rather quickly. The baby at this point is still attached by its umbilical cord to the placenta (afterbirth) in the mother. Two clamps are placed on the umbilical cord and the cord is then cut between them. Upon being born, the child is held by its heels to help drain out any fluids that it may have in its mouth and throat. The child usually cries and inflates its lungs for the first time and begins to take care of its respiratory needs. The stump of the umbilical cord that remains ultimately dries up and drops off, leaving the navel or umbilicus as its mark of birth. The baby is cleaned and an identification bracelet is usually placed on it. It will also have a 1 per cent solution of silver nitrate placed in its eyes to avoid possible infection.

In the third stage of labor there is the expulsion of the placenta from the uterus. This takes place within fifteen or twenty minutes after the birth by contractions of the uterus or at times by pressure applied by the physician.

Caesarean Section

Birth by Caesarean section is the surgical removal of the baby from the uterus. This is not the preferred manner of birth and is used when, for one reason or another, normal delivery through the birth canal is not possible or advisable. This method is employed when the child is too large to pass through the pelvic opening of the mother. In other cases, the mother with a heart, lung, or kidney condition may be a poor candidate for the vigorous second stage of labor, which is physically demanding.

The Breech Birth

Normally, the child in the birth process moves down the birth canal head first. In about 4 per cent of the cases, there is a breech presentation with the baby's buttocks, shoulders, or feet appearing first. These deliveries are invariably more difficult and sometimes more hazardous to the child. The experienced obstetrician, however, can effectively deal with the situation.

Natural Childbirth

In recent years, there has been a great deal of discussion about natural childbirth. The aim of this method is to effect the birth of the child without the use of drugs. The woman is prepared for this event by following a regimen of exercise, good health practices, and by psychologically preparing herself.

The latter is accomplished by increasing her understanding and acceptance of childbirth, thereby eliminating tension and fear.

There is great variation in the way drugs may be used in childbirth, ranging from general anesthesia to the injection of drugs to make specific parts of the body insensitive. Some advocates of natural childbirth have displayed a missionary zeal and feel that *all* childbirth should be drug-free. Obstetricians generally feel that this is an irresponsible attitude. The decision of whether to use a drug, when, what kind, and how, should be that of the trained obstetrician. Many women suited for natural childbirth physically and psychologically report great exultation in experiencing childbirth. Herein lies the contribution made by this method and its advocates. It has tended to blunt the stories of horror about childbirth told by those who would enshrine themselves in martyrdom. Somewhere in between these two extreme sweeps of the pendulum lies the average woman's thinking. She is inviting neither unwholesome fear of childbirth nor adolescent enthusiasm. When a woman feels that the fewer drugs used the better, an obstetrician can be found to be guided by the principle. A competent physician, however, does not want his actions dictated before the fact. When circumstances demand that drugs or other actions be taken to save child and/or mother, he does not want to have his hands tied by misplaced enthusiasms.

THE PREMATURE CHILD

A child that is born before 36 weeks after conception is regarded to be premature, 40 weeks being considered full term (slightly more than 9 months). Another criterion for determining prematurity is that of weight. Any child born weighing less than 5 lbs. 8 oz. is classified as premature. The closer to full term the fetus is, the bigger and more highly developed will be its organs and body systems. Its chances for survival, therefore, are proportionately increased.

Those born within the 32- to 36-week period will usually weigh from 3½ to 4 pounds. The infant will be weak, but can manage to cry for its food when hungry. Careful supervision and nursing care are needed if the baby is to live. When birth occurs 28 to 32 weeks after conception the fetal infant will weigh about two pounds. An infant of this size and maturity would require constant medical supervision for survival, because it cannot nurse and has particular difficulty maintaining a constant body temperature. A fetal infant born sooner than 28 weeks after conception is not given any chance for survival.

One of the several handicaps that the premature child must overcome is the difficulty of regulating body temperature. This difficulty results from the large body surface in proportion to its weight, a lack of insulating fat, and an incompletely developed sweating mechanism. The nutritional needs of a normally rapid growing fetus are high. Yet its sucking and swallowing reflexes are weak or absent, and the ability of its digestive tract to handle and absorb foods is often lacking. The premature are also more vulnerable to infectious diseases.

The greatest problem the premature baby will encounter, however, is the respiratory difficulty caused by hyaline membrane disease (HMD). When babies are born, the inner surface of the lungs contain a surfactant which lubricates these surfaces. After one breath is forced out, this surfactant allows the lungs to expand again to let the next breath in. Premature babies born with hyaline membrane disease are born *without* this surfactant or lubricating device. Their lungs do not inflate enough, and a struggle for oxygen develops. If the baby lives for three days, he will usually begin to produce surfactant and may survive. The problem, then, has been to prevent brain damage from oxygen deprivation in those first critical days. New medical approaches are now being used to produce a higher survival rate for the baby with hyaline membrane disease.

More than half of the neonatal deaths (within a month after birth) are due to prematurity. Some of the causes of prematurity revolve around the mother, with injury, malnutrition, infectious disease (tuberculosis, syphilis), cardiac or diabetic disorders, and toxemia with multiple pregnancy as the most common. Those causes that are related more closely to the child include malformation of the fetus, premature separation of the placenta, Rh factor difficulties, as well as a large group of undiagnosed causes. It must be noted that a number of the factors causing premature births are also related to the incidence of stillbirth (birth of a dead child). Prevention of prematurity is considered the basic research aim. In the meantime, good prenatal care properly utilizing medical information already known is the best guarantee of a healthy child.

ABORTION

Man has struggled for centuries with the complex multifaceted social, medical, legal, and moral problems related to abortion. In recent years there has been a great deal of public discussion centered on these issues. The more recent discussions do not differ to any great extent from the following discussion that took place between two physicians in another century. "About the terminating of a pregnancy, I want your opinion. The father was syphilitic. The mother tuberculous. Of the four children born, the first was blind, the second died, the third was deaf and dumb, the fourth also tuberculous. What would you have done?" "I would have ended the pregnancy." "Then you would have murdered Beethoven."[12]

[12] Norman St. John Stevas, *The Right to Life* (New York: Holt, Rinehart & Winston, 1964), p. 16.

Abortion refers to the separation of the fetus from the uterus during its first twenty-eight weeks of prenatal life. After the twenty-eighth week it is termed a premature birth. When this occurrence is precipitated by natural causes, it is referred to as a *spontaneous abortion.* The term "miscarriage" is often used in referring to this kind of abortion. It is believed that the improper implantation of the fertilized egg, hormonal imbalance, or imperfections in the fetus are the primary causes of the occurrence. In the 1940s and early 50s, obstetricians in an attempt to correct the hormonal imbalance administered (estrogenic) hormones to women with histories of spontaneous abortion. Recently, however, a warning to discontinue the use of synthetic hormones during pregnancy has been circulated because of the possible link to vaginal cancer in the female offspring born to women so treated. The mother often relates the spontaneous abortion to a fall, a bumpy ride, or similar incident. However, these are considered to be at most secondary causes. Most spontaneous abortions occur in the first three months of pregnancy.

A *therapeutic abortion* is one that is induced by a physician. There are several methods that have been widely used by physicians because of their practicality and safeness. The criterion for the choice of method is usually the length of the pregnancy. Prior to twelve weeks of pregnancy a dilatation and curettage (more commonly known as a D & C) is the preferred method. Under local anesthesia the cervix of the uterus is dilated, and with the use of an instrument called a curette the lining of the uterus is scraped free of all embryonic material. A variation on the D & C is the vacuum aspiration technique. The cervix is dilated and a small tube that is attached to a vacuum pump is inserted into the uterus. The fetal matter is drawn off in this manner. It has been determined from initial studies in New York with therapeutic abortions, that 77 per cent were done either by a D & C or a suction curette. If the pregnancy has continued to the 16th through 24th week the amniotic fluid is drawn from the amniotic sac and a saline (salt) solution is substituted for it. This foreign solution kills the fetus. Within 24 to 72 hours a miniature labor begins until the fetus is expelled. When sterilization of the mother is indicated in addition to a therapeutic abortion, physicians may remove the pregnancy by hysterectomy, which is the removal of the entire uterus. This is, however, rarely done.

The Legal Aspects of Abortion

The legislative developments relative to abortion laws in the United States during recent years have been nothing short of revolutionary. Although women have sought and found abortion since the beginning of time, it is only now in this period of rapid social change that we have shed the Victorian cloak of silence to witness the pendulum swinging full arc to "abortion-on-demand!"

In 1973 the United States Supreme Court handed down a precedent-setting decision on abortion. The decision in effect legalized abortions desired by the mother and recommended by a physician during the first trimester of pregnancy.

The state may regulate abortion procedures after the first trimester to the extent that the procedures relate to the preservation and protection of maternal health. The court saw the state interest in potential life during the last ten weeks of pregnancy when the fetus could survive outside the womb. Four states, Alaska, Hawaii, New York, and Washington were not affected by the Supreme Court decision. Fifteen states had to rewrite their existing abortion laws in accordance with the court decision, whereas the rest of the states found their antiabortion laws invalidated by the new federal law and had to write new laws.

The Morality of Abortion

The liberalization of the abortion laws is not a complete answer to this dilemma. There are those who feel that an abortion results in the destruction of a human life. A very real moral issue needs, then, to be dealt with. There is also a difference of opinion at what point the destruction of the unborn is morally right or wrong. Some feel abortions can be permitted before the fetus resembles a child and others feel it is permissible before the mother feels movement of the fetus (quickening). Another point of view is that the abortion should not take place after the time when the child would live if it were born at that moment. This usually refers to a seven-month-old fetus or older. Others feel that life begins at birth and the destruction of the unborn child at any time before that is capable of moral justification. Then there are those who state that a woman cannot be half pregnant. She is either pregnant or she is not. If she is pregnant, then she is bearing a life. The destruction of that life, this group feels, is as morally wrong as the murder of an older person. Birth is only the separation of one phase of development of a human being from another. Each individual, then, needs to develop values upon which to base his thinking on this issue.

The reasons why abortions may be sought must be considered in this decision. A pregnancy that results from rape or incest is a case in point. Should a woman who has been violated suffer the further indignity of bearing the child? There are responses to this query to the effect that you cannot correct one crime by performing another. Yet, is it not criminal to expect a woman to bear a child she cannot love? It is not the intent of the author to confuse the reader, but merely to indicate the complexities involved in the issues. The woman who contracted German measles during her first trimester of pregnancy has a similar decision to make. This unfortunate occurrence means that her unborn child has a significantly increased chance of being born with a deformity. Many women would seek an abortion on these grounds. Yet, there is a chance that the abortion would result in the destruction of a normal child. The decisions here do not come easily.

Many public health experts point out that we have exerted great efforts to reduce infant mortality. There have been the development of vaccines for diphtheria, tetanus, poliomyelitis, whooping cough, measles, and improvements in nutrition, prenatal care, obstetrics, and other areas. At the same time, estimates indicate that over a million fetal lives are lost in abortions. The two facts stand in contradiction to each other. The more effective use of known birth control methods, it is felt, could make a preventive contribution to this problem.

Many a hospital nurse who has been trained morally and professionally to preserve life is revolted at having to discard a human being in development like so much refuse. On the other hand, there are those who accept abortion with a disdainful casualness, and a callousness inconsistent with humaneness. At best, abortion should be regarded as a distasteful correction for a situation that in most instances should not have occurred in the first place. If abortion is accepted as a primary birth control method, or an unqualified adult right, some fear that it may serve as the basis of a greater problem than those it is seeking to correct. Abortion should therefore be used as a reluctant last resort.

SOME ASPECTS OF INFERTILITY

While many young married couples are preoccupied with keeping the size of their families small, there are about 15 to 20 per cent of married couples who are faced with the possibility of never having children born to them. The reasons for infertility vary and are equally shared by either the husband or the wife. In the male the numbers of sperm produced may not be sufficient, the amount of seminal fluid may be scant, there may be an obstruction somewhere in the pathway from the testes to the end of the penis, or there may be some difficulty in maintaining an erection. In the female the infertility may arise from the ovaries not producing mature ova, or a malformed uterus that is not responding to the hormones in the bloodstream. There sometimes occurs, as a result of infection or disease, a blockage of the fallopian tube so that the egg cannot pass through. In addition, the vaginal environment may sometimes be overly hostile to the sperm. Through medical detection once the problem is identified in either or both partners, therapy can begin. It is estimated that $\frac{1}{3}$ to $\frac{1}{2}$ of infertile or subfertile couples can be helped to have children by either surgical or medical means.

The therapy most people are aware of is artificial insemination (AI). This is the process of transferring sperm-filled seminal fluid from the male to the female by artificial means. If the male whose sperm is used is the husband, then the process is called AIH (Artificial Insemination–Husband). If a donor other than the husband is used, as in cases where the husband is irreversibly sterile or carrying an undesirable genetic trait, then the process is termed AID (Artificial Insemination–Donor). Couples may choose artificial insemination as a more desirable alternative to a childless marriage or to the adoption of a child.

GENETIC COUNSELING

There was a time when being a "carrier" meant that a person was harboring a dread communicable disease. In these days of greater sophistication, the term can now mean that the person is a carrier of a defective gene. Such a person could have offspring with a genetic disease, i.e., Down's syndrome, sickle-cell anemia, Tay-Sachs disease.

The worst genetic mistakes are usually aborted early during pergnancy, sometimes before the mother even knows she is pregnant. Nature's correction of its own mistakes, however, is not foolproof, and genetic mishaps do occur. Many persons are unaware that they are carrying defective genes until they have a child born to them with a genetic disease. Where there is such a family history, genetic counseling can offer a couple some hope for the future. Through genetic examinations of both parents, physicians can indicate what the risks are of having an abnormal baby. Some alternatives available to a couple running a high risk of producing a defective child may well be to remain childless, adoption, or artificial insemination.

As a result of a medical technique called *amniocentesis,* physicians can now for a number of diseases accurately predict whether the fetus is the victim of a genetic disease. This involves microscopic examination of the chemical composition of the amniotic fluid or the cells found in the amniotic fluid surrounding the fetus. Ideally the fluid sample is drawn during the 14th to 18th week of pregnancy and will clearly detect over 70 genetic faults. A family alerted through an amniocentesis that they will bear a hopelessly defective child may either seek an abortion or carry the child to full term and care for it as best they can. In some instances, techniques have been developed to aid the fetus in spite of his genetic weakness. The physician thus alerted to the problem may act to correct it or minimize its effects. In counseling parents, only information is given. All decisions on planning or terminating a pregnancy are left to them.

One problem in developing genetic disease prevention programs is the difficulty in identifying high-risk pregnancies. For example, if amniocentesis would be performed in all women over 35 years of age who became pregnant, the estimates are that the rate of occurrence of Down's syndrome (mongolism) would be cut in half. When a woman has already borne a child with a genetic disease, we have a second justification for amniocentesis in future pregnancies.

It has been suggested that if prenatal diagnosis and selective abortions were coupled with screening programs to find carriers of genetic diseases, very significant reductions could be effected in these diseases. If the screening program discovered those families where *both* parents were carriers, the monitoring of all their pregnancies would result in the detection of many cases of genetic disease. It would then be possible to offer selective abortion for

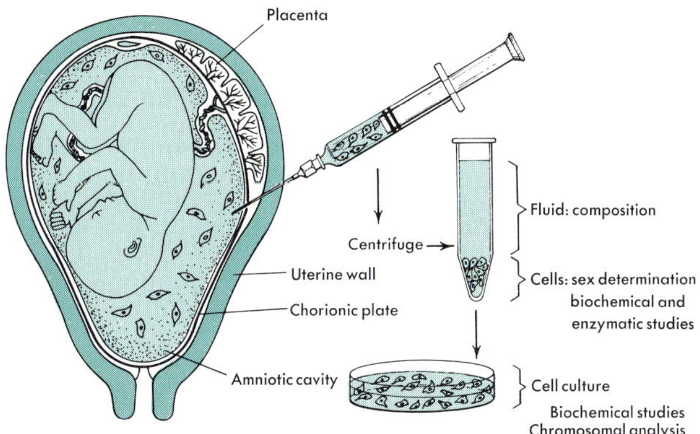

Figure 5–7

Diagram of aminiocentesis.

those fetuses affected. Since it is estimated that it costs $250,000 to care for each infant born with Down's syndrome, it would be *economically* feasible to conduct such a program of detection and prevention. The greater issue that surfaces here goes well beyond the economics of things. Man is entering an era where he can control the quality of life born to him. It is time to review the ethics upon which such profound determinations are to be made.

REVIEW QUESTIONS

1. What are the influences of the culture on concepts related to masculinity and feminity?
2. What changes have taken place with regard to the role of women in our society? What are the implications of these changes for the men and their concepts of masculinity?
3. What constitute some of the wrong reasons for sexual involvement? Why do they fail to serve the individual properly?
4. Why do many consider sex to be in the most desirable context when it is part of a love relationship?
5. What will probably be some of the outcomes of the feminist movement?
6. How have societal attitudes toward masturbation been changing? What kinds of concerns are *now* expressed with regard to this practice?
7. What can be the varied motivations for petting? Why is it important to recognize the nature of these motivations in oneself as well as one's partner?

8 Distinguish between premarital and nonmarital sexual intercourse.

9 How do premarital relations complicate the breaking off of a relationship, should this decision be reached?

10 The terms *homosexuality* and *heterosexuality* should not be viewed as absolutes. Explain.

11 Why is maturity an essential quality for a successful marriage?

12 What are some of the negative motivations for marriage? Why are they poorly based?

13 Love has been defined in many ways. How do you interpret the term?

14 How has the greater equality of the sexes in our society created some conflicts in the marital roles of the husband and wife?

15 Discuss the importance of an economically stable marriage.

16 Why should religious viewpoints be discussed before marriage even if both parties are members of the same religion?

17 What are the potential problems that need careful discussion by a couple contemplating an interfaith marriage?

18 What are the advantages of an informal engagement period before the declaration of a formal engagement?

19 What are the purposes served by the engagement period?

20 Describe the functions served by the premarital physical examination.

21 How have changes in our society affected attitudes related to having children.

22 What factors must a couple consider in deciding upon parenthood?

23 How significant is the role of the father in successful child rearing?

24 "Man can initiate life, but he cannot create it." Explain.

25 Abortion should not serve as a birth control measure. Explain.

26 How has good prenatal care made childbirth safer for mother and child?

27 What are the major factors to be considered in determining if the baby will be breast-fed or bottle-fed?

28 Describe the three stages of labor in childbirth.

29 Define: (1) Caesarean section, (2) breech birth, (3) natural childbirth, (4) premature child, (5) abortion.

30 What are some of the measures that can be taken to prevent the birth of the premature child?

31 What are the medical, social, and moral issues in the discussion about liberalizing abortion laws in the country?

32 How can amniocentesis prove helpful in the area of genetic counseling?

6. Health & the Consumer

A PERSON BECOMES a health consumer when he first buys a product or service related to his health. In a competitive society it seems inevitable that commercial companies would attempt to *oversell* their health products and services and the financial health of the company sometimes is deemed more important than the health of the consumer. In addition, there are those who sell worthless products and services that prove to be harmful or at the very best a waste of money. How can the consumer protect himself and his resources from those who would exploit him? What are the responsibilities of government in the protection of the consumer? If we are not to lose our money or our health by our own ignorance, then we must be prepared to be wise health consumers.

QUACKERY: A PRODUCT OF AN UNINFORMED PUBLIC

The judgment of the American as a consumer of health products and services is extremely poor. The National Health Test given by CBS television in 1966 confirmed this with test results indicating that basic health knowledge was generally inadequate in this country. A study conducted by the Food and Drug Administration in 1972 confirmed that Americans have some strange ideas about maintaining their health. They expect vitamins to give them added energy and even prevent cancer and arthritis. Many carry on self-medication based on ignorance. There is a lack of health education either as courses of study in our schools or as part of public education programs which has resulted in a woefully uninformed American. This fact, coupled with the misrepresentation of health products and services, has created the most lucrative con game in this country. It has now reached such proportions that it is causing concern and alarm among physicians and other health professionals. An amount of $250 million a year is spent on quack devices for arthritis alone and this is just a small part of the "market."

Research has not provided medical science with treatment that will result in the complete cure of all cases of arthritis. Medical treatment in its present stage can, however, relieve pain associated with the condition and prevent a great deal of crippling, particularly where arthritis cases are treated early.

Because arthritis is a painful condition and a complete cure is not available, many arthritics reach out for the "miracle" cures offered by the quack. It has been found that 14 out of 100 arthritics have been sold vibrating devices that are either useless or harmful, as well as glorified aspirin at extremely high prices. Arthritis often follows an unpredictable course. There are times when no pain is felt and it appears the disease has gone away. This is called a remission. Just as mysteriously as the pain went away, so it will return. Such remissions and recurrences are typical of the disease. When a remission follows the use of a fake product, the arthritic is misled into thinking that he has found an effective treatment.

Fraudulent practices in the area of cancer "cures" are also many and varied. The delays they cause in reaching legitimate treatment often make the difference between life and death. When the person with a terminal case of cancer seeks out the quack, the only thing that disappears is his money.

Probably the oldest form of cancer "treatment" is the use of a salve or similar concoction that is supposed to draw the cancer right out of the body. For the cancers that are deep inside the body, pills or injections are offered by the quack. In this way he tries to imitate modern medical procedures. Some of the pills or injections sold have been found to contain substances that actually speed up cancer growth. Others have been found to contain laxatives. A widely used quack treatment is giving injections of plain water to cancer victims. The fees for the injections are usually several hundred dollars. Other frauds sell "shots" that are supposed to be vaccines. In recent years a number of "cancer curing" diets have also evolved. To add to the fraud, a variety of mechanical devices that give off varied colored lights and make impressive noises have been sold as cure-alls. The fleecing of ailing older people who have limited savings is undoubtedly the cruelest of hoaxes.

How difficult it is to determine what is fraudulent was exemplified by the Krebiozen case. Dr. Andrew Ivy, a well-known physiologist, was scientific adviser for the Krebiozen Research Foundation, producers of the drug Krebio-

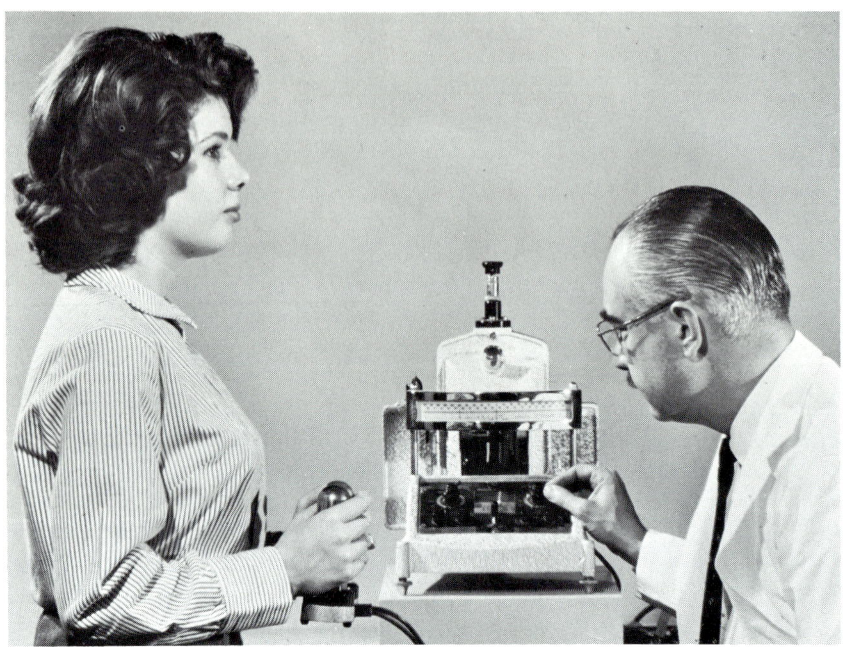

Figure 6–1

A nationwide drive launched by the FDA has resulted in the seizure or voluntary destruction of 1,093 Micro-Dynameter devices to date. This "improved" model was represented as capable of diagnosing cancer, tuberculosis, rheumatism, nephritis, etc. During a court trial, evidence was introduced which showed that the Micro-Dynameter was incapable of distinguishing between a cadaver and a living body. These devices sold for as much as $875 each. Some are still in use.

(FDA photo)

zen. Claims were made that the drug could cure cancer, resulting in its wide use and sale. Government analysis of the drug showed that Krebiozen contained creatine, a common body substance that had no effect on cancer.

"Doorbell doctors" are busy selling vitamins and mineral supplements and a wide range of devices with flashing lights and ozone-generating mechanisms that promise to cure just about everything. They incorporate in their sales talk professional-sounding terms and are usually quite free in giving medical advice. They are too often successful in selling needless dietary supplements. It is estimated that about 50,000 such salesmen prey upon the American public with misleading information and needless products.

The sales of so-called health foods have been increasing. Examples of these are yogurt, which has the same nutritional value as milk, or blackstrap molasses, which consists of the impurities gathered from the refining process of sugar.

The iodine that is found in kelp tablets is supplied in adequate amounts in natural seafoods and iodized salt. Producers of so-called health foods try to imply that the American food supply does not have the necessary nutrients to keep us healthy. This is obviously not true. Other fraudulent products include air purifiers that are supposed to treat diseases such as tuberculosis, pneumonia, and influenza. "Tired blood" tonics are supposedly sold for iron deficiency anemia, whose symptoms resemble a large number of other conditions. A number of cosmetic preparations have been sold with the promise that they will restore youthful attractiveness.

In addition to the money lost to these practices, the health of many people is being endangered. Fraudulent devices and services often keep a patient from the legitimate, early diagnosis and treatment that would have saved his life had he gone to a doctor in the first place when he did not feel well.

Testimonials represent a basic means of selling nostrums (quack medicines) and services. They are often written by deluded people who were told they had a dread disease and were subsequently "cured" by a quack device or treatment. Such diseases are easy to cure when the person does not really have them in the first place. The person's account of a situation connot be described as being scientifically accurate; he is merely reporting his impressions.

Legitimate health services do not rely on testimonials to justify the worth of their services, but on well-established research procedures and their resultant scientifically accurate findings. Ulcer cures, wrinkle removers, royal jelly (for the restoration of sexual potency), seawater, kidney remedies, high blood pressure treatments, various hormones, and hazardous diabetes treatments are all part of a moneymaking, dangerous business called quackery. It is unfortunate, if not disgraceful, that this problem exists to the extent that it does in our society. We have for too long a period of time tolerated practices that are wasteful and a threat to the health of the American people.

STRETCHING THE TRUTH AND SHRINKING THE CONSUMER DOLLAR

In addition to the outright quackery that we have just discussed, there is a more subtle form of quackery that exists today. It does not take one long to find out that advertisements in television, radio, newspapers, and the magazines make a real attempt to lead the consumer into the practice of self-diagnosis and self-medication. They also seduce the consumer into buying products that are either of questionable value or are downright dangerous to one's health. What of the tobacco industry spokesmen who continue to insist that smoking is safe, or the automobile manfacturers who resist building safer cars? What of the book publishers who produce "health" books when recognized medical authorities denounce the theories these books are based on?

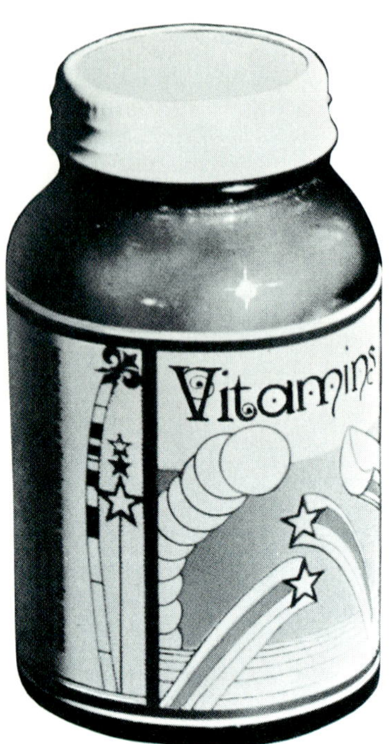

Figure 6–2

It's not a bottle of magic! Over the past decade the fantastic claims that vitamin-mineral pills are going to make you healthier and give you extra energy has turned thousands of consumers into pill poppers. The excessive and indiscriminate use of vitamins could be dangerous.

(*FDA Consumer,* December 1973–January 1974)

The mass media have been quite successful in selling the public on the habitual use of unnecessary drugs that take the form of alkalines, laxatives, pain relievers, vitamins, tonics, and so forth. Millions of dollars a year are spent in this country on drugs that advertisers are leading people into using excessively and indiscriminately. It is time that we asked why this kind of situation exists? What of the drug industry? Does it not have a responsibility not only to label its product properly but to advertise it honestly as well?

Let us take a look at some of the malpractices. A mouthwash advertisement implies that the product will help prevent the common cold by destroying the bacteria found in the mouth. The fact is that the common cold is *not* caused by *bacteria* but by viruses.

One gargle product is advertised as being effective for the treatment of sore throats and bleeding gums. The ineffective treatment of a sore throat caused by a streptococcal infection could delay legitimate treatment and possibly result in the development of nephritis or rheumatic heart disease.

Aspirin is sold under various brand names as well as guises. In some cases it is buffered; in others caffeine and phenacetin are added. False claims with regard to its speed of absorption by the body or its pain-relieving effectiveness are then made. Adding other substances has a doubtful effect on the performance of the drug. Aspirin is aspirin! Then to make it still worse the prices are raised.

Many eyewashes are advertised as relievers of that "tired eye feeling." They also imply that the eye should be cleansed periodically for further relief. The eyes do not need to be cleansed any more than the digestive tract does. Human tears, the fluid layer that covers the eye, not only soothe it best, but also have mild antiseptic qualities as well. Again, should the person experiencing eye discomfort be reaching for an eyewash or finding out what is wrong?

The amount of sound information that reaches the American public is very small compared with the great amount of misinformation they read, hear and see. Radio and television are often sources of misleading and false health information. Books on health topics found on best-seller lists sometimes contain invalid information. The person who relies on his physician for health information finds that he sees him all too seldom or only *after* he becomes ill. Many of our schools add to the problem by omitting from their curricula health instruction that is concerned with the many vital health issues of our society. The school, which should serve as a major source of health information, often fails to do so. It is no wonder that the health consumer is conned into doing or buying some inappropriate things concerning his health.

PRESCRIPTION DRUGS AND THE DRUG INDUSTRY

Few industries, if any, are more useful to society than the ethical drug industry.* Its leaders have emphatically and often stated its concern for the public welfare. In recent years, however, a number of questions have been raised concerning the drug industry that we must examine.

The drug industry has been the most profitable in the United States. Its profits after taxes are about twice the national average for all industries. While it has never been a crime to make money in this country, complaints about drug prices and other practices of the drug companies prompted the late Senator Kefauver and his Senate subcommittee to look into the matter in 1960. One of the factors related to drug price was the manner in which prescription drugs were sold. When a drug is purchased under a brand name, its price is many times higher than if the same drug were bought by its generic name. (The "generic name" refers to the chemical ingredient in the drug. The brand name refers to the name given to a drug by a particular company. Thus several brand name drugs of different companies can all contain the same generic drug.)

Buying a drug by its generic name, however, is not simple. Getting the family physician to prescribe drugs by generic name is not easy. The drug industry campaigns vigorously to get the physician to write brand names on

* The ethical drug industry refers to those manufacturers producing prescription drugs. It does not include drug products sold over the counter (OTC) without a physician's prescription.

prescriptions rather than generic names. A drug is put out in many forms, combinations, and brand names. As a result the busy physician finds it difficult to keep up with them all. He finds it easier to follow the leads given by the drug industry via its medical advertisements and detail men (drug salesmen), and to prescribe the more expensive brand name drug. It is estimated that out of every ten dollars spent on a drug, three dollars goes for pharmaceutical advertisements aimed at physicians.

The American drug industry has claimed that the high cost of drugs is due in great part to research that they conduct. Investigation has shown that most new drugs are developed in other countries or by independent or governmental efforts. Many drug industries find research too costly. Though they do some, they would rather concentrate on marketing a new product or developing variations of it. Very often research is nothing more than copying another company's successful drug, developing new forms of an old drug, and packaging it differently in order to get a "new" drug on the market.

The Senate subcommittee questioned the safety and effectiveness of drugs being marketed. Side effects of drugs were not being properly reported to physicians by the drug industry, and testing procedures of the drug compounds for new drugs were also found faulty.

After thorough Senate committee hearings on the drug industry, the Kefauver-Harris Drug Amendments Act of 1962 was proposed. These amendments seemed to have no chance of adoption by Congress until the news of the thalidomide tragedy broke. Thalidomide was a drug used in Europe to prevent nausea in early pregnancy. The drug, it was found, caused deformed births. Babies were being born without parts of limbs and, in some cases, no limbs at all. Dr. Frances Kelsey of the FDA prevented a major medical tragedy in this country by refusing approval for the sale of this drug in the United States and asking for more testing information on it for further assurance as to its safety. In the interim, the tragic qualities of thalidomide became known. The public demanded stronger drug legislation. Consumers had every reason to hail the passage of the Drug Amendments of 1962 as a major advance in the cause of safe, effective, and honestly promoted drugs.

Senator Kefauver's committee first started the drug industry investigation in an effort to determine why drug prices were so high. While the legislation stimulated by Senator Kefauver and his group resulted in major reforms with regard to insuring drug safety, the part of the bill dealing with drug prices was omitted. Senator Kefauver also wanted to check into the prescription and the over-the-counter drug prices. The committee hearings indicated that a few large drug companies seemed to have undue influence on drug costs. Drug prices in Europe, it found, were well below those in the United States; this included those drugs sold in Europe made by American drug companies. Senator Kefauver's untimely death in the early sixties interrupted his work. In this day of increasing medical care costs, the question of drug prices remains very much at issue.

THE HIGH PRICE OF DRUGS ON THE LEGAL MARKET

"For years the American people have been forced to pay the highest prices for drugs—prices which fall most heavily on those who are least able to afford them—the sick, the poor, and the aged."[1] In hearings held by Senator Nelson, he found that the Eli Lilly Company sold 100 tablets of Darvon to druggists in the United States for $7.02. The same product was sold in Ireland for $1.66 and to pharmacists in England for $1.92. The Ciba Pharmaceutical Company charged druggists $39.50 for 1000 tablets of Serpasil, a drug used to lower blood pressure. The same drug ordered by the U.S. Defense Department under the generic name of Reserpine, cost 60¢ per thousand. Pfizer charged $20.48 for 100 tablets of Terramycin (an antibiotic) in this country, $4.63 in Brazil, and $3.68 in New Zealand.

> One of the most outrageous examples of price gouging is the tranquilizer meprobamate, a widely prescribed drug sold under the trade names of Miltown and Equanil. The holder of the patent on this drug is Carter-Wallace, Inc., a pharmaceutical manufacturer based in New York City. Although this firm sells meprobamate under the trade name, Miltown, it does not and never has produced its own meprobamate either in bulk or in final dosage form. Carter-Wallace buys the bulk material from foreign manufacturers for resale to U.S. manufacturers and for use in the meprobamate tablets it sells under its own name. Carter-Wallace was buying this drug in bulk at 87 cents a pound and selling it to domestic manufacturers at $23.80 a pound, a markup of about 2,600 percent.[2]

Of added interest is the case described in *Consumer Reports* of Osco Drug Inc., a retail chain of 178 pharmacies in 17 states. Osco Drug Inc. took the unprecedented action of posting the prices of prescription drugs in their drugstore windows. "The Illinois Board of Pharmacy began proceedings to suspend the licenses of Osco pharmacists on charges of 'gross immorality.' Rival pharmacists telephoned Osco's director of professional services and called him a 'prostitute' and a 'traitor.' Pharmacy associations spoke out publicly against the Osco program and, in several states, threatened to demand revocation of Osco pharmacy licenses."[3]

The American Pharmaceutical Association has taken the position that the posting of prices of prescription drugs is inconsistent with its code. It denies

[1] *Parade* Magazine, January 21, 1973.

[2] *Congressional Record,* Proceedings and Debates of the 93rd Congress, Omnibus Drug Bill S. 966, February 21, 1973.

[3] "Drug Pricing and the Rx Police State," *Consumer Reports* (March 1972), p. 137.

that its motivation is economic gain and insists that the public health and welfare are its sole concern.

Part of the Osco Drug Company's motivation to post its prices came from a Department of Health, Education, and Welfare report from its Task Force on Prescription Drugs, which stated in part, "If a patient is to maintain the right to select a pharmacy, he also has a right to know the prices it charges and to compare these with other prices."[4]

OTHER ISSUES CONCERNING THE DRUG INDUSTRY

The ethical drug industry has at times been accused of nonethical behavior. Back in 1966 Dr. James L. Goddard, the then newly appointed commissioner of the FDA, spoke bluntly of the drug industry's practice of submitting slipshod data on new drugs to the FDA. He said:

> I have been shocked at the materials that come in. . . . In addition to the problem of quality, there is the problem of dishonesty in the Investigational New Drug stage. . . . I will admit there are gray areas in the IND situation.
>
> But the conscious withholding of unfavorable animal or clinical data is not a gray-area matter.
>
> The deliberate choice of clinical investigators known to be more concerned about industry friendships than in developing good data is not a gray-area matter.
>
> The planting in journals of articles that begin to commercialize what is still an Investigational New Drug is not a gray-area matter.
>
> These actions run counter to the law and the ethics governing the drug industry.[5]

The drug industry's response to the charge was that Dr. Goddard was overemphasizing "isolated instances without acknowledging the integrity and responsibility which our industry has consistently demonstrated."[6]

A few years later a scandal in drug testing which involved prison inmates of several southern states precipitated some legislative actions by Senator Gaylord Nelson of Wisconsin. It seems an enterprising physician, who had no formal education or training in pharmacology, was hired by several drug companies to carry on testing of new drugs. In fact it was estimated that this doctor had made between 25 and 50 per cent of the initial new drug testing in the United States, with little or no medical supervision of the studies. The

[4] Ibid.

[5] Speech before Pharmaceutical Manufacturers Association, 1966.

[6] "Rx for Drug Industry," *New York Times,* April 10, 1966.

National Communicable Disease Center released its extensive investigation of this physician and made known the records attributing an epidemic of viral hepatitis to blood plasma programs that were operated by him in the prisons of Alabama, Arkansas, and Oklahoma. Outraged by this scandal, Senator Nelson proposed legislation to impose more rigorous tests on experimental drugs and to make mandatory that these tests be carried out by the federal government, and *not* by the drug companies. While drug companies would have to pay the costs of federal testing, they would have no jurisdiction over the selection of scientists who were testing their product.

More recently Ralph Nader's Health Research Group developed a report that had some disturbing allegations. It "criticized FDA's practice of allowing drug-company officials free access into FDA offices, and using "consultants" with possible conflicts of interest to perform duties identical to those of line officers."[7] The report continues:

> It is well known to medical officers that drug company officials are constantly in the corridors of FDA, walking into the scientific staff offices expecting immediate attention. The reason for industry's presence in FDA halls is similar to that of detail men in doctor's offices: to persuade doctors to make drug decisions on the basis of factors other than the scientific evidence before the doctor. Drug men's freedom of access to FDA personnel not only contributes to a division backlog, but is a potential danger to the scientific judgment of the medical officers responsible for the safety of the American drug supply.[8]

The great number of drugs marketed by the drug industry continues to add confusion and problems to the scene. At the present time there are some 21,000 drug products on the market. This duplication of drugs exists because of the many brand name drugs that are marketed containing the same generic drug. Dr. Walter Modell one of this country's great pharmacologists has stated,

> Simply because a drug is new, it is not necessarily better than those already available, safer or even just as good. Often, it is even less effective and sometimes more hazardous than the parent drug. But they also do harm by their very existence in the drug market. I take the stand that as a general principle everything that adds to the difficulty in dealing with and understanding drugs also makes drugs more dangerous. Thus, the excessive number of needless drugs constitutes a present danger. We can make the useful drugs both less dangerous and more efficient by weeding out the useless, the ineffective and the duplicates, and by so doing, make it possible for the physician to learn in depth about the potent drugs he will prescribe for his patients. We must add only those new drugs that really add something more than their mere presence.[9]

[7] *U.S. Medicine,* April 15, 1972, 1601 18th Street N.W., Washington D.C. 20009.

[8] Ibid.

[9] *Drug Industry Antitrust Act:* Hearings, Subcommittee on Antitrust and Monopoly; Committee on the Judiciary, 87th Congress, 1st Session; Part I, AMA and Medical Authorities, p. 320.

An added problem is identified by HEW's Task Force on Prescription Drugs.

> Upon entering private practice, the average physician, knowingly or unknowingly, becomes the key figure in drug marketing strategy.
>
> He must choose from a very large number of competitive and often duplicative products.
>
> He must deal with a very large amount of advice, biased or unbiased, from detail men, advertisements, and other forms or promotion.[10]

In order to correct the problems related to drug production, safety, testing, advertising, sales, research, and labeling, Senator Nelson proposed legislation (Omnibus Drug Bill) that would provide the following.

I—Sets up a National Drug Testing and Evaluation Center which will be responsible for the testing of all drugs, both prescription and over-the-counter, that are now or will be marketed in the United States.

II—Provides for the publication of a compendium [a comprehensive summary] which will list all drugs available in the United States by both generic and brand names.

III—Establishes a committee which will compile a formulary of drugs necessary for good medical practice, for purposes of direct procurement by the Federal Government and reimbursement for all Government financed programs, indicating the best drug available for each therapeutic category, in order to assist the physician in his prescribing of medication.

IV—Gives the Secretary of Health, Education and Welfare the authority to require batch-by-batch certification of all drugs—when needed—which will include provisions prescribing standards and identity of strength, quality and purity, tests and methods to determine compliance with such standards, and other measures necessary for the public good.

V—Prohibits the distribution of sample drugs without the written request of the physician.

VI—Is a general section providing that (1) potentially dangerous drugs will be labeled with the appropriate warning; (2) labeling of drugs will be required so that all active ingredients will be clearly labeled; (3) no drug salesman shall make any oral presentation regarding any drug until he has placed before the physician or pharmacist an FDA approved document about the drug; and (4) the Secretary of HEW shall approve all advertising in advance that appears in either the electronic media, or in any publication or advertising circular, for any drug. The Secretary will approve only advertising which does not mislead or misrepresent the product, either in text or layout.

[10] *Congressional Record,* Proceedings and Debates of the 92nd Congress, Vol. 117, No. 166. November 4, 1971.

VII—Is designed to protect the American public against excessively high and discriminatory prices for drugs through mandatory licensing of drug patents at a reasonable royalty.[11]

Needed reform is always difficult to achieve. There are those who have vested interests, while the uninformed and the complacent are always ready to make their peculiar contributions. There is considerable doubt whether the Kefauver-Harris Drug Amendments would have become law without the "help" of the tragic thalidomide incident in Europe.

In 1937, when the sulfanilamide drugs were first introduced, a chemist at the suggestion of a salesman tried to put the drug out in liquid form. He used diethylene glycol as a solvent, which proved to be deadly and killed 108 people. A few simple tests would have proven the toxicity of the compound. The law at that time did not require even these kinds of simple testing procedures. An outraged public moved its representatives to put into effect the Federal Food, Drug and Cosmetic Act of 1938. It is disquieting to realize that a supposedly sophisticated society such as ours still relies on tragedy and disaster as a stimulant for progress. How long can we afford to do so?

CONSUMER PROTECTION

Years ago when the marketplace was simple and uncomplicated, when bartering of services and produce was in order, the slogan "Let the buyer beware!" was the only protection one had. It was the individual's responsibility to make a good bargain. Today, the individual has less and less control over matters concerning his purchase of health products and services. As stated by Dr. James L. Goddard, all the consumer has is a great deal of faith.

> "If the doctor is not qualified, they wouldn't let him practice."
> "If the medicine is no good, they wouldn't let it on the market."
> "If the lab is not accurate, they wouldn't give it a license."
> "If the insurance doesn't cover it, they wouldn't allow the policy."
> "If the records are wrong, they wouldn't put them into the machine."
>
> "They" constitute the vast and highly sophisticated teamwork upon which the individual now instinctively relies because he has no alternative. This is especially so in the field of public health. The quality and integrity of his life, along with the lives of his unborn children and his aging parents, are intimately entwined with "them." "They"—and I suggest we include all our health professionals in this category—"They" are making decisions, setting standards, adjusting the environment, controlling production, forming judgments, and otherwise surrounding the individual citizen so that "consumer choice" is worthy of more careful examination.[12]

[11] Omnibus Drug Bill S. 966, op. cit.

[12] James L. Goddard, M.D., "Public Health and the Consumer." Delivered at the 63rd Annual Health Conference, May 24, 1967.

Let us look more closely at "They," namely the governmental and private organizations that endeavor to protect the consumer.

The Food and Drug Administration (FDA)

The major function of the Food and Drug Administration is the enforcement of the Federal Food, Drug and Cosmetic Act, which is designed to protect both the consumer and law-abiding manufacturers and dealers.

In 1970 there was a major administrative reorganization of the Department of Health, Education and Welfare. The Public Health Service was reorganized into three functioning units which consisted of the National Institutes of Health, Health Service and Mental Health Administration, and the Food and Drug Administration. The FDA, as one of the three operating agencies of that service, itself began reorganization and evolved with six major Bureaus and two additional functioning units.

1. *Bureau of Foods* is responsible for the purity, safety, and wholesomeness of foods, food additives, colors and cosmetics. It conducts research designed to improve the detection, prevention, and control of contamination which might cause illness or injury conveyed by foods, colors, and cosmetics. It samples and tests for pesticide residues in food and enforces those tolerance levels that have been established by the Environmental Protection Agency.

2. *Bureau of Radiological Health* is concerned with the protection against unnecessary human exposure to radiation from electronic products and in the healing arts.

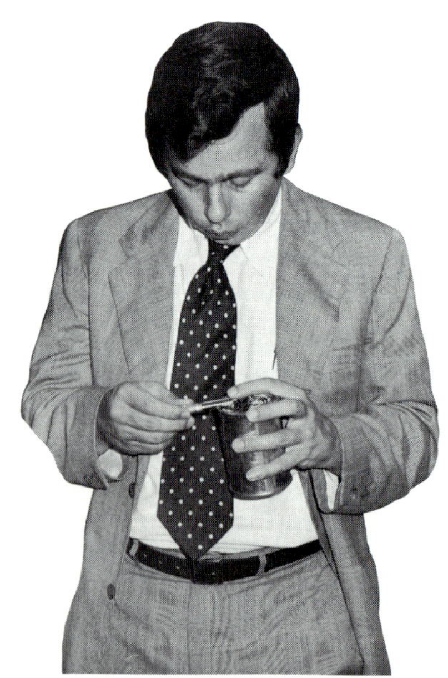

Figure 6–3

The seam thickness of a sealed can is measured with a micrometer by a Bureau of Foods inspector.

(*FDA Consumer,* December 1972–January 1973)

3. *Bureau of Drugs* has the responsibility for overseeing the safety and effectiveness of the nation's drug supply both prescription and over-the-counter (OTC) products. This bureau monitors the clinical tests of new drugs before they are put on the market and follows up the drug after its release for any unexpected side effects. Inspectors investigate drug plants to be sure ingredients are pure and facilities are complying with sanitation regulations, as well as the other facets of good manufacturing procedures which prevent errors in the drug production, labeling, and distribution. All batches of insulin and antibiotics for human use are tested for purity and potency. The FDA has authority over the advertising of prescription drugs only. These drug advertisements that are aimed at physicians must be truthful and fully informative. *Advertising* of OTC drugs on television and radio or in magazines and newspapers falls under the jurisdiction of the Federal Trade Commission.

4. *Bureau of Veterinary Medicine* requires that veterinary drugs devices and medicated foods be safe and effective to ensure the health and safety of the animal and to ensure the wholesomeness of the food derived from treated animals. Particular attention is given to residues of drugs found in the tissues of slaughtered animals.

5. *Bureau of Biologics* is responsible for assuring the safety, purity, and potency of biologic products which include vaccines, antitoxins, blood and blood products for human use.

6. *Bureau of Product Safety.* As of this printing, the Bureau of Product Safety will be separated from the FDA as a result of the signing of the Consumer Product Safety Act on October 28, 1972. The new agency will have jurisdiction over former FDA programs of the Hazardous Substances Act and the Child Protection and Toy Safety Act, the Flammable Fabrics Act, as well as the National Electronic Surveillance System (NEISS).

7. *Executive Director for Regional Operations* executes direct authority over all the nineteen FDA regional offices. It serves as the liaison for activities between FDA, state, and local agencies.

8. *National Center for Toxilogical Research* is not a bureau but a multiagency facility that will provide a national resource for projecting through animal studies the effects on man of an increasing array of chemicals in his environment. The FDA will administer the new facility but the Environmental Protection Agency and a number of other government agencies will utilize the center for assessing potential health hazards from chemicals in foods, drugs, and from environment sources.

In 1972 the Food and Drug Administration announced a massive and unprecedented review program to ensure that the many thousands over-the-counter drugs (OTC, those sold without a prescription) were safe, effective, and had fully informative labeling for self-treatment of minor, symptomatic conditions. The FDA was concerned that many formulations did not have the claimed effect, or adequate instructions for effective use by the consumer. They were also concerned about those drugs that were promoted in deceptive

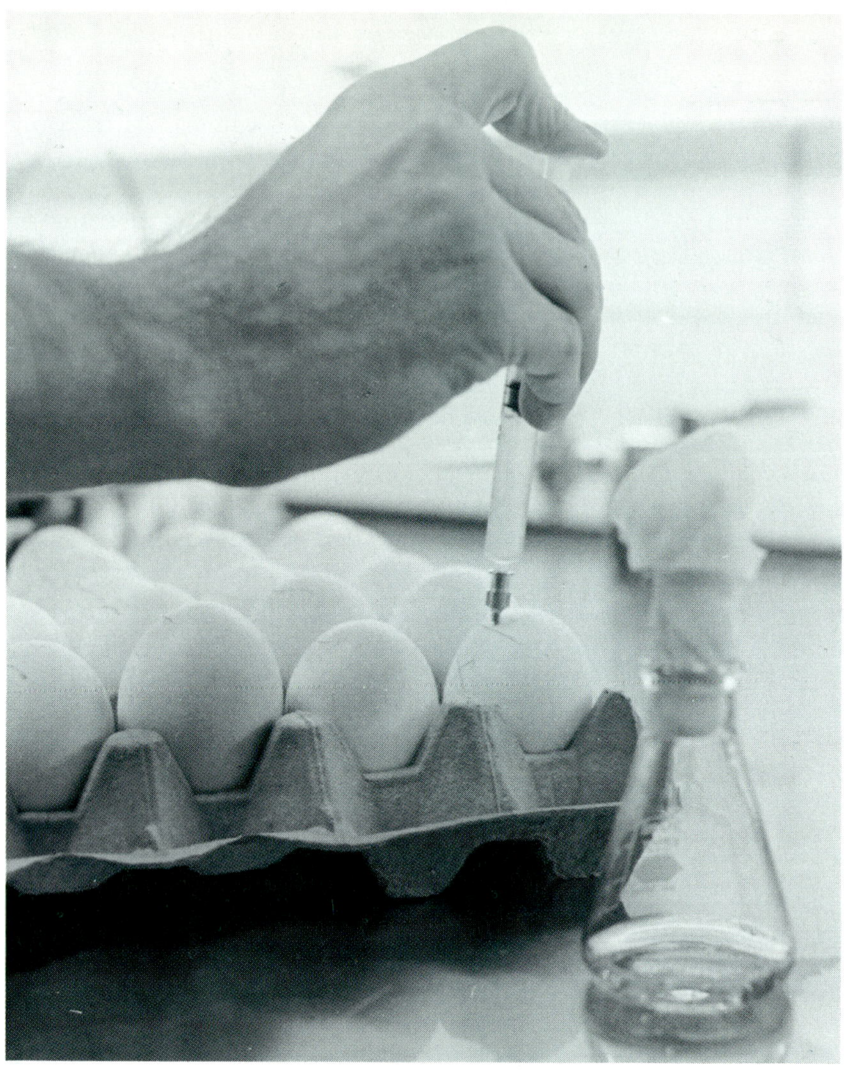

Figure 6–4

The flu vaccine is produced in fertilized eggs (chick embryo inside) that have been inoculated with flu virus. The embryo becomes infected along with the membrane surrounding it. The egg is then opened and the fluid removed. This infected fluid becomes the starting material for the vaccine. The virus is then killed before it is given to people so that it cannot produce the disease but still has the power to prevent it. The fever and body aches that some people experience following the "flu shot" is believed to be an allergic reaction to the nonvirus proteins from the chicken's egg. The Bureau of Biologics of the Food and Drug Administration sets standards of quality and safety for vaccine production.

(*FDA Consumer,* February 1973)

and indefensible ways. These included such preparations as antacids, cough remedies, stimulants, laxatives, and analgesics.

This new investigative program was unprecedented in scope and intensity. It was designed to build a permanent system of offering all American consumers the best possible assurance that every OTC drug not only was safe and adequately labeled but that it did what the manufacturer claimed it would do for the relief of minor illnesses and discomfort.

The Federal Trade Commission (FTC)

The Federal Trade Commission has the responsibility of enforcing the Federal Trade Commission Act of 1938 and the Wheeler-Lea Amendment of 1938. It was the Wheeler-Lea Amendment that empowered the Federal Trade Commission to control false or misleading advertisements of foods, drugs, cosmetics, and devices via the mass media. It attempts to review advertisements that are beamed out over 4,000 radio and television stations as well as those that appear in published material.

This agency has been notoriously understaffed and lacks a realistic operating budget for the massive assignment that it has. Advertisements are not reviewed by the Federal Trade Commission *before* they are used. The understaffed commission must not only *find* the misleading or false advertisement; it has the additional task of proving it false.

When the FTC wants to question a pseudoscientific claim in an advertisement, it must develop a sound medical-legal case against it. Studies need to be conducted to disprove claims that the manufacturers have backed up by "tests" and often self-styled "research studies." When the FTC has finally prepared its case, it issues a complaint to the advertiser. The advertiser has thirty days to respond to the complaint while the selling of the product via fraudulent advertising goes on. The advertiser often appeals the complaint, which means that a hearing must now be scheduled on a busy FTC calendar. If the decision at the hearing goes against the advertiser, he can appeal the decision to the FTC—another delaying tactic. If the FTC denies the appeal and issues an order to cease and desist, the advertiser can now appeal to the courts. The court decision can be appealed all the way up to the Supreme Court. If the advertiser finally loses, he is fined up to $5,000, which represents a drop in the bucket for a firm carrying on a nationwide operation. Though the misleading advertisement is now stopped, the advertiser by this time has developed a new approach, which, if misleading, could start the cycle all over again. For years Carter's Little Liver Pills were being sold with the suggestion that they helped the liver. The case took 16 years before the company was made to drop "liver" out of the name. In the meantime, practically a generation of Americans grew up thinking Carter's Little Liver Pills were good for the liver, when in fact it was simply a laxative.

More recently the Federal Trade Commission came under close investigation by three young men who were dubbed "Nader's Raiders"[13] by the newspapers and in 1969 a presidential commission recommended to the President of the United States that, indeed, drastic reforms were needed in the FTC. In 1970 with a new chairman, the commission underwent some administrative reforms and structural overhauling. In some newer cases the commission called on the *manufacturers* to substantiate claims of safety, performance, and therapeutic value instead of assuming the burden of proof. The commission's tough new policy was demonstrated again in the spring of 1972 when Anacin, Bayer Aspirin, Bufferin and Excedrin were accused of misleading the public with false advertisements. Not only were the advertisements to "cease and desist" but the commission "called for two years of corrective advertising to remove the heavy veil of deception from the public eye."[14]

Another example of the FTC's more vigorous policy has been its battle against the J. B. Williams Company, makers of Geritol. This governmental agency concluded that the advertisements for Geritol were deceptive because most people suffering vague, tired feelings were not helped by the product. The Geritol makers violated a series of "cease-and-desist" orders while the case seemed hopelessly stalled in the courts. After almost 14 years of battling, a Federal judge in 1973 fined the Williams Company $812,000 for deceiving the public into thinking that their product was a cure-all for that "tired blood" feeling. These are excellent examples of how constructive, intelligent criticism can bring about changes within our institutions.

The Federal Communications Commission (FCC)

The Federal Communications Commission is charged with the responsibility to see that the airways are used in the public interest. Although this kind of mandate implies almost limitless powers to prevent commercial abuses, it is rarely used. It has not only permitted misleading advertisements but also recognized quacks who reach the public through these media.

The realization that the television commercial as the country's biggest drug pusher is beginning to take hold. In 1972, the FTC urged the FCC to develop regulations mandating "counter-advertising" and "to provide free time for broadcasting replies to commercials that raise issues of current public importance."[15] Heretofore, this had been done only with cigarette advertising until 1971 when cigarette commercials on radio and television ended. Now, however, enlightened consumer groups are demanding honest advertising for all products as well as issues. For Example:

[13] Edward F. Cox, Robt. C. Fellmeth, and John E. Schultz, "The Nader Report" on the Federal Trade Commission (New York: Richard W. Baron, 1969), p. ix, Preface by Ralph Nader.

[14] "Aspirin: A Bitter Pill for the Ad Men," *New York Times,* April 23, 1972.

[15] *National Clearinghouse for Smoking and Health,* February 1, 1972.

> a Washington-based consumerism group called the Stern Community Law Firm filed a complaint with the FCC after the three networks rejected a counter-commercial dealing with the 1971 recall of some 2 million Chevrolets with defective engine mounts. The Stern-produced spot lists recalled models and warns: "If you have one of these Chevrolets, it could cost you your life. Get it to a Chevrolet serviceman . . . slowly."[16]

Another countercommercial displays samples of six top-selling pain-relieving products while the commentator says, "The American Medical Association has found remedies like these to be either irrational, not recommended or unsound."[17]

Hopefully, the countercommercials will force the advertiser to rid his ads of the misleading and deceptive information. However, some advertisers are threatening to withdraw their advertising from television rather than have their product attacked by countercommercials, as did the tobacco industry.

The Post Office Department

The Post Office Department's Division of Fraud and Mailability can act against parties attempting to use the United States mail for the purposes of fraud. The Fraud Statute empowering the Post Office to take action in these cases was enacted by Congress in 1872. The Post Office can issue a fraud order to a company that is sending through the mail materials with the intent to defraud. The aged legislation on the basis of which the Post Office operates inhibits it from taking consistently effective action because of its many loopholes. The Post Office may be successful in stopping the sale of a fraudulent product through the mails and yet be unable to prevent a mail circular from going through announcing where the product is available.

Consumer Action Groups

In recent years a consumer movement has arisen. Ralph Nader started the movement to help the consumer get his dollars worth in the marketplace. Many factors have created a concern and a consumer militancy not seen before. One big factor is the product guarantee that protected the manufacturer rather than the consumer. Other factors are poor workmanship, misleading advertisements, and the rising costs of health care. Therefore a number of consumer action groups have been created. A consumer will be able to take his complaints to such a group and get some action.

Professional Organizations

The American Medical Association, the American Dental Association, as well as others set standards of education and performance for their members.

[16] *Newsweek,* June 5, 1972, p. 65.

[17] Ibid.

They also concern themselves with fraudulent practices with regard to services and products in their areas. The American Medical Association's Department of Investigation checks on practices in medical quackery. Its Council on Foods makes studies of manufactured foods. The Council on Physical Medicine reports on nonmedical devices and apparatus that are sold to the public, physicians, and hospitals. The Council on Dental Therapeutics sets standards and approves dental products. These professional organizations work closely with the federal agencies in their efforts to control fraudulent practices.

EVALUATING HEALTH INFORMATION

Making judgments with regard to advertisements and claims for health products and services is not easy. Some questions a person might ask in the evaluation of health products and services are:

1. Do they lead one to self-diagnosis and self-medication?
2. Are services being sold on the basis of personal testimonials?
3. If research findings are quoted, who did the research? Were they done by qualified and unbiased people?
4. If authorities are quoted, who are they?
5. If literature is presented, is it acceptable to medical, dental, and public health professionals?
6. Does the sales appeal play on fears, or superstitious beliefs?
7. Is the sponsor of the product or services a recognized, bona fide organization?
8. Is the product offered as a cure-all or as a sure cure for cancer, arthritis, or heart disease?

Where doubts exist with regard to health products and services, they should be checked out with the family doctor, the local health department, Consumer Action Groups, or the school or college health educator. Well-recognized organizations occasionally put out publications evaluating certain kinds of health information that is of value to the consumer. For example, the Arizona Dietetic Association, Inc.,[18] has made available a publication to help individuals choose reliable books on nutrition. The American Medical Association and the American Dental Association have all kinds of information booklets concerning one's health.

Consumers Union is a nonprofit organization with the consumer's interest at heart. In its monthly publication, *Consumer Reports,* all kinds of consumer

[18] *Nutrition Books for Lay Readers: Recommended, Recommended for Special Purposes, Not Recommended,* The Arizona Dietetic Association, Inc., Education Section, Compiled 1972.

commodities are evaluated. These products, ranging from vacuum cleaners to contact lenses, are rated after careful laboratory and use tests, thus enabling the consumer to get the best product for his money. Medical doctors serve as consultants to Consumers Union and make judgments on matters of health and medicine. Their comments are based on the study and findings of many research scientists and research institutions. The Consumers Union publication, *The Medicine Show,* is concerned with health-related products and services.

Many articles and editorials in *Today's Health* magazine evaluate health products and services. Innumerable publications of this type are also available from the Food and Drug Administration, the United States Public Health Service, official health agencies, and various voluntary health agencies (American Heart Association, American Cancer Society, National Mental Health Association, and others).

HEALTH CARE PROFESSIONALS

Preparation to become a doctor of medicine requires four years of college work and an additional four years of medical school. This is followed by a one- or two-year internship. All doctors must be liscensed by the State Board of Medical Examiners before they can practice within that particular state. A physician may refer a patient with a complex problem to a medical specialist who has additional training in a particular area of medicine.

To check the credentials of a physician, one need only refer to the American Medical Association Directory found in any local library. The AMA Directory will indicate if the physician involved has a membership in the local medical society and the AMA, and if he is certified by the appropriate specialty board (be it for the area of pediatrics, internal medicine, obstetrics, or any of the others). The Directory will also indicate fellowship in the American College of Surgeons or the American College of Physicians. In choosing a family physician, another criterion to be considered is whether the doctor is continuing postgraduate work in his area of specialization to help him keep up with current developments in his field.

Types of Medical Specialists[19]

Allergist. One who treats and diagnoses body reactions which show hypersensitivity to drugs, pollens, foods, animals, or other things (a subspecialty of internal medicine).

[19] Definitions of medical specialists have been adapted or quoted from *Stedman's Medical Dictionary,* 20th ed. (Baltimore: The Williams & Wilkins Company, 1961). *Today's Health* (January 1963), pp. 12–13: W. W. Bauer, ed., *Today's Health Guide* (Chicago: American Medical Association, 1965); *Health Careers Guidebook* (Washington, D.C.: U.S. Govt. Printing Office, 1965).

Anesthetist or Anesthesiologist. One who administers an anesthetic to effect a loss of consciousness (general anesthesia) or a loss of sensation in a specific location (local anesthesia).

Cardiologist. One having special knowledge and experience in the diagnosis and treatment of heart disease (a subspeciality of internal medicine).

Dermatologist. A practitioner who specializes in the diagnosis and treatment of cutaneous lesions and the related systemic diseases; a "skin specialist."

Endocrinologist. One who deals with the internal secretions of the ductless glands and their physiologic and pathologic relations.

Epidemiologist. One who specializes in the study of the determinants and distributions of disease prevalence.

Family Physician. One who specializes in a new area called Family Practice. This area of specialization deals with preventive medicine for the entire family.

Gastroenterologist. A specialist in the diseases of the digestive system.

Gerontologist or Geriatrician. One who specializes in the science of the physiologic and pathologic changes that take place in old age.

Gynecologist. The physician who specializes in the branch of medicine which has to do with the diseases peculiar to women, primarily those of the genital tract, as well as female endocrinology and reproductive physiology.

Internist. A physician trained in internal medicine, which is the medical specialty concerned with illnesses of a nonsurgical nature, mainly in adults.

Neurologist. A specialist in the nonsurgical treatment of diseases of the nervous system.

Neurosurgeon. A specialist in the diagnosis and surgical treatment of the nervous system.

Obstetrician. One who is skilled in the medical care of a woman during pregnancy and in childbirth and the interval immediately following.

Ophthalmologist or Oculist. A specialist in diseases and refractive errors of the eye.

Orthopedist or Orthopedic Surgeon. One who specializes in the branch of surgery that has to do with the treatment of chronic diseases of the joints and spine and the correction of deformities.

Otolaryngologist. A specialist in the diseases of the ear and larynx.

Otologist. A specialist in the diseases of the ear.

Otorhinolaryngologist. A specialist in the diseases of the ear, nose, and larynx.

Pathologist. A specialist in the identification of disease through the analysis of body tissues, fluids, and other body specimens.

Pediatrician. A medical practitioner who specializes in the prevention, diagnosis, and treatment of diseases in children.

Plastic Surgeon. The physician who specializes in the branch of operative surgery that corrects or repairs deformed or mutilated parts of the body.

Proctologist. A specialist in the science that deals with diagnosis and treatment of the colon, rectum, and anus.

Psychiatrist. A specialist who deals in the interpretation and treatment of mental and personality disorders.

Radiologist. A physician who is skilled in the diagnostic and therapeutic use of X rays and other forms of radiant energy.

Rhinologist. A specialist who deals with the disorders of the nose.

Surgeon. A specialist who treats diseases through operative measures.

Urologist. The physician who specializes in the study, diagnosis, and treatment of diseases of the genitourinary tract.

Dental Specialists

Dentists are individuals trained to care for the health of the mouth, teeth, and supporting tissues. The degrees of DDS (Doctor of Dental Surgery) or DMD (Doctor of Dental Medicine) are awarded after completion of a course of study at approved dental schools. The dentist today is becoming more and more allied with the field of medicine. His early training parallels that of the medical student, with great emphasis on the basic sciences. This background is necessary because of his key role in the detection of oral cancer and in the dental treatment of patients with diabetes, hemophilia, or allergies. Because he is licensed to prescribe drugs, he needs to have a background parallel to that of the medical student.

State board examinations must be passed in order for a dentist to practice. Graduate schools offer specialization in particular areas of dental medicine. Following are a few of the dental specialists with a brief description of each:

Endodontist. One who specializes in the diagnosis and treatment of diseases of the pulp (or nerve) of a tooth. This specialty embraces methods of pulp conservation as well as tooth retention once infection at the root has developed.

Orthodontist. The dental specialist who is concerned with the correction and prevention of irregularities of the teeth and malocclusion of the jaw.

Pedodontist. One who specializes in the treatment of dental ills of children.

Periodontist. A dentist who specializes in the treatment of the supporting tissues of the teeth.

Prosthodontist is concerned with the construction of special appliances (dentures, bridges, crowns) to compensate mechanically for oral deficiencies such as tooth loss and cleft palate.

Osteopathy

Osteopathic Physician (Doctor of Osteopathy, D.O.). A practitioner licensed to practice medicine and surgery who includes in his treatment some elements of manipulative therapy, which must not be confused with the adjustments and manipulations practiced by the nonmedical chiropractor. Today the osteopathic physician is recognized as having training comparable to the medical general practitioner. He is licensed to practice osteopathic medicine and surgery in all states. In some states the osteopathic and medical associations have merged. The American Osteopathic Association has resisted such a move on the national level for fear that it would merely be absorbed by the larger American Medical Association and lose its distinctive recognition of the function of the musculoskeletal system in health and disease.

Initially, osteopathic practice was based on the theory that malfunction was related to disalignment of the body. It has since developed philosophy, training, and practices that are more closely related to the medical profession. Osteopathic medicine encompasses all phases of medicine, for example, anesthesiology, dermatology, internal medicine, neurology, and so forth. There are 6 osteopathic colleges in the United States. In addition to the provision of four years of training, the student serves a year of internship in one of 263 osteopathic hospitals, and has the option of specializing in any of the specialties with postgraduate training.

Nonmedical Specialists

Optician. A craftsman who is skilled in the grinding of lenses according to the prescription of the oculist or optometrist, and properly sets these lenses in the frames.

Optometrist. A graduate from a school of optometry and licensed in all fifty states to measure visual acuity and to prescribe glasses and other nonmedical measures.

Orthoptist. A technician trained to correct defects of the ocular muscles through eye exercises and visual training as prescribed by the oculist.

Podiatrist. One who engages in the specialty that includes the diagnosis and treatment (either medical, surgical, mechanical, or physical) of the diseases, injuries, and defects of the human foot. A number of podiatrists are affiliated with hospitals and are generally recognized as being a paramedical profession. The National Association of Chiropodists in 1958 decided to change its name to the American Podiatry Association. While Podiatry (Podiatrist) and Chiropody (Chiropodist) are synonymous terms, Podiatry is now the preferred one.

Psychologist. An individual without a medical background who concerns himself with applying scientific methods to the study of human behavior. He may be a *School Psychologist* and perform such duties as testing, classifying, and counseling of students. If he is a *Clinical Psychologist,* he has earned a Ph.D. and has completed a supervised internship at a psychiatric clinic. If the clinical psychologist meets the standards set by the American Psychological Association, he is then qualified to diagnose and treat behavior disorders, usually through testing and other psychological diagnostic devices, without the use of medication.

THE CHIROPRACTIC CONTROVERSY

One of the most controversial groups in the health care field in the United States is that of chiropractic. Most medical doctors view them as akin to quacks; chiropractors view themselves as being the professional equals of medical doctors; others view their status as somewhere in between the first two assessments. Basic to the issue is the theoretical basis of chiropractic practice. As stated in *Your Health and Chiropractic:*

> These four principles make up the bedrock of chiropractic practice.
>
> 1. Anatomical disrelation can create functional disturbances in the body.
> 2. Disturbances of the nervous system are primary factors in the development of many disease conditions.
> 3. Spinal subluxations (minor displacements of spinal bones) are a specific cause of nerve irritation or interference.
> 4. The viscero-spinal principle: nerve irritation at the spine may lead to a disturbance in the function of one or more internal organs of the body.[20]

While chiropractors accuse physicians of inflexibility in not recognizing chiropractic, physicians are equally dismayed at chiropractors who refuse to recognize the value of eminently successful medical procedures such as immunization programs. Epidemics of smallpox, diphtheria, and polio have been reduced to almost zero incidence, not through the spinal manipulations to reduce subluxations, but through programs of immunization. As stated by Dr. Andrew V. Friedrichs of the Department of Pathology and Bacteriology at Tulane University: "the chiropractors advocate . . . that all immunization and inoculation for polio, tetanus, typhoid, smallpox, diphtheria, to name a few, and many other diseases which are combatted by immunization and inoculation, be discarded, to be replaced by manipulation of the spinal column, to normalize the flow of nerve impulses."[21]

The Department of Health Education and Welfare developed a Report on chiropractic. Some of their conclusions include:

> 1. There is a body of basic scientific knowledge related to health, disease, and health care. Chiropractic practitioners ignore or take exception to much of this knowledge despite the fact that they have not undertaken adequate scientific research.

[20] Thorp McClusky, *Your Health and Chiropractic,* (New York: Pyramid Books, 1962), p. 17.

[21] Ralph Lee Smith, *At Your Own Risk: The Case Against Chiropractic* (New York: Trident Press, 1969), p. 151.

2. There is no valid evidence that subluxation, if it exists, is a significant factor in disease processes. Therefore, the broad application to health care of a diagnostic procedure such as spinal analysis and a treatment procedure such as spinal adjustment is not justified.
3. The inadequacies of chiropractic education, coupled with a theory that de-emphasizes proven causative factors in disease processes, proven methods of treatment, and differential diagnosis, make it unlikely that a chiropractor can make an adequate diagnosis and know the appropriate treatment, and subsequently provide the indicated treatment or refer the patient. Lack of these capabilities in independent practitioners is undesirable because: appropriate treatment could be delayed or prevented entirely; appropriate treatment might be interrupted or stopped completely; the treatment offered could be contraindicated; all treatments have some risk involved with their administration, and inappropriate treatment exposes the patient to this risk unnecessarily.
4. Manipulation (including chiropractic manipulation) may be a valuable technique for relief of pain due to loss of mobility in joints. Research in this area is inadequate; therefore, it is suggested that research based upon the scientific method be undertaken with respect to manipulation.[22]

THE CHANGING NATURE OF HEALTH CARE

Anyone who has ever watched television is familiar with the character "Doc" from the western "Gunsmoke." "Doc" was a trusted friend in the community. His mere chin-rubbing presence assured everyone that needed help was at hand. In addition to his ability to probe for bullets in human beings (a Dodge city avocation!), he also delivered babies and treated a variety of folk for a variety of ailments aided only by the pitiful few aids he carried in his little black bag—a kind of nineteenth-century "trick or treat" medical approach. It was an era when a great many people died of "natural causes," with equal numbers recovering from their ailments for the same reasons. With the advent of the twentieth century, medical research produced great amounts of new medical information. Since no one man could master such great amounts of knowledge, this resulted in physicians' specializing in specific areas of medical care as well as the development of varied allied health professional groups who became part of the health care team. The twentieth century also brought forth sophisticated (and expensive) diagnostic and therapeutic equipment that the individual doctor could not afford to buy.

In the last few decades, there has therefore been a definite trend toward increased medical group practice. With the increased sophistication in respect not only to knowledge but to diagnostic techniques, there has been emphasis

[22] HEW Report of Chiropractic, pp. 196–197.

on laboratory and technical procedures in the prevention, diagnosis, and treatment of disease. Not only did group practice make it easier to obtain expensive equipment but it also facilitated hiring of allied health staff. The sharing of this equipment and staff is not only an economical move but makes available to each physician a greater capacity for quality medical care. In group practice, there seems to be a greater emphasis on preventive medicine. There is greater opportunity for comprehensive physical examinations to catch disorders in their early stages before they are dangerous, or through health education to prevent them in the first place. Such practice also provides more free time for the doctors involved. Vacation time, as well as time for further study, can be scheduled much more easily because there are others to cover for the missing physician. In addition, it provides the doctor with the professional stimulant of working closely with other branches of medicine and leads to some healthy exchanges of information as well as philosophy. A possible disadvantage in this kind of arrangement is that some medical men find it difficult to work as part of a team. In addition, from the physician's point of view solo practice is usually a more lucrative one and can often produce greater monetary benefits than group practice. There are also dangers with regard to the doctor-patient relationship. Where a number of physicians are involved in the care of the patient, a more impersonal doctor-patient relationship may develop.

There are many variations of group practice. These might include groups of a few doctors or many doctors, with varied combinations of general practitioners and specialists. The majority of the groups operate on a fee-for-service basis (the patient attends the clinic for a particular medical service and upon receiving it pays the fee). The Mayo Clinic in Rochester, Minnesota, and the Lahey Clinic in Boston exemplify this kind of arrangement. Other group practice is financed by the prepayment insurance plan that involves comprehensive coverage. The New York City Health Insurance Plan (HIP) exemplifies this kind of group practice. The original purpose of HIP was to care for the

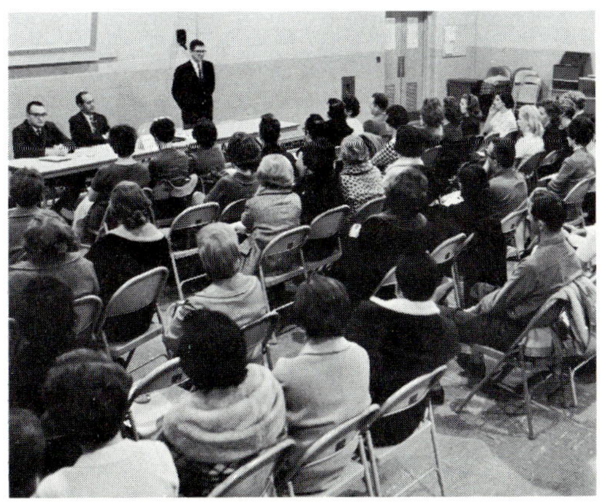

Figure 6–5

Increasingly health education is being made a part of preventive health care. It promotes health and tends to reduce health care costs.

[Health Insurance Plan (HIP), East Nassau Medical Group]

municipal workers in New York City; however, others may now join the plan. It has some thirty-two medical centers. People who join this plan have a choice of physicians within each of these groups. A number of them work for HIP on a part-time basis with a private practice on the side. This organization boasts a department of health education stressing education as one of its aspects of preventive medicine.

Recent scientific advances as well as socioeconomic developments indicate that there will be a further growth of medical group practice. This form of medical practice is increasingly acceptable to both physicians and the general public.

FINANCING COSTS OF HEALTH CARE

There have been dramatic increases in the cost of health care in this country. In 1950 the average health care expenditure for an individual was $79 a year; by 1970 this amount rose to $324. At the present time approximately $70 billion a year is spent on health care, more than five times spent two decades ago. While 50 per cent of the rise in costs reflects an increased population and greater utilization of health services, the other 50 per cent in increased costs reflects higher prices.

Through the years it has been noted that *direct* payments for medical costs have been reduced as a result of broader health insurance coverage. In 1950, 9.7 per cent of medical costs were covered by insurance benefits; by 1960 this rose to 24.2 per cent. The objective is to have this kind of coverage extend to 90 per cent of health care costs.

Voluntary Health Insurance

There are five basic types of health insurance policies that are generally offered by insurance companies. These are:

HOSPITAL EXPENSE INSURANCE. Coverage provides to some degree for room and board in addition to drugs, anesthetics, and the use of the operating room. General nursing care is also covered. Coverage may be for maximum periods of 60, 90 or 100 days. Hospital expense insurance is the most popular one, with more people being covered by this kind of protection than any other type.

SURGICAL EXPENSE INSURANCE. This type of coverage pays part or all of the surgeon's fee for a given operation. The policy will usually list various kinds of operations and the amount it will allow for each. There are variances in the amounts allowed for operations and these, of course, are covered by varying insurance premiums. This type of insurance is often combined with hospital expense insurance.

GENERAL MEDICAL EXPENSE INSURANCE. This type of coverage will pay part or all of the physician's bills other than for surgery. It will cover a doctor's call at the hospital or the home or for patient's visits to the physician's office. Often this kind of policy will include diagnostic, X ray, and laboratory fees. The policy will indicate the amount that is payable as well as the maximum number of calls that it will cover.

MAJOR MEDICAL EXPENSE INSURANCE. This type of coverage is to provide payment for exceedingly heavy medical and hospital bills. It is intended to prevent the wiping out of a persons' savings and the possibility of being thrown into debt. This type of policy picks up where hospitalization and surgical plans leave off. Costs in excess of these plans are covered by major medical policies taking care of physicians' fees, hospital bills, nursing care, drugs, and any other expenses arising out of treatment in or out of the hospital. These policies may pay up to 10,000 dollars or more in medical expenses. In order to keep the premiums of major medical insurance within reasonable limits, they may contain a deductible provision similar to deductible auto insurance whereby the policyholder will pay a certain amount before the policy takes over. In some instances, the deductible feature of the policy may be combined with a coinsurance clause. The policyholder in this case may pay 25 per cent of costs past the initial deductible amount, with the insurance company paying the remainder or 75 per cent of major medical costs. Major medical insurance is the most recent type of health insurance as well as the fastest-growing one.

LOSS OF INCOME INSURANCE. This type of insurance helps to replace income that is lost during a period of illness or disability, and is usually written for the family breadwinner. It permits the family to pay its rent, buy its groceries, and cover its basic costs of living. Its benefits usually begin a week or two after the illness or disability occurs. Some policies, however, call for 30-, 60-, or 90-day waiting periods before payments start. Insurance of this type that provides 50 per cent of regular salary is considered good. Many families plan to pay the costs of minor illness out of their regular income and rely on health insurance for coverage for longer disability periods.

Federal Health Insurance Programs

Medicare (Title 18), enacted in 1966, is a health insurance program for older people. The *basic* part of this plan is financed through social security payments during a person's working years. At the age of 65, the person is eligible to receive medicare benefits that include hospital and nursing home care, home visits by nurses, and limited out-patient services in hospitals. The purpose of the program is to provide paid-up health insurance for older people for the time in their lives when they need it most.

The *voluntary* portion of Medicare is financed by a modest monthly premium payment by the individual. This part of the program helps to defray costs of doctor bills, X rays, and other diagnostic tests, surgical supplies, and various therapeutic appliances, iron lungs, or artificial limbs, physical therapy, and drugs.

When an aged person with Medicare cannot pay his portion of medical costs under this plan, he may be helped by the Kerr-Mills Medical Assistance program (Medicaid). This program is operated by the states and subsidized by the federal government. Criteria to determine if a person is in need of financial assistance vary from state to state. If a state decides that a patient is very poor, it would under this plan pay for the patient's portion of Medicare costs.

Title 19 of the Social Security Act established a federal-state program for health care of the needy and medically indigent. Persons eligible for medical aid under this program would include the aged, the blind, the disabled, and medically poor children under 21. It also provided that states participating in the Kerr-Mills program must provide, as a minimum, five kinds of services:

1. Inpatient hospital services. (patient remains in hospital)
2. Outpatient hospital services. (patient visits hospital for services)
3. Doctor's services.
4. Nursing home services.
5. X ray and other laboratory services.

Title 19 serves as a supplement to Medicare by providing the states with additional assistance to pay for the premium of the voluntary portion of Medicare for those aged who are in need. It may also pay for the patient's share of the Medicare bill.

AVAILABILITY OF HEALTH CARE

In the United States we have groups who do not have access to adequate medical care. They include the unemployed, the disabled, and their families. There are also the "medically indigent," a group who are otherwise self-

Figure 6–6

The increased costs of health care and the shortage of health professionals have seriously affected the availability of health care services.

(New York State Health Department)

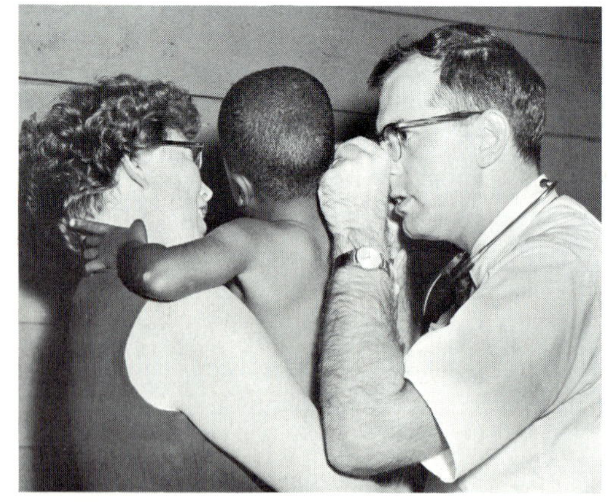

supporting but who cannot afford the added costs of medical care. It is ironic to note that those groups most in need of health services are also least capable of purchasing them. The poor people and those in rural areas do not get the quality service that some people in the cities get. This is partly because there are not enough doctors and other health personnel and facilities in rural areas and among the poor.

> The national average physician-to-population ratio is 150 to 100,000. This is the number once cited by a Surgeon General as that necessary to protect the health of the people. But in many areas of our Nation, mostly in inner-city and rural areas, there are far fewer than 150 physicians per 100,000 people. In the Kenwood area of Chicago, for example, there are five physicians per 100,000 people. And in the South Bronx in New York City, in East Los Angeles, and in central St. Louis, the ratios are less than 50 to 100,000. In the rural areas similar situations prevail. In all of Kansas there are only 108 physicians per 100,000 population. In one five-county area, this decreases to less than 45 to 100,000. In Mississippi the figures are 88 to 100,000, with certain areas decreasing to less than 20 to 100,000. The facts are then quite clear—health care is simply not available to many Americans.[23]

Though the major medical centers will continue to be located in high population urban areas, a system of primary treatment needs to be developed for all population groups. In addition, a system for referring those in need of the more sophisticated services of the medical centers must be made available.

ORGANIZING FOR COMMUNITY HEALTH ACTION

Some new concepts in medical care delivery have been evolving in the last decade. The dire health needs of the poor have heretofore been inadequately served by present health department and hospital facilities. The long lines at hospital clinics and the great distances the rural poor must travel in order to get medical care have been discouraging. The impersonal handling of patients oftentimes reflects a lack of "Establishment" acceptance of minority groups. In response, there has been a developing movement to establish health care facilities that are neighborhood or community oriented. They have involved people from the community as members of governing councils and boards. This has represented a "reaching-out"—in essence the provision of health services where the people are. In some instances, however, where militant neighborhood groups have decided to have a dominating voice in the manage-

[23] William R. Roy, M.D., *The Proposed Health Maintenance Organization Act of 1972.* Sourcebook Series Volume 2, Science and Health Communications Group, 1730 Rhode Island Ave., N.W. Washington, D.C. 20036.

ment of the health care facilities without the professional expertise that is essential, programs have failed. Where health professionals *and* neighborhood groups have worked together in developing policy and program, the chances of success have been greatly increased. Where they have been successful, these health care facilities or clinics

> have gained a wide popularity by respecting the needs and the imperfect humanity of their patients. They have revitalized the doctor-patient relationship and shown its relevance in modern, computerized medicine. They have demonstrated the desirability and practicality of minimizing red tape in dealing with people. They have pioneered the use of paramedical volunteers and staff workers in a country faced with a severe shortage of doctors and professional personnel.[24]

At the same time the neighborhood or community-based health center may be criticized by those who are threatened by changes in the paternalistic doctor-patient relationship, who are more obsessed with bureaucratic procedure than people, who see security in the shortage of doctors and health personnel, and who see paramedical volunteers as invaders of their professional turf.

The forms that these health care facilities have taken vary considerably, depending on the community being served. The Whitney M. Young, Jr., Community Health Center is funded by the Department of Health, Education and Welfare, and policy for the center is determined jointly with a nearby medical center and an advisory council. This neighborhood health center is able to offer continuous family-oriented care, which is often more personalized than clinic situations at hospitals. Patients seeking treatment are assigned a nurse who remains with that patient for the length of the treatment. The patient may also request the same physician at each of the health center visits. In this way, some physician-patient rapport may be established. Although the health care involves emergency treatment as well as health-related services, a concern for preventive medicine is also apparent. Lead poisoning and sickle-cell anemia detection, as well as nutrition education, obstetric, and pediatric care, are such preventive areas. Paraprofessionals from the community have been trained at the Center to follow up patients who have missed or canceled appointments or have no phone or other means of communicating with the Center. A listing of local pharmacists who agree to charge fixed fees for medications is available to the patient who must be medicaid-eligible in order to be a regular member of the Health Center.

Another neighborhood health center located on New York City's lower East side is the NENA (Northeast Neighborhood Association) Health Center. The structure of this center varies somewhat from the first in that it is a much larger operation employing over 100 persons and handling approximately 12,000 registered patients. Its community is an integrated one where economic

[24] David E. Smith, M.D., and John Luce, *Love Needs Care* (Boston: Little, Brown, 1971), p. 370.

levels vary and where many ethnic groups are represented. The large numbers of elderly people living alone and the young Spanish-speaking families with many children tend to require special consideration in this neighborhood, where the median income is the lowest in New York City. Policy for the center is determined by a Health Council whose members must be residents of the area served. The concept exemplified here is that the consumer must participate in determining health policy while he remains accountable to his "neighbors."

In the late 1960s, when the Haight-Ashbury drug scene was at its height, there was a critical need for an on-the-spot medical facility which was available 24 hours a day—a place where drug abusers could be treated for acute drug crises, detoxified, and counseled and where education about drugs, nutrition, and proper hygiene could take place. The emergence of the Free Clinic in this section of San Francisco was fashioned somewhat after the Watts Clinic, which began providing medical care for the poverty-stricken of that area after the riots of 1965. The infectious diseases ran rampant in the young people of the Haight-Ashbury district who were generally weakened from poor eating and hygienic habits. A variety of dental problems and parasitic infestations flourished, to say nothing of the incidence of venereal diseases, hepatitis, and skin disorders. Dr. David E. Smith, founder of the Haight-Ashbury Free Clinic, envisioned the clinic as a new medicine and health-care delivery system that was urgently needed in this country. During the year 1968, 20,000 people were treated at the clinic's Medical Section. For these many thousands, the clinic was their only source of medication, treatment and health education. As stated by Dr. Smith and John Luce:

> the free clinics have proven their ability to reach alienated economic, racial and philosophic minorities. They have advanced the goals of community medicine by seeking out patients in their own environment and by regarding the environment as an organism capable of being healed. They have provided an outlet for idealism and social frustration. And they have served as a conscience for the country.[25]

Presently there are over 200 free clinics in the United States with 1 to 2 million patient visits yearly, at an average cost of $2 per visit.

The health needs that free clinics meet are obvious. In a pluralistic society, facets of the health care delivery system must be flexible enough to meet the varying health care needs unique to a particular community.

Ironically, criticism of the free clinics often comes from the members of the communities being served. Their complaint is that free clinics propagate a two-layered system of health care and that the existing medical care system is not pressured to change its health care delivery approach to include *all* members of society. Perhaps what is needed is the merging of the free clinic movement with the established health care delivery system. This would result

[25] Ibid, p. 370.

in the added resources necessary and greater equality in the health care received by all.

A major factor inhibiting the availability of medical care has been its skyrocketing costs. In the decade 1960–1970 the costs of hospital care rose 170 per cent and physicans' fees 60 per cent, as compared to an average rise of 30 per cent in consumer prices during that same period. Some have concluded that the rising costs of medical care have even made the middle- and upper-middle-income Americans incapable of purchasing medical care.

The problem has been further aggravated by shortages of physicians and other health personnel. As both voluntary and government health insurance plans proliferated, greater demands for health care have placed added strains on an understaffed health care system.

In addition, the manner in which some health insurance is written causes the inappropriate use of already strained medical care facilities. For example, an individual in need of an X-ray series finds that the cost of this procedure will be covered by his health insurance only if he is hospitalized for it. If the X rays are done on an outpatient basis, then he has to assume the costs. He naturally seeks to be hospitalized for the X rays, resulting in not only the inappropriate use of the hospital but the unnecessary costs of a hospital stay. There is need therefore to redesign the organization of medical care delivery *and* the way it is financed.

HEALTH MAINTENANCE ORGANIZATION (HMO)

A community-based group of medical and allied health specialists with complementary skills and a concentration of preventive diagnostic and therapeutic facilities has a great potential for high-quality medical care. It is this kind of thinking that has led the federal government to give impetus to the development of a new medical care delivery system with the above ingredients.

The new medical care delivery system of the United States will consist of a series of Health Maintenance Organizations.

> An HMO, in addition to accepting payment for health care, assumes responsibility for actually providing health care services to its members. This is the major difference between an HMO and traditional indemnity health insurance such as Blue Cross/Blue Shield and Aetna. Indemnity insurance pays for health care if it can be found; an HMO provides the services itself. Since it controls the delivery mechanism itself, an HMO, unlike indemnity insurance, is in a position to quarantee the availability, accessibility, and continuity of care.[26]

[26] *The Proposed Health maintenance . . .*, op. cit., p. 13.

The Health Maintenance Organizations will be in the form of prepaid health insurance financed by a varied combination of individual, employer, and government contributions. They will also feature group medical practice. Changes in medical care delivery have been stimulated by governmental activity in the form of legislation as well as finances.

With the developing philosophy that medical care is not a privilege but a right of the citizen, increased governmental activity in this area seems inevitable.

A LOOK TO THE FUTURE

We are entering an era that will be marked with a level of health consciousness and action that is unprecedented. It will be accentuated with an increasing intolerance for preventable disease and infirmity and an increased desire for higher levels of health. There will be greater and more widespread demand for high-quality medical care. Some rather startling changes are already taking place, not only in the practice of medicine, but in the manner in which it is organized and financed.

The practice of medicine as an individual enterprise is being transformed into one involving highly organized teams of health personnel operating in groups and/or in hospitals with the latest of modern equipment. Open heart surgery, for example, is not undertaken by an individual doctor, but by a team of physicians, nurses, and technicians in a hospital where a heart-lung machine is available as well as other facilities and equipment needed for this advanced operative procedure. Those who advocate that medical group practice be related to medical or hospital centers appear to be responding to the dictates of advancing technology and knowledge. The highly expensive and complex preventive diagnostic and therapeutic equipment and personnel can no longer be duplicated in each doctor's office, but must be centrally located in the community.

Specialism in medicine is also resulting in the development of a large number of allied health professions. They include medical librarians, statisticians, health educators, social workers, and dieticians, among others. This broad development of allied health professional personnel is partially due to a reduction in the number of physicians in proportion to our growing population. It is expected that the population will continue to outgrow the number of doctors who will be graduated from our medical schools. Increasing emphasis on comprehensive care and preventive medicine is another reason for the expected proliferant development of the allied health professions. The physician already represents less than 10 per cent of the health personnel in a developing "health industry."

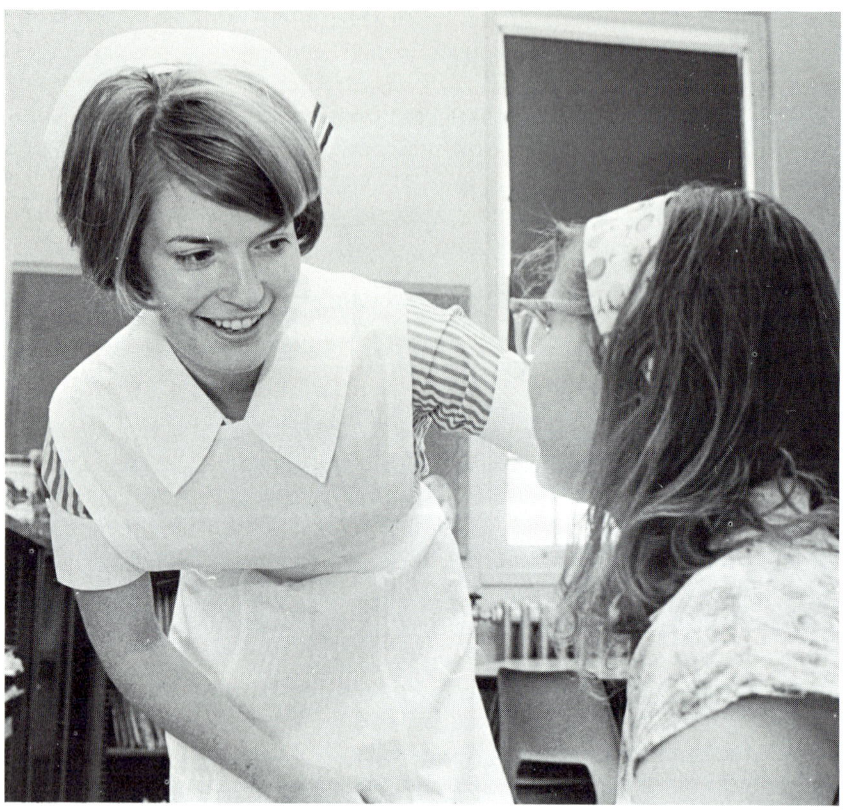

Figure 6–7

A variety of health professionals work with the doctor as a health team to provide better health care.

(New York State Department of Mental Hygiene—Julian A. Belin).

The concept of comprehensive care is one that has been gaining momentum. It refers not only to diagnosis, treatment of disease, and rehabilitation, BUT *to the promotion of health and the prevention of disease as well.* This approach is in sharp contrast to that in which a person would seek out a doctor only *after* illness has occurred and oftentimes when the illness has reached a terminal stage. The increase in the number of allied health personnel gives the physician more time for patient care, thus compensating somewhat for the doctor shortage. It also escalates the potential in the area of preventive medicine. It makes possible testing by the technician, for example, counseling by a social worker, educating by the health educator. These are functions that the overworked physician has less and less time for. Preventive medicine is on the threshold of universal acceptance.

REVIEW QUESTIONS

1 How does one explain the extensive quackery problem prevalent in the United States?

2 Why does the Food and Drug Administration firmly enforce the federal regulations governing the testing of new drugs or vaccine, even when they are being used on terminal cases?

3 What can be identified as some of quackery's areas of gray? Why may this problem be of greater concern than outright quackery?

4 What is the role of the Food and Drug Administration in the protection of the consumer?

5 What are the responsibilities of the Federal Trade Commission? How is this federal agency handicapped in its efforts to carry out its assignment effectively?

6 What were the significant issues raised by the late Senator Kefauver's Senate subcommittee investigation of the drug industry?

7 What criteria should be used in the evaluation of health information and products? Identify those organizations that help the consumer in their evaluation.

8 Describe the professional preparation of the medical doctor. What kind of examination must he pass to practice in a state to become a specialist?

9 Why is the osteopathic physician generally recognized as comparable to the medical doctor who is a general practitioner?

10 Identify the various areas of specialization in dentistry. Describe the functions of each.

11 Define: (1) optician, (2) optometrist, (3) orthoptist, (4) podiatrist, (5) psychologist.

12 What have been some of the questions raised with respect to the quality of training of chiropractors?

13 What are the significant changes taking place in the organization of medical care?

14 What are the basic types of coverage found in health insurance policies?

15 Describe the factors that have resulted in the inequities of health care in this country.

16 How have the advances in the medical sciences actually resulted in greater medical care needs?

17 Describe the basic and voluntary portions of Medicare (Title 18).

18 What are the trends in medical care administration and practice? How do you envision the future practice of medicine in the United States?

7. Our Drug-Oriented Society

THERE IS EVIDENCE that drugs were used before 2100 B.C. as a way of casting out the evil spirits which were then believed to cause pain or disease. Man has not yet outgrown this era of the medicine man. He still looks for the magic potion that will cure all his ills. Just as primitive man looked with awe at his pain-relieving drugs, so modern man reflects this attitude by calling antibiotics the "miracle" drugs. Though some "primitive" medicines have been proven useful in modern-day treatment of disease (digitalis—blood vessel dilator; ephedrine—a stimulant; and reserpine—a tranquilizer) there were many of the early drugs used by man that had no real effect on the ailments they were supposed to relieve. People using them felt better simply because they thought they were being helped. This is still true today where many of the self-prescribed drugs are not effective for the ailments they are used for. Many patients pressure doctors into prescribing drugs because they feel that they "need something." They find it hard to accept that what they need is perhaps a day of rest rather than an ineffective pill. A recent report has indicated that doctors are overusing antibiotics on such a massive scale, that the so called "miracle drugs" may now be doing more harm than good. The overuse of these drugs is producing resistant strains of bacteria that in turn are responsible for thousands of deaths. Man has always had the fond dream of finding a drug that would take care of every disorder that plagued him. He would rather be told that there is a vaccine or drug that will prevent or cure a disease than be asked to follow practices related to diet, exercise, or rest that would accomplish the same thing.

The easy availability of drugs has no doubt served to provoke drug abuse. Both illegal and legal drugs have been readily available for those who have sought them. It must also be pointed out that the number of drugs made available by the pharmaceutical industry in recent decades runs in the thousands. Drugs have also been sold through television commercials as solutions to all of life's problems. They put you to sleep, wake you up, speed you up, slow you down, help you to compose yourself, take care of headaches, overeating, family problems, and so forth. In fact one advertisement indicated that they had invented a new disease. They then described some vague general symptoms and indicated they would not have invented a disease if they did not also have the cure—namely their product. The result of all this huckstering has been the development of a drug-oriented culture seeking a pill for every ill.

We have in essence turned loose in our society thousands of potent chemicals without any real attempt to inform the public *or* professionals what makes up proper use of those substances. They were in fact pushed on the public as cure-alls. Add to this the mystique that surrounds some of the illegal drugs such as LSD and marihuana and the huge profits associated with heroin-trafficking and the stage has been set for massive drug abuse.

Perhaps most curious of all are the adult drugstore junkies whose purses, pockets, and medicine cabinets are lined with a wide variety of drugs but who are so terribly concerned about the drug abuse problem amongst their youth. On the other hand we have young people who think they are doing their own thing by taking drugs without realizing how establishment-oriented they really are!! An age of technology and mass media has also been an age of noncommunication.

Figure 7–1

Drugs have often been sold to TV's captive audience as solutions to all of life's problems.

(*FDA Consumer,* December 1973–January 1974)

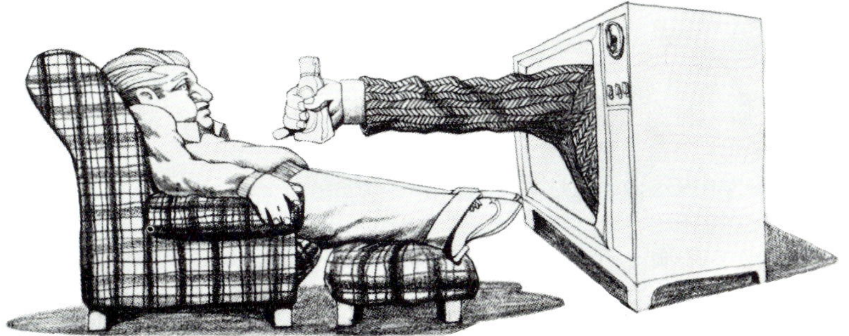

DRUGS ARE NOT ALL BAD

Significant advances have been made in the discovery of a number of chemical substances that have proved to be quite helpful in the prevention and control of many diseases. Antibiotics like penicillin destroy disease-causing bacteria. Other drugs control conditions such as arthritis or convulsions related to epilepsy. Pain-relieving drugs range from fairly simple substances like aspirin to the powerful opiates. Mood drugs such as stimulants can help individuals out of depressive states, while the tranquilizers can have a quieting effect. Other drugs help the body to get rid of excess fluids, and antihistamines are used to control allergic reactions. The effect of all this has been a major contribution to life expectancy, which has increased from 47 years in 1900 to approximately 70 years in 1966. It is estimated that more than 5 million Americans are alive today as a result of the changes in the mortality rate in the last three decades. More than 90 per cent of the prescriptions that are now written are for drugs that did not exist 25 years ago. Approximately 800 to 900 drugs are extensively used by the general public in the United States at this time.

The nature of drugs varies considerably. A number of them come from plants. Penicillin, reserpine, and quinine would serve as examples. Others are obtained from animals, as in the development of vaccines. Most drugs, however, are chemical compounds that are developed in the laboratory.

The human body is, in essence, a chemical factory that produces drugs of its own in the form of hormones and enzymes. These substances have the function of controlling various body processes such as growth, digestion, and activity. The introduction of "foreign" drugs into this chemical factory often results in unexpected reactions called *side effects* that can many times prove harmful. Side effects can be as mild as a slight rash and as severe as convulsive death. How a drug will affect a particular person can never be completely predictable, because each person's body chemistry varies. A physician's supervision in the use of more powerful drugs is naturally a wise idea. These more powerful drugs are usually classified as prescription drugs.

Prescription Drugs

Prescription drugs, also referred to as *ethical* drugs, are those that can be bought only with a prescription from a medical doctor, a doctor of dentistry, or an osteopath. The Dunham-Humphrey Amendment of the Federal Food, Drug and Cosmetic Act forbids the filling of a prescription not authorized by these professionals. Dosages of prescription drugs are based on the person's age, height, weight, and his condition of health, among other things. In essence, the drug in this case is a rather personal thing. The giving of a prescription drug to someone else because he appears to have the same or a similar ailment in effect constitutes the practice of medicine without a license.

It is at best foolhardy to attempt to diagnose an ailment when even the well-trained physician is hard put at times to accomplish this task.

Nonprescription Drugs

Nonprescription drugs are those that are sold "over the counter" or without a prescription. They are sometimes referred to as OTC drugs. The law requires that these types of drugs have directions on the label with regard to their use. These directions should be followed carefully because any drug, if misused, can have dangerous effects. Typical warnings that may appear on the label would refer to:

1. Its safe use.
2. When *not* to use it.
3. When it should be discontinued.
4. When to see a doctor.

They usually read as follows:

> Don't apply to broken skin.
>
> Do not exceed recommended dosage.
>
> Do not drive or operate machinery while taking this medication.
>
> Discontinue use if rapid pulse, dizziness, or blurring of vision occurs.
>
> WARNING
>
> If pain persists for more than 10 days or redness is present, or in conditions affecting children under 12 years of age, consult a physician immediately.

Nonprescription drugs should be used for minor and short-term ailments. Any continuing illness or symptoms should be referred to a physician. It is wise never to become a steady user of *any* drug unless it is recommended by a doctor.

DRUG ABUSE

Drug abuse refers to the inappropriate use of drugs taken without medical advice, obtained illegally, or used in amounts that constitute a danger to the individual as well as the community.

The scope of drug abuse is an ever-widening one as the number of new drugs keeps increasing. An inherent danger in the improper use of these drugs is the development of drug dependence best described in terms of drug addiction or habituation. The World Health Organization has defined these terms as follows:

> *Drug Addiction* is a state of periodic or chronic intoxication produced by

the repeated consumption of a drug (natural or synthetic). Its characteristics include:

1. an overpowering desire or need (compulsion) to continue taking the drug and to obtain it by any means;
2. a tendency to increase the dose;
3. a psychic (psychological) and generally a physical dependence on the effects of the drug;
4. an effect detrimental to the individual and to society.

Drug Habituation (habit) is a condition resulting from the repeated administration of a drug. Its characteristics include:

1. a desire (but not a compulsion) to continue taking the drug for the sense of improved well being that it engenders;
2. little or no tendency to increase the dose;
3. some degree of psychic dependence on the effect of the drug, but absence of physical dependence and hence of an abstinence syndrome;
4. a detrimental effect, if any, primarily to the individual.[1]

It is significant to note that a number of drugs that were hailed as safe when first discovered and introduced were later found to be addictive, strongly habituating, or harmful in other ways. Drugs demand a respect for their beneficial effects when properly used and for the dangers they present to health and life itself when abused. A healthy respect for drugs is not present in our society as indicated by increased drug dependence, drug misuse, and drug-related deaths.

WHO ARE THE DRUG ABUSERS?

It is often assumed by the older segments of our population that drug abuse is associated only with the young. At the same time younger groups in the population see obvious widespread instances of drug abuse among their elders. In order to draw attention to our drug-oriented society Dr. Alton Dohner identified drug abusers as follows:

> They are not all young. Neither are they all hippies, nor all hippies drug abusers. Drug abusers are physicians who recklessly prescribe amphetamines and tranquilizers rather than helping individuals learn to cope adequately with normal anxiety, frustration, depression and fatigue. Drug abusers are pharmaceutical companies who advertise their products to deal with "the everyday problems of anxiety and tension."

[1] "Report of the Task Force on Addictions," Section on Mental Health, New York State Planning Committee on Mental Disorders. June 1965.

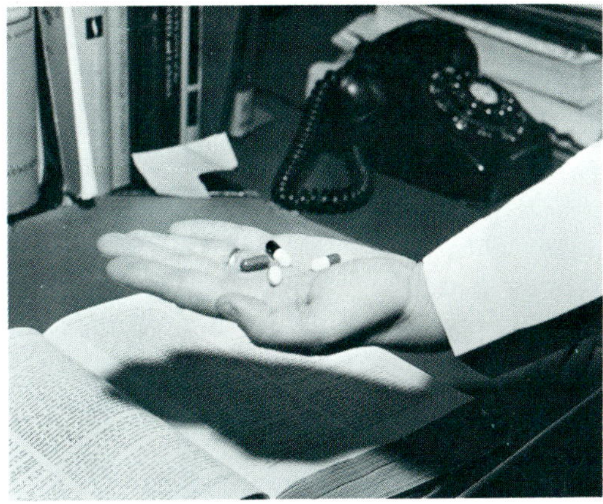

Figure 7–2

An offer of medical help or an invitation to disaster?

(New York State Health Department—M. Dixon)

> Drug abusers are truck drivers who take amphetamines for long runs; they are workers who use amphetamines to stay awake for night shifts or a second job. Drug abusers are students who use amphetamines to stay awake for studying.
>
> Drug abusers are housewives who use amphetamines to give them the energy to complete everyday chores or allegedly to cut appetite and enable them to lose weight. Drug abusers are housewives and workers who live on tranquilizers and sleeping pills. Drug abusers are parents who give tranquilizers and diet pills to their children without a physician's prescription.
>
> Drug abusers are businessmen who must have a martini with lunch; they are fathers who need a drink immediately upon returning home from the day's routine. Drug abusers are "the hidden alcoholic"—the housewives who drink several times each day.
>
> Drug abusers are persons who smoke one or more packs of cigarettes per day. They are persons who drink 10 to 16 cups of coffee or endlessly consume cola drinks each day. Drug abusers are persons who take 20 to 40 aspirin tablets daily strictly for a mood effect.
>
> Drug abusers are children and adolescents who sniff glue, gasoline, thinners and solvents. They are young people who try spices, their parents' medicines, nitrous oxide or unknown tablets in search of a high.
>
> Drug abusers are high school and college students who continue to smoke pot or take LSD, mescaline and STP for alleged consciousness-expansion. Drug abusers are social dropouts who shoot heroin or amphetamines. They are businessmen, doctors, lawyers, etc., who daily take morphine or Demerol to avoid pain. This pain may be real or imagined, social, vocational, physical or psychological.[2]

It is interesting to note that many of the motivations for drug abuse are common to young and old alike. Neither does it make much difference (from

[2] V. Alton Dohner, "Drugs Are Not the Problem," *Compact,* Vol. 4, No. 3 (June 1970), p. 21. Published by the Education Commission of the States.

a health point of view) whether a drug is a legal or illegal one. Drugs are all potentially harmful ranging from marihuana to heroin among the illegal drugs, and from aspirin to barbiturates among the legal ones. The issue of drug abuse has often been emotionalized by an attempt to identify some drugs as being those of the young (i.e., marihuana) and others associated with the adult, (i.e., alcohol). Yet surveys have shown the drug most commonly used and abused by young people is alcohol, whereas marihuana has been increasingly tried by adults. It is important to note that the issue at hand is not always drugs. In recent years the phenomenon of alienation has played a significant role in the drug scene. Groups of young people questioned and rejected the established institutions of our society such as the church, schools, government, industry, and marriage, among others. Hair styles and manner of dress differed greatly from those of the establishment. These groups also sought out drugs for use that were different from those of the establishment. Drugs such as marihuana and LSD thus became a part of new subcultures.

STIMULANT DRUGS

The *amphetamines* are usually referred to as "pep" pills. Their intake serves to stimulate the central nervous system. Because they act as body stimulants and depress appetite, they are sometimes used by overweight people. They are also used in inhalers because they help to reduce the swelling of mucous membranes when one is suffering from a common cold. The stimulant drugs help develop a sense of well-being in people suffering from feelings of depression. Overdoses of amphetamines can result in the loss of judgment. People under their influence many times feel capable of performing impossible and oftentimes dangerous feats. Students often use "pep" pills to stay awake in order to cram for an upcoming examination. The feelings of well-being developed by the drug often give the student the impression that he has done well in the exam. This is, unfortunately, too often not substantiated by the grade received. How efficient study can be under these circumstances of masked fatigue is questionable. The numbers of students who have fallen asleep during exams or missed the exam because they overslept indicate other problems that are related here. Continued abuse of the drug can also result in hallucinations and a psychotic state. It has been found that truck drivers who habitually use these drugs to stay awake on long trips will occasionally have hallucinations. They imagine that they are being attacked by animals or experience other frightening episodes and become involved in severe and tragic highway accidents. Some people who have little understanding of the potentialities of drugs will often use barbiturates to sleep and amphetamines to wake up. The alternate use of these drugs often leads to an overdosing with both, which can result in serious mental illness or barbiturate poisoning. Though the amphetamines are not addicting drugs, they are habit forming.

Thousands of women using amphetamines as a means of reducing weight often find the drug may create more problems than it solves. Because the drug reduces appetite and gives the person a feeling of well-being as an extra added reward, it can appear to be a pleasant way to lose weight. However, once the person stops taking amphetamines she usually goes back to the same old overeating and underexercising habits with a resultant weight gain. The real problem starts when that feeling of well-being becomes *the* reason for taking the drug, and the weight problem used as the excuse for needing the "medication." The question that inevitably comes to mind is if the person does not have the willpower to restrict food intake and increase physical activity, how can he have the willpower to control the use of powerful amphetamines?

The Harris-Dodd Act (an amendment to the Federal Food and Drug Act) in an attempt to control this abusive practice forbids the excessive refilling of dangerous drug prescriptions. The amphetamines and barbiturates are classified as dangerous drugs. This legislation also requires that records be kept of the manufacture, sale, and distribution of these drugs.

THE HALLUCINOGENIC DRUGS

The term *hallucinogenic* refers to a group of drugs that can affect the mind, causing visions and hallucinations. They are sometimes referred to as consciousness-expanding drugs. Some can have comparatively mild effects, but others can precipitate a psychotic state. They range from marihuana to LSD.

Marihuana

The strength of marihuana varies considerably. It is comparable to the alcoholic beverages ranging from beer to hard liquor. The active ingredient in marihuana is tetrahydrocannabinol (THC). The amount of it present determines the potency of the marihuana. The variety of marihuana (bhang—India) generally found in this country is of low potency. Ganja (India) is a higher grade of marihuana obtained from the flowering tips and leaves of the plant and is of somewhat higher potency. When the pure resin is removed from the leaves of the female *cannabis sativa* plant (a weed of the hemp family), a more potent source of THC is derived. This gummy-like substance is what *hashish* (Charas—India) is made up of and is 5 to 10 times more potent than the strongest marihuana generally found in this country.

Most of the marihuana entering the country comes from Mexico, although the plant can be grown in the United States. Marijuana is usually smoked in the form of cigarettes, causing degrees of intoxication. It creates feelings of pleasant drowsiness, visual distortions, and greater suggestibility. The person may believe he is experiencing increased sexual desire. The latter is considered related to the drug's lowering of inhibitions. In other instances, the drug may cause nervousness and anxiety.

It has been noted that marihuana will adversely affect reaction time, visual and time perception, and intelligence test scores. It also causes a reddening of the eyes. Since this is a means of identifying the marihuana smoker, dark glasses have often been used to hide this reaction. There have been instances where a person developed "pink eye," an infection of the eye and found himself in more difficulty than anticipated. Current research also indicates that marihuana apparently does not affect hearing acuity, memory, verbal or musical abilities. To date, there appear to be no long-term physical effects from marihuana smoking except for respiratory tract irritation. Those who have studied the effects of tobacco in terms of broad-scale incidence of emphysema and lung cancer predict that chronic smoking that involves inhalation will inevitably cause damage to sensitive lung tissue. They feel that this may be particularly true as related to the enforced inhalations of the marihuana smoker. Research is obviously needed to substantiate these predictions.

The psychosocial implications of marihuana use have more substantive concern related to them than the physical implications of the drug. While marihuana is not *physically* addicting, it can for some be psychologically addicting. *It is not so much the drug that has this property as it is the personality that seeks and needs a chemical escape.* At the present time there are some 9 million people who have used alcohol and ensuing alcoholism as an escape from their problems. The fear is that broad-scale unrestricted use of marihuana will exact a societal price in the form of 9 million potheads.

The stepping-stone theory has been one idea that has persisted in the minds of some people who believe that marihuana leads to the use of harder drugs. Pharmacologically there is nothing in marihuana that would lead to heroin use. It may be that those who seek chemical solutions to personal problems are unsatisfied with marihuana and thus seek out harder drugs. One positive correlation that does exist is that those buying marihuana place themselves in contact with the illegal drug market who have harder drugs as part of their wares.

Laws related to marihuana have in recent years become more lenient, helping to break it away from its undeserved categorization with drugs as potent as heroin. In 1972 the National Commission on Marihuana and Drug Abuse recommended that legal penalties be exacted only for those selling the drug and eliminating penalties for the user. There are some groups who take the stand that the only alternative is the legalization of marihuana. The latter does not appear to be an action that will be taken until more extensive short- and long-term research on marihuana and its more potent cousin, hashish, have been conducted. The liberalization of marihuana laws to make them more compatible with the pharmacological effects of the drug will probably be a continued trend.

Mescaline, Psilocybin, LSD: The More Potent Hallucinogens

The sources of the more potent hallucinogens vary, although their effects are similar. Mescaline is derived from the buttons or tops of the peyote cactus found in the southwestern part of the United States and in Mexico. Psilocybin, a somewhat more potent drug, comes from the Mexican mushroom (Psilocybe Mexicana). Some of the people of Mexico and Central America have used mushrooms during religious ceremonies, just as southwestern Indians have the peyote buttons. The purpose of the drug in these ceremonies is to bring the person into closer contact with these peoples' concept of God.

LSD (lysergic acid diethylamide tartrate) is a derivative of ergot, a rye fungus, and can also be produced synthetically. Though tasteless, odorless, and colorless when dissolved in water, it is one of the most powerful chemical agents known to man. One ounce of LSD can serve as an average dose for 300,000 people. The drug was discovered by Dr. Albert Hofmann, a Swiss chemist, in 1938. It was not until 1943 that Dr. Hofmann accidentally ingested some of the drug and experienced, as a result, fantastic visions which included a kaleidoscopic array of vivid colors, with objects appearing wavy and deformed. Occasionally he felt as though he were outside his own body. Other descriptions of the drug's effects include the following:

> The marked heightening of the sensation of color is usually one of the first manifestations, so that ordinary reds and blues, for example, become astoundingly vivid and flowing. New colors, difficult to put into appropriate words, are seen. They swirl around the individual with great vividness. Fixed objects fuse and diffuse; there is often a perpetual flowing of geometric designs and one sensation merges into another and one sense into another so that the individual may say he can taste color; touch sound. The body image is distorted and ordinary sounds increase profoundly in intensity. There is a sense of intense isolation and depersonalization so that "me" as an individual disappears and the user feels he is fused with all humanity and with his environment.[3]

Some regard the experience as an erotic one, while others attach religious meanings to it, claiming a better understanding of God, the universe, life, and death. Under the influence of the drug there appears in some instances to be the ability to look into one's unconscious. In experimental work that is being done, psychiatrists are attempting to use this phenomenon as a way of helping mental patients and alcoholics to develop greater insight into their emotional problems. To date the use of LSD in treating emotional problems has not proved promising.

Although some LSD reactions are pleasurable others are not. Some people have experienced the most terrifying of hallucinations, mental disorganization,

[3] Donald Louria, M.D., *Nightmare Drugs* (New York: Pocket Books, 1966), pp. 45–46.

and overwhelming feelings of panic. The unstable personality seems to be most negatively affected by the drug in uncontrolled situations. It also appears to be this kind of personality who is most attracted to the illicit use of LSD or other hallucinogens. The result may be a prolonged psychotic condition in the user. The effects of the drug may also recur weeks later without the taking of additional amounts of the substance. One user suddenly became a flying horse a month after an LSD episode. Fortunately, the users of the drug have generally been the immature, who do not have serious responsibility for others. One shudders at the thought of having one's surgeon or airline pilot suddenly become preoccupied with kaleidoscopic swirls of vivid colors, touch sound, taste color, and feel literally beside himself. If we were to become a society of "acid heads" (LSD users), who would be left to watch the store?

The illicit use of LSD has alarmed health authorities and legislators alike. The result has been that Congress has passed legislation providing strong penalties for the manufacture, sale, or possession of the drug. A number of states, including New York, California, and Nevada, have enacted similar laws. An unfortunate effect of the sensationalism that has surrounded LSD is the suppression of research. Researchers often do not want to "get involved" when this kind of interest is associated with a drug. The federal government is currently serving as the LSD source for a small group of highly qualified researchers.

THE ADDICTING DRUGS

Barbiturates

Barbiturate drugs are sedative, prescription drugs that are used medically to help people to relax and sleep. (The names of these drugs usually end in "al," as in phenobarbital, luminal, nembutal.) In larger doses than would be normally prescribed they can cause an intoxication similar to that caused by alcohol. Continued unsupervised use of barbiturates has been found to lead to addiction. Related to its misuse has been an increase in the incidence of barbiturate poisoning, which is a leading cause of death by poisoning. A person intoxicated with barbiturate drugs is irresponsible and capable of swallowing a handful of pills that will cause his death. Many such deaths are listed as suicides. It has also been discovered that barbiturates and alcohol make a dangerous combination. The taking of a moderate dose of barbiturates after a few alcoholic drinks may cause death. Because of the relatively easy access to these drugs, some authorities fear that barbiturate addiction may be more widespread than realized in our society. The number of barbiturate addicts that we have in this country is unknown. Estimates indicate that they may be in the many thousands.

The AMA has categorized abusers of barbiturates into four groups:

1. Those who deal with emotional stress by sedating themselves, sometimes right out of this world.
2. Those who have developed a tolerance for the drug and can tolerate large doses which produce feelings of excitation rather than depression. The reaction is similar to that experienced with amphetamines.
3. Those who use the drug to counteract the effects of other drugs such as LSD or amphetamines.
4. Those who use the drug with other depressant drugs such as alcohol or heroin. The combined use of depressants produces a more instant "high." This combination of drugs is particularly dangerous. One must question the presence of the conscious or unconscious motivation to commit suicide or the influence of blatant ignorance.

The withdrawal illness associated with barbiturate addiction is more severe than with any of the opiate drugs. The sudden withdrawal of barbiturates from an addicted person will usually result in convulsions and a temporary psychosis. It may even result in death. The addicted person who attempts to withdraw from the drug on his own is risking his life. Withdrawal from the drug even under medical supervision is tricky and may take as long as two months.

Methaqualone

Methaqualone is a drug that is not a barbiturate but produces similar effects on the body. It appears on the market under the brand names of Quaalude, Sopor, and Optimil, among others. Medically, methaqualone is prescribed for sleeplessness. The *Physicians' Desk Reference,* which publishes drug information provided by drug companies, described it as a drug which only occasionally caused psychological dependence with physical dependence rarely reported. Drug companies' advertising depicted the drug as nonaddicting and the fact that it is not a barbiturate caused thousands to use the drug for recreational purposes, resulting in a widespread faddish use. Abuse of the drug, however, soon demonstrated it to be a dangerous addicting drug. It is now described by pharmacologists to be chemically different from barbiturates but pharmacologically the equivalent.

The heavy abuser of methaqualone who abruptly stops the intake of the drug will go into convulsions. As stated by Dr. Craig Whitehead of the Haight-Ashbury Clinic, "If convulsions aren't treated, you risk status epilepticus developing. That means one grand mal seizure after another—and if they aren't broken, the body will expire of exhaustion."[4]

Methaqualone, like barbiturates, can be particularly dangerous when taken in combination with alcohol. Many of the fatalities attributed to the abuse

[4] *Connection,* "Bigger than Marijuana Methaqualone: Dangerous New Abuse Fad Sweeping West?," Institute for Social Concerns, Oakland, Calif., p. 4.

TABLE 7–1

Common Drugs—Used and Abused

	Drugs	General information	Medical use	Signs and Symptoms of drug abuse
STIMULANTS	Amphetamines	Called pep pills, bennies and co-pilots. Can cause distorted images. Disguises fatigue. Methamphetamine (Methedrine) referred to as "Speed," often taken by injection.	Appetite suppressant	User will exhibit a great deal of nervous energy and will have difficulty sleeping. When effects of the drug wear off, the individual will have a feeling of depression which is referred to as "post amphetamine depression" or the Crash.
	Cocaine	Very strong stimulant. Extracted chemically from the leaves of Coca bush in South America. Can cause excessive excitement and uncontrollable behavior.	Local anesthetic	Cocaine is an extremely strong stimulant but is not used very often by the drug dependent person because of its high cost.
HALLUCINOGENS	LSD	Lysergic acid diethylamide. Most potent hallucinogen. Made in the laboratory. Causes different reactions in different people. A very unpredictable substance. No known way of knowing who will react badly and who will not. Harmful effects can be prolonged and sometimes permanent.	None	Effects of the hallucinogens are unpredictable. Reaction to use of these drugs ranges from mild nausea and hallucinations to prolonged insanity.
	Mescaline	Derived from the Mexican cactus Peyote. Causes hallucinations.	None	
	Psilocybin	Derived from certain mushrooms found in Mexico. Causes hallucinations.	None	
	DMT	Dimethyltryptamine. A new hallucinogen. made synthetically. Also found within certain plants.	None	

	Marijuana	Classified as a mild hallucinogen. Made from the flowering tops and leaves of the female plant. Main ingredient THC (tetrahydrocannabinol) synthesized recently. Much research is taking place concerning its effects. Resin extracted from the Marijuana plant (Cannabis) is called Hashish.	None	Effect of this drug depends on the individual, the parts of the plant used and climate in which it is grown; stronger varieties of marijuana can produce hallucinations.
DEPRESSANTS	Barbiturates	Referred to as "Goof Balls." Named for its color—"Yellow-Jackets," "Pinks," and "Rainbows" etc.	To induce sleep	The effect of depressants resemble alcoholic intoxication. Behavior is one of confusion and drowsiness and the thinking process is quite dull. Muscular control is uncoordinated; walking and reaching for objects becomes difficult. Staggering like a "punch drunk" person can become a permanent effect.
	Non-barbiturate sedatives	Doriden, Noludar, Methaqualone Developed as substitutes for Barbiturates.	To induce sleep	
	Tranquilizers	Miltown, Valium, Librium, Thorazine.	Relieve nervous tension and treat mental illness	
	Glue and others	Generally abused by young people. Brain damage likely with continued use.	None	
OPIATES	Morphine	Extracted from Opium. Used as a standard by which the other pain relievers are measured.	Pain relief	Drowsiness, restlessness, nausea and loss of weight accompany the effects of opiate abuse. Personal neglect, malnutrition and infection are signs that occur after extended use of opiates. Frequently you will find needle scars from repeated injections—particularly with heroin.
	Heroin	A derivative of morphine and a source of hard core drug addictions. Illegal in U.S.A. under all circumstances.	None in U.S.A.	
	Codeine	Extracted from Opium. An ingredient of some cough syrups.	Pain relief	
	Demerol	Synthetic. Used widely in medicine. Effective pain reliever.	Pain relief	
	Methadone	Synthetic. Used in the treatment of addicts.	Pain relief	

 Drug chart appears in *Decision* (Junior High Edition) and *The Drug Society* (Senior High Edition).

of this drug have occurred when the drug was used with alcoholic beverages. Research has also found the drug to cause skeletal abnormalities in the offspring of rats given the drug. Its use by pregnant women is therefore discouraged. More recently even the medicinal value of the drug has been questioned by physicians.

Tranquilizers

Tranquilizers were first introduced about 20 years ago. Their initial use was for the treatment of the mental patient. The tranquilizing effect of the drugs made the patient more receptive to psychotherapy, as well as blunting agitation caused by his emotional problem. In recent years there has been proliferate use of these substances with approximately a half million pounds of tranquilizers used each year in the United States. This is no doubt reflective of a great deal of self-doting, of the inability of people to "endure" normal nervousness. This "sick" national attitude is often aided and abetted by the family physician too willing to prescribe such drugs.

To date, six tranquilizers have been found to be capable of addiction. The biggest problem related to these drugs is their strong habituating quality. The lethargic, tranquil attitudes and lack of coordination often induced by the drug have been responsible for many automobile accidents. The intake of large amounts of alcohol in combination with tranquilizing drugs can pose a serious threat to the health of the individual. In fact, it may precipitate an unplanned eternity of tranquility; this combination has in some instances caused death.

Tranquilizers provide the same dangers to the individual as do the barbiturates. They are addicting when abused, and withdrawal from them can prove deadly. Their massive use indicates the extent to which we have as a society attempted to avoid normal anxiety and stress. Where anxiety and stress are reflective of deep-seated problems, the drug merely masks the symptoms without resolving the causative factors. The physician who overprescribes the drug has also ducked the needed therapy. The busy, harried physician does not have the time to discuss one's personal problems. It simply becomes easier to prescribe a "miracle drug."

Opiates

Opiates are obtained from the milky juice of the unripe seed pod of the opium poppy. All drugs derived from opium are addicting and tend to have a depressant effect on the central nervous system. Though they have no curative value, they can serve to relieve pain. *Morphine* is the opiate most commonly used medically for this purpose. It is given under careful medical supervision if addiction is not to take place. As with the other opiates, a tolerance can be developed for the drug, requiring larger and larger doses to obtain the same effect. Morphine is sometimes used by addicts; however, the more "popular" opiate used for this purpose is heroin.

Heroin is a white powder that is made from morphine. When first developed, heroin was thought to be nonaddicting. Actually, however, it is so powerful and addicting that it cannot be used even for medical purposes in the United States. One grain of the drug taken over a two-week period can cause addiction. The addict injects the heroin into a vein in order to produce its desired effects. The use of unsterilized needles by the addict often results in the transmission of such serious diseases as malaria, hepatitis, and syphilis. The strength of the adulterated heroin that reaches the addict cannot be predicted. The underworld dilutes the heroin with milk sugar to the extent of 95 per cent. If the drug reaching the addict is less dilute than usual and is too strong, the user's "normal" dose may kill him. If, on the other hand, it is too weak, it will not relieve the addict's developing symptoms of withdrawal illness. The addict is essentially at the mercy of the underworld in what has become his most important commodity. The physical dependence on the drug causes the body to react in its absence. The symptoms of the withdrawal illness that follow resemble those of the flu, with the person experiencing chills, tearing eyes, running nose, aching and twitching arms and legs, followed by diarrhea and vomiting. Severe cramps develop in the arms, legs, stomach, and back, which cause the person to assume a curled-up position. The peak of the withdrawal symptoms is reached in 24 to 30 hours. A dose of the drug is good for only 4 to 8 hours; the addict lives in constant fear of the withdrawal illness. He is therefore strongly motivated to steal or, in the case of women, to resort to prostitution for sources of income. Maintaining the heroin habit may cost as much as $50 to $100 a day.

Poor social conditions appear to be a breeding ground for heroin addiction. They create the climate for anxiety, frustration, and broken homes. The social pathology produces underdeveloped personalities, lacking discipline and dreaming of unrealistic goals. The euphoric effects of heroin, therefore, become very attractive. Once hooked on heroin, the addict centers all his activities on getting his next needed supply.

DRUG TRAFFIC

Raw opium is gathered by Turkish farmers and is converted into a morphine base before being shipped to Italy and France. There it is converted to heroin and then smuggled into the United States. Approximately two pounds of raw opium can be bought for about $350 from Turkish farmers. After it has been converted into heroin and diluted, it is then sold to addicts for a half million dollars. The price of heroin is many times that of gold. The Federal Bureau of Narcotics, which is a part of the United States Treasury Department, has stationed agents around the world in its attempts to reduce the heroin traffic into the United States. This country is the principal target of the illegal narcotics trade, with New York City being the largest addiction center. The United Nations has made attempts to establish a controlling agency for all opiate drugs in world trade. Small countries that produce opium, however, receive a large income from the illegal sale of these drugs. This vested interest has been an inhibiting factor in the development of an international control agency. More recently the United States has made attempts to work with individual countries to effect a reduction in heroin traffic. Farmers are being encouraged to substitute other crops for the poppy.

In this country, participation in illegal drug trade carries heavy penalties, particularly where sales to a minor are involved. The sentence may run from 10 to 40 years' imprisonment and up to $20,000 in fines. A special penalty for the sale of heroin to a minor may include life imprisonment or even death if a jury so decides.

A great deal of concern, talk, and action has been precipitated by illegal drug traffic, with the greatest focus on heroin. At the same time comparatively little concern has been expressed about those drugs produced by the American pharmaceutical industry, such as amphetamines and barbiturates, that find their way into the illegal market. Some estimates indicate that only 10 per cent of the amphetamines produced in the United States is needed for medical reasons; the rest either finds its way into the illegal market or is overprescribed by physicians. Since amphetamines and barbiturates can be even more harmful than heroin, controlling their traffic becomes at least as important.

Approximately 8 billion amphetamine pills are manufactured in the United States each year. This is equal to 40 pills for every man, woman, and child. Senator Claude Pepper, Chairman of the Crime Committee, has suggested that the Attorney General with the advice and counsel of the Secretary of Health, Education and Welfare set production limits on this drug. In October of 1972, Senator Pepper managed to get his proposal through the Senate but it was killed in the House of Representatives. Senator Pepper blamed this on drug industry lobbying. He reported that the American Pharmaceutical Association has a 70-member staff in Washington and a budget of over $3.5 million.

The AMA Committee on Alcoholism and Addiction has reported that the current production of all sedatives far exceeds medical needs, with over 6 billion capsules a year being produced. These drugs are often taken by individuals in a weakened psychological state which makes them more vulnerable to abuse such drugs. Large amounts of both amphetamines and barbiturates are shipped out of the country only to return as part of the illegal drug market.

DEALING WITH THE DRUG PROBLEM

A traditional approach to a health problem has been to wait for the person to become ill, then attempt to treat and rehabilitate him. The drug abuse area has been no different even though little is known about effective treatment. The rehabilitation of the heroin addict requires much more than removing him from his physical dependence on the drug. The addict is a person who is often a product of a poor social environment and who has spent all his time "hustling" (stealing) and "shooting up" (injecting heroin). His rehabilitation therefore hinges on his acceptance and preparation for a new life-style. He must develop a marketable occupational skill and discipline himself to accept the regimen of a working society. His desire for a new way of life must be strong enough for him to view heroin addiction as a threat to a good thing. Effecting that kind of dramatic change is not easy. The success rates of treatment and rehabilitation programs have therefore been understandably poor.

Methadone Maintenance Programs

Methadone is an addicting, synthetic, narcotic drug. Its pharmacological properties are quite similar to those of heroin. Methadone has the ability to block the euphoric high the addict gets from heroin as well as to prevent withdrawal symptoms from heroin. Methadone thus blocks the physical need for heroin. With this as a crutch, time is provided to help the addict develop psychologically, socially, and vocationally. Where successful, the addict finds a steady job, supports his family, and becomes a productive member of society.

Since methadone is itself addictive, the addict is really switched from heroin addiction to addiction of a more manageable drug. He must, however, take a daily dose of methadone usually dissolved in orange juice or a similar beverage. Some people have compared the addict maintained on methadone to the diabetic who needs a dose of insulin daily to maintain his normal functioning.

The long-term effects of methadone use is as yet undetermined. Evidence indicates that alcohol use in combination with methadone can cause liver damage as well as other toxic effects. Since many addicted to heroin also abuse alcohol, screening out such individuals from methadone programs is imperative. Some researchers report that studies of brain tissue of methadone users (whose causes of death have been attributed to drug overdose) have shown abnormalities indicating early senile changes usually found in much older people.

A problem on the increase is the rising incidence of methadone-addicted babies born to mothers on a methadone maintenance program. Indications are that withdrawing these infants from methadone may be more difficult than withdrawal from heroin. This presents an additional facet to an already complex problem.

The shifting of a person's addiction to what is considered a less harmful drug can be viewed as progress, but it certainly is an incomplete answer to the problem. The success rate for the treatment of drug addiction has been highly questionable, with a small percentage truly rehabilitated. Methadone maintenance may prove to be a step forward in this area. It is hoped, of course, that continued research will bring more adequate answers to the problem. Prevention, however, still remains as the best *cure* to any problem.

Drug Abuse: A Social-Health Problem—Not a Legal-Moral One

In the United States we have viewed the drug abuse problem as a legal-moral problem rather than the social-health problem that it is.

A young person (preferably bearded) in possession of marihuana may be legally incarcerated, whereas the person (preferably white, older, middle-class) becoming addicted to a legal drug such as a barbiturate is on the verge of self-destruction with no one about to intercede. The societal judgments in the drug field appear to be made on the basis of legality and the particular values and life-style of the person in question. The effect on the health of the person appears to be a most secondary consideration.

An example of this is the expectant, heroin-addicted woman who enters the hospital without revealing her addiction. Shortly after having the child she leaves the hospital to seek out heroin before the withdrawal symptoms set in. Estimates are 50 to 90 per cent of children born to addicted mothers will exhibit withdrawal symptoms. It is also estimated that deaths among the untreated drug-dependent newborn runs as high as 96 per cent. It would seem that it was neither the intent of the mothers in these cases or society to so punish these innocent newborn. Does the legal-moral approach, then, have the opposite effects than intended? Does it also produce a hysterical environment with people feeling that crime is rampant but not knowing what the crime is, who is performing it, and where it is being performed? It would seem important to define the problem carefully so that it is understood and can be reacted to objectively and constructively.

This means that schools and universities need to develop programs that focus in on the motivations for drug abuse and the psychosocial issues surrounding it. Communities need to become much more knowledgeable of the *real* issues in the drug abuse field and the individual and societal responsibilities each person has in helping to develop an environment in which constructive action *can* take place. This means recognizing the problems of legal drugs, and adult drug abuse, among others. It also means a more responsible news media who are interested in accurate reporting rather than sensationalism that sells newspapers and air time. It also means putting to eternal rest the political rhetoric that daily declares war on drugs as though these inert substances were "the enemy." It is time that each of us began to really understand the underlying causes of drug abuse and, more important, to recognize constructive alternatives for ourselves and others.

Despite the criticisms we may level at the mismanagements of the drug problem by government, by news media, by industrial self-interest, and by a variety of inept community groups, when all is said and done, Pogo, the comic strip character, probably summarized the situation best when he stated, "We have met the enemy, and they is us!"

ALCOHOL

Man has been using some form of alcoholic beverage since the beginning of history. The natural fermentation of fruit and vegetable juices and cereal mashes provided him with his first sources of such beverages. Brewed beers and fermented wines have been a part of Western culture for over two thousand years. Distilled beverages (whiskeys) were first introduced in Europe about A.D. 1500.

There is evidence that the Romans gave their victims wine before executing them as a way of dulling the agony and anticipation of death. This was referred to as the "wine of the condemned," and was considered a merciful use of the beverage. Its use has more often been related to important occasions such as weddings and births, and to religious ceremonies. For some people it is simply a beverage that is part of the family meal; for some others, however, it is a means of escaping life's problems.

The attitudes of people toward alcohol are as varied as the nature of its uses. Some view any use of alcohol as being highly immoral, whereas others see nothing wrong with its use in moderation. Inebriation is alternately viewed as something humorous, disgusting, or as a sign of illness (alcoholism). Our attitudes with regard to alcohol and its use become rather personal in nature and are dependent on our experiences, what others close to us think, and what we know about it.

WHY PEOPLE DRINK

While millions of people can drink alcoholic beverages without apparent harm to themselves or others, there are approximately 19 million people in the United States (10 per cent of the American work force) who have serious drinking problems. Why some people get into difficulty with alcohol while others do not has been a question for which there have not been clear answers. While research is looking for the answers it seems ironic that most people who drink alcohol do not know that they are drinking a potentially addicting drug.

The importance of this simple fact is underscored by sociological research that points out, "countries with a high overall consumption of alcohol have high rates of alcoholism and countries with a low overall consumption have low rates of alcoholism."[5]

[5] Report on the Governor's Conference on Alcohol Problems (November 1971), p. 45.

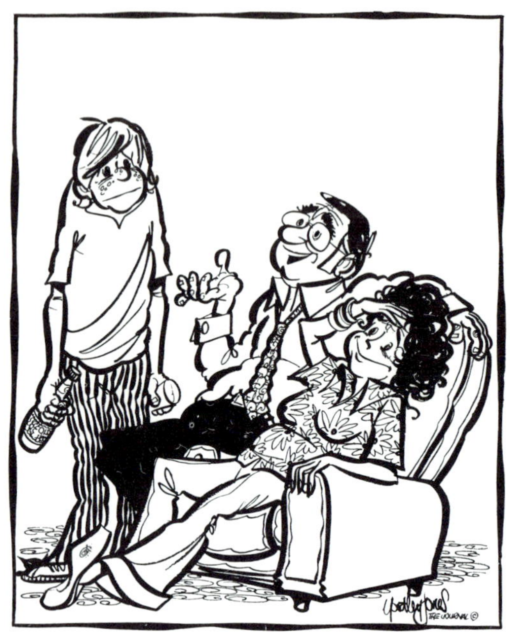

Figure 7–3

"Thank heavens son! When you said you had an addiction problem we thought it was drugs."

(The Journal, October 3, 1973. Published by The Addiction Research Foundation, Toronto.)

The rate of alcoholism in France is ten times that of Finland, Norway, or the Netherlands. The consumption rates of alcohol are also comparable. If alcoholism were to be regarded as the result of emotional disturbance and personality disorder, then the incidence of these conditions should be ten times higher in France than in the other countries. It clearly is not.

It would seem important to view patterns of alcohol use in the United States from the point of view of frequency of use and amounts of alcohol consumed.

> The United States is one of the world's chief consumers of alcoholic beverages. Beer, this nation's most popular alcoholic beverage, is consumed at a rate approximating 22 gallons per person annually. Distilled spirits, with a consumption rate of almost 2 gallons per person per year, makes wine the third choice of Americans. Here the rate is less than 1.51 gallons. The rate of consumption for absolute alcohol, regardless of the beverage in which it is contained, is a little over 2 gallons per year for each person over 15 years of age in the United States.[6]

In some cases many have concluded that the use of alcoholic beverages with meals is a wholesome practice. In accepting a dinner invitation it is not unusual to find oneself exposed to several predinner drinks, several wines during dinner,

[6] Marvin A. Block, *Alcohol and Alcoholism,* Basic Concepts in Health Science Series (Belmont, Calif.: Wadsworth, 1970), p. 9.

an after-dinner drink and as many after, after-dinner drinks as one cares to attempt to handle. It would seem appropriate at any social gathering where alcoholic beverages will be served that nonalcoholic beverages also be available. The person choosing the nonalcoholic beverage should not be made to feel defensive about his choice as though he were selecting the much less desirable kind of drink.

If one travels and flies first class, he will find himself treated to four ounces of liquor on each leg of his trip. If there are enough legs on the trip, one could very well arrive without one to stand on. An increasing cause of concern is whether the automobile ride home at the end of the plane trip isn't becoming the most dangerous part of the trip because of the degree of drinking on the plane.

Additionally an increasing number of people have invested a significant amount of space and money to build a bar in the home. Some of these have been motivated by Hollywood films that depict a "bar in the home" as the possession of the wealthy, and therefore becomes a sought-after status symbol. In other instances people relate alcohol use to pleasure and bring it to closer proximity with all the fixings. And eventually some use the bar in the home as the vehicle for becoming the neighborhood pusher.

The drinking patterns of the United States seem to be a combination of those found in Europe and other parts of the world. Some Americans drink alcoholic beverages with their meals as do the French and Italian. Others seek intoxication as do the Irish and Finns. In addition, we have made drinking a part of a round of golf, the closing of a business deal, a way to pass an afternoon or evening, to celebrate an occasion, to mourn an occasion, to greet a friend, to say goodbye to a friend; in essence drinking has become a part of many of our everyday activities significantly increasing the number of occasions for alcohol use. As an extra added attraction, whiskey-flavored toothpaste and rum-flavored pipe tobacco are now available.

Despite the great amount of drinking in our society, it is estimated that approximately one-third of our adult population does not drink. The reasons for this abstinence usually include religious convictions, feelings that drinking will injure health, and also that alcohol can present many different kinds of personal problems these adults would just as soon avoid.

Another group includes the moderate drinkers whose drinking would range from an occasional drink for a family celebration to fairly frequent drinking with meals and at social occasions several times a week. The reasons given for drinking in this group include a desire for relaxation, the need for a mealtime beverage, and the belief that drinking acts as a social relaxant. Most are seeking the pleasant glow and release from tension that moderate amounts of alcohol intake can produce. How often, how persistently, and with what intensity some pursue the use of alcohol as a social relaxant determine their dependence on, or their independence from, this drug.

In an additional group is the drinker who feels he cannot have a good time without an alcoholic beverage. He also accords to drinking a certain status. It makes him feel important. He looks forward to the time when he can drink because of the satisfactions it brings him, whether the drinking be with friends or alone. This person is not an alcoholic and he may possibly never become one, but he could be identified as a type of prealcoholic. This person has woven some of his basic psychological needs around alcohol, which forms a rather unstable structure.

> In general, research has shown that for groups that use alcohol to a significant degree, the lowest incidence of alcoholism is associated with certain habits and attitudes:
>
> 1. The children are exposed to alcohol early in life, within a strong family or religious group. Whatever the beverage, it is served in very diluted form and in small quantities, with consequent low blood-alcohol levels.
> 2. The beverages commonly although not invariably used by the groups are those containing relatively large amounts of non-alcoholic components, which also give low blood-alcohol levels.
> 3. The beverage is considered mainly as a food and usually consumed with meals, again with consequent low blood-alcohol levels.
> 4. Parents present a constant example of moderate drinking.
> 5. No moral importance is attached to drinking. It is considered neither a virtue nor a sin.
> 6. Drinking is not viewed as a proof of adulthood or virility.
> 7. Abstinence is socially acceptable. It is no more rude or ungracious to decline a drink than to decline a piece of bread.
> 8. Excessive drinking or intoxication is not socially acceptable. It is not considered stylish, comical or tolerable.
> 9. Finally, and perhaps most important, there is wide and usually complete agreement among members of the group on what might be called the ground rules of drinking.[7]

ALCOHOL AS A DRUG

Scientists classify drugs according to the effect they have on the body.

Sedative. This type of drug has a quieting effect, relieving tension.

Analgesic. Analgesics relieve pain without producing sleep (aspirin).

Anesthetic. This type of drug will bring about the loss of sensation to pain.

[7] *Alcohol and Alcoholism,* National Institute of Mental Health Public Health Service Publication No. 1640, 1970, p. 28.

Alcohol can act as a sedative in small amounts and as an analgesic in even smaller quantities, with its most characteristic effect being that of an anesthetic. Describing a person who has had too much to drink as "feeling no pain" is apparently quite apt.

ALCOHOLIC BEVERAGES

Three basic types of alcoholic beverages are used, namely beers, wines, and distilled liquors.

Beer is made by boiling a broth of cereal grains such as barley, wheat, or corn. In these cereal grains, sugar is in the form of starch. Malt is first added to the broth, and this has the effect of changing the starch to sugar. Yeast is then added so that the sugar can be fermented into alcohol. The fermentation process in the making of beer is interrupted, with the result that beer has approximately a 4 per cent alcohol content in this country. Hops, which are a small bitter fruit, are added to the beer to add to its flavor.

Wine is made from the juices of vegetables, fruits, or berries whose taste and color vary to a great extent. Most wines, however, are made from grapes. Because fermentation usually stops at about 14 per cent, most wines will have about that level of alcohol in them. Some wines are referred to as fortified wines when additional alcohol is added to bring the alcoholic content up to 18 or 20 per cent. Those wines that contain no sugar are called "dry." Sparkling wines are those that contain CO_2 gas produced in the fermentation process. Producers permit some of the CO_2 to remain in order to produce this bubbling effect.

Distilled liquors are made through the process of distillation. It is known that various liquids have different boiling points; therefore, alcohol in solution with water can be separated out by heating the entire solution. Alcohol, having a lower boiling temperature, would evaporate off first. If this vapor is then passed through a cooling tube, the alcohol vapor is condensed back into a liquid that is pure alcohol. Whiskey is distilled from fermented cereals or grains such as rye, corn, and barley. Rum can be distilled from fermented molasses; brandy is distilled from wines. Gin is nothing more than alcohol flavored with berries, and vodka is plain, diluted alcohol. Distilled beverages contain from 40 to 50 per cent alcohol. This is usually expressed in terms of degrees of proof. In other words, a 90 proof beverage would contain 45 per cent alcohol. The type of alcohol found in beer, wine, and distilled spirits is ethyl alcohol. There are, of course, many other kinds of alcohol that are used for commercial and industrial purposes such as methyl, butyl, and propyl. These types of alcohol are poisonous to drink and if taken internally may result in death, blindness, or other tragic outcomes.

THE EFFECTS OF ALCOHOL ON THE BODY

The effects that alcohol will have on the body are variable and dependent on many factors. For example these will vary depending on whether the beverage is taken on an empty stomach or with food, or whether the individual is a light drinker or a heavy drinker. The same amount of alcohol will have differing effects on a person as compared to another and may even differ in the same individual from week to week. The absorption of alcohol takes place quickly from the stomach and continues mostly from the small intestine. The level of alcohol in the blood (or blood-alcohol concentrations) thus absorbed will depend on:

1. *Presence of food in the stomach.* The presence of protein and fat in the stomach, particularly, slow down the absorption of alcohol.
2. *Alcohol concentration.* The highest blood-alcohol levels are produced most rapidly by undiluted, distilled spirits (particularly vodka and gin), whereas the alcohol in wines and beers is absorbed more slowly. This is due to the fact that wines and beers contain additional chemicals or food substances. If a beverage is diluted with water or juice the rate of absorption is diminished. However, the presence of carbon dioxide in the stomach, such as in sparkling wines, champagnes, soda, or ginger ale, increases the rate of absorption.
3. *Speed of Drinking.* Sipping or drinking moderate amounts will keep blood-alcohol concentrations lower than if the beverage is consumed in one gulp.
4. *Body Weight.* If a standard amount of alcohol is consumed by two men, one weighing 200 lb and another weighing 140 lb, the blood-alcohol concentration in the heavier man will be less than that in the smaller man.

If a person of average height and weight were to quickly ingest three ounces of whiskey, this would result in a .06 per cent level of alcohol in the blood. This level of alcohol would begin to affect the judgment of the person, and signs of sedation, and tranquility would take place. The feeling of warmth that ensues is due to the dilation of the body's surface blood vessels. While this causes a feeling of warmth on the surface of the body it also results in a loss of body heat. Those who take alcoholic beverages to keep warm during outdoor, winter activities are actually causing the opposite effect than desired and will ultimately feel colder. If the person were to continue to drink, he would then reach the next level of impairment. This would include slurred speech and poor muscle control, and the person would probably stagger,

TABLE 7-2

Some Effects of Alcoholic Beverages*[1]

Amount of beverage	Concentration of alcohol attained in the blood	Effects	Time required for all alcohol to leave the body
1 highball (1½ oz. whisky) or 1 cocktail (1½ oz. whisky) or 3½ oz. fortified wine or 5½ oz. ordinary wine or 2 bottles (24 oz.) beer	0.03%	Slight changes in feeling	2 hrs.
2 highballs or 2 cocktails or 7 oz. fortified wine or 11 oz. ordinary wine or 4 bottles beer	0.06%	Increasing effects with variation among individuals and in the same individual at different times Feeling of warmth—mental relaxation, slight decrease of fine skills—less concern with minor irritations and restraints	4 hrs.
3 highballs or 3 cocktails or 10½ oz. fortified wine or 16½ oz. (1 pt.) ordinary wine or 6 bottles beer	0.09%	Buoyancy—exaggerated emotion and behavior—talkative, noisy or morose	6 hrs.
4 highballs or 4 cocktails or 14 oz. fortified wine or 22 oz. ordinary wine or 8 bottles (3 qts.) beer	0.12%	Impairment of fine coördination—clumsiness—slight to moderate unsteadiness in standing or walking	8 hrs.
5 highballs or 5 cocktails or 17½ oz. fortified wine or 27½ oz. ordinary wine or ½ pt. whisky	0.15%	Intoxication—unmistakable abnormality of gross bodily functions and mental faculties	10 hrs.

*Source: Rutgers Center of Alcohol Studies.

[1] Based on a person of "average" size (150 pounds). For those weighing considerably more or less, the amount would have to be respondingly more or less to produce the same results. The effects indicated at each stage will diminish as the concentration of alcohol in the blood is reduced by being oxidized and eliminated.

possibly fall and have difficulty rising. If the alcohol level in the blood were then to reach a .40 per cent level, the person would lose consciousness and would be regarded as being "dead drunk." It takes more than a pint of whiskey for the average person to reach this stage. If the concentration of alcohol were to reach .50 per cent, the person would be in a deep coma and in serious danger of death. As the level of alcohol in the blood approached 1 per cent the breathing center of the brain would become paralyzed and death would follow.

Once the alcohol is absorbed by the blood, the rate at which the body uses or gets rid of the alcohol will depend on the actions of the liver. It can use up approximately one ounce of 80 proof whiskey in an hour or one-half ounce of pure alcohol in that period of time. If the alcohol intake is progressing at a faster rate than the liver can use it up then the level of alcohol in the blood would naturally rise.

The effects of alcohol on the liver are complex and not well defined. Cirrhosis of the liver occurs in about 10 per cent of alcoholic patients, or about eight times as frequently among alcoholics. Though it is a frequent result of excessive drinking, it does occur in nondrinkers, and is related to diseases like hepatitis. It has been observed that heavy drinking causes the cells of the liver to become enlarged and unable to handle fat metabolism. This normally leads to a fatty degeneration of the liver, a forerunner of cirrhosis of the liver.

The hangover is the most common and infamous effect of alcohol on the body. The exact biochemical explanation for its occurrence is not known, nor is satisfactory treatment for its symptoms available. "There is no scientific evidence to support such popular remedies as coffee, raw egg, oysters, chili peppers, steak sauce, "alkalizers," vitamin preparations, or such drugs as barbiturates, thyroid, amphetamine, or insulin. For general treatment, physicians usually prescribe aspirin, bed rest, and ingestion of solid foods as soon as possible."[8]

ALCOHOLISM

Alcoholism, a progressive illness that is now epidemic in nature, affects men and women from both rural and urban areas. It has little regard for educational, religious, cultural, or financial status. One of the reasons for our slowness as a society in attacking problems like this is a lack of concern for the people affected. They are often not recognized as being "ill people" and to date the usual reaction has been to punish them rather than to treat them. Broader understandings with respect to alcoholism must be universally accepted before progress can be made in its control through prevention and treatment.

[8] Ibid, p. 23.

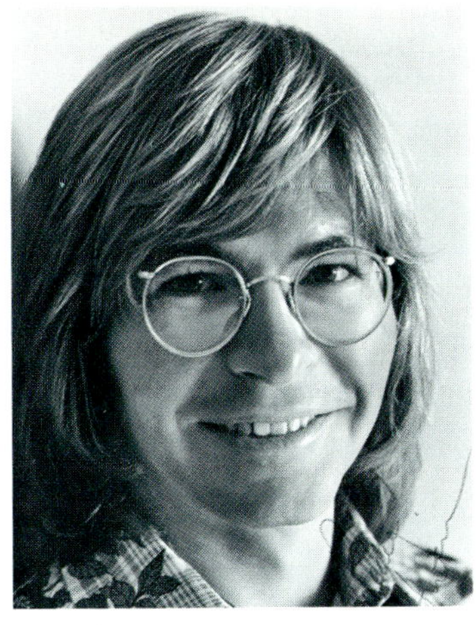

Figure 7–4

Please, Daddy, don't get drunk this Christmas
I don't wanna see my mama cry. . .

John Denver's musical plea illustrates the extent to which children are also affected by alcoholism.

(PLEASE, DADDY, Don't Get Drunk This Christmas by Bill Danoff and Taffy Nivert. © Copyright 1971, 1973 by Cherry Lane Music Co. Used by Permission—All Rights Reserved.)

The specific causes of alcoholism are not well understood as yet. Research seems to support the multiple cause theory of disease in this case, and evidence suggests that there are physical or biological causes, psychological factors, as well as social considerations—all contributing in varying combinations to this illness. Typical of many alcoholics is a low frustration threshold and an inability to face everyday problems. They usually start out by relying on alcohol to get them over difficult aspects of life. More and more they need to fortify themselves with a drink before they can face their problems. They ultimately retreat from them completely, utilizing the alcohol as a crutch. It is rather ironic that the person who takes a drink because he feels it will help him to function more efficiently is actually using a substance that will undermine his ability to perform both professionally and socially. He also finds out too late that alcohol does not solve his problem; it merely irrigates as well as aggravates it.

Other alcoholics, when they feel overwhelmed by their problems, use alcohol as a means of reaching a state of oblivion. It represents a panicky flight from a responsibility they cannot face. Many alcoholics will complain that they have difficulty sleeping, although members of their families will indicate that they sleep as much as the average person. This desire for continual sleep is another indication of their need to escape.

Some alcoholics have a compulsion to drink. This is a form of compulsive behavior they cannot control and invariably results in their addiction to alcohol.

Many people feel that alcohol is the cause of all alcoholism. Actually, alcohol is a neutral agent that can be used or abused. The following case history gives an indication of how the escape agent can be transferred from one substance to another and how, in the absence of alcohol, other substances may often be used.

> . . . I was able to stay dry for several months at a time. But inevitably, after dry periods of from three to six months, I would wind up terribly drunk.
>
> Eventually I began to recognize the symptoms that preceded a drinking episode and realized that I needed help. I went to a neighborhood physician since the problem did not seem important enough for my family doctor. I explained that I was an alcoholic, that I was getting jittery and that I did not want to drink. I asked the doctor if he could give me something for my nerves.
>
> The doctor was sympathetic. Since I had not had a drink in six months, the doctor maintained that I was not an alcoholic. He also prescribed half-grain tablets of phenobarbital, three tablets to be taken during the day and two at bedtime.
>
> Needless to say, like so many alcoholics who attempt to prescribe sedatives for themselves, I found myself in a very short while taking fifteen pills a day.
>
> I had completely transferred my dependency from alcohol to barbiturates. I began to carry a supply of pills in my vest pocket. When something disturbing occurred at the office, I would make a trip to the water cooler and pop several pills into my mouth. After that, whatever had been disturbing me no longer would seem important.
>
> Because of the tolerance that I was developing to the drug, it is doubtful whether the phenobarbital had much effect on me physiologically. But I had definitely developed a psychological dependence that became more compulsive over a period of four years.
>
> There was one occasion when I remember taking three pills but actually took forty-five. I have absolutely no recollection of taking the other forty-two. By the time the doctor reached me I had virtually no pulse. My life hung in the balance for hours as my wife spooned hot, strong, black coffee into me throughout the night.
>
> Both personal experience and observation have convinced me that an alcoholic cannot safely take "the first pill" any more than he can take "the first drink."[9]

Treatment of the Alcoholic

The first step in the treatment of the alcoholic is to withdraw him from alcohol. With a long-term or chronic alcoholic, the condition known as delirium tremens may occur as a result of alcohol withdrawal. Trembling and hallucinations of a terrifying nature characterize this disorder. With appropriate medical help, patients are helped to keep this activity under control, recover promptly, and are ready to start other forms of treatment.

Because the large intake of alcohol impairs the desire to eat, various nutritional problems must be corrected as part of the therapy. Nutritional deficiency diseases can be easily corrected with proper food intake and the addition of

[9] "Tranquilizers, Sedatives and the Alcoholic," Alcoholics Anonymous World Services, Inc., 1961.

vitamins to the diet. After the alcoholic has been withdrawn from alcohol and is physically rehabilitated, the important job of preventing his future drinking begins.

Drugs such as disulfiram and calcium carbimide have been used in efforts to discourage the patient from drinking. An alcoholic on these drugs finds that any contact with alcohol produces nausea, vomiting, palpitations of the heart, and loss of breath. This method of treatment requires close medical supervision because of the severe physical reactions.

Psychotherapy is often the method used to help the individual to self-examine his motivations for drinking, to counsel and guide him, and ultimately to change his feelings and behavior so that he may live effectively without his drug dependence. Psychotherapy may take many forms: it may be done in groups or alone; it may include hypnosis or role playing; it may include a conditioned-response[10] approach; or it may include the patient's family.

Supportive organizations, such as Alcoholics Anonymous, a voluntary organization made up of former or recovered alcoholics, stand ready to help. Their sole purpose is to help the alcoholic to overcome his problem. Former alcoholics, having gone through the ordeal, understand the feelings and temptations that beset the individual with his alcohol dependence. People who seek help from Alcoholics Anonymous receive no preaching, are not asked to sign a pledge, and are not scolded for their past behavior. Other organizations offering special family aid are Al-Anon and Al-Ateen. Al-Anon was established to help wives and husbands, friends, and other relatives of alcoholics better understand the problem. An attempt to improve the environment to which a rehabilitated alcoholic must return would seem essential. Al-Ateen was established to help children of compulsive drinkers understand their parents' problems, to understand that alcoholism is not inherited, and to help develop in themselves better alternatives in coping with emotional and social stresses. They learn that their situation is not unique and try to find ways to adjust to them.

The Revolving Door

In all the jails throughout our country, the number of prisoners with a drinking problem serious enough to result in arrest or imprisonment is very high. The jailing of people with an alcoholic dependence does not serve to solve the problem. The jailing represents nothing more than the setting up of a revolving door through which the alcoholic migrates from community to jail and back again. The jailing of a person for any crime or disorder represents on the part of society a kind of frustration. Being unable to prevent

[10] *"aversion,"* or *"conditioned response,"* is described by Marvin A. Block as a technique whereby in a controlled environment a patient is given whatever alcoholic beverage he wants. The beverage is modified, however, to make him ill. If the technique is repeated over an extended period, the patient will become ill when he even thinks of taking a drink.

or cope with the situation, we seek correction through restraint. We have the knowledge and means for the correction of alcoholism; our continuing to jail the alcoholic renders us guilty of a kind of thinking that lacks logic.

MAN'S USE OF TOBACCO

Contrary to popular opinion stimulated by current cigarette advertisements, cigarette smoking did not start with the cowboy, but with the Indian. Tobacco was used by the New World natives even before Columbus' voyage. The thought that the burning of the curious leaves and the inhalation of the smoke was to be the basis of a major industry apparently did not occur to the Indian. The Indian smoked not only for enjoyment and ceremonial purposes, but for the curative powers he believed tobacco possessed. Smoking, as well as the misconceived notion that tobacco had curative powers, spread to Europe and there is evidence that in the seventeenth century tobacco was used in attempts to cure cancer and to ward off the plague.

During the 1920s and early thirties, all prohibitory laws with regard to cigarettes were repealed. The sale of cigarettes began to boom from this time on. The United States is now the world leader in tobacco production, exportation, and consumption. Americans spend approximately $8 billion dollars a year on tobacco products. This country, in addition, exports annually approximately 25 billion cigarettes.

WHY PEOPLE SMOKE

The reasons why people smoke are as varied as the individuals themselves, with each person seeking satisfaction in one form or another. Much has been written on the subject of why young people start smoking. Some scholars state that the oral satisfactions derived from smoking are reminiscent of the suckling time in one's life, with all the security that went with the mother's breast. Whether the smoking habit stems from this subconscious motivation or from the very real pressures from one's own peers, it is obvious that this is a complex problem.

One of the most important factors related to teenage smoking is whether or not the parents or older siblings smoked. If the family attitude toward smoking is one of acceptance, then smoking becomes a part of "growing up." There is also a higher incidence of smoking when the young adult does not enjoy peer group status. The smoking in these instances becomes a form of compensatory behavior. The smoking may therefore be symptomatic of emotional problems.

In further exploring why people smoke one cannot overlook the multimillion dollar advertising campaign of the tobacco industry as a causative factor in initiating cigarette smoking.

The reasons the veteran smoker offers for smoking are pleasure, sociability, relief of tension, self-assurance, stimulation, and nicotine craving. The question of whether smoking has addictive qualities is being less debated, as confirmed smokers experience definite withdrawal symptoms when they attempt to stop smoking. The term *addicted smoker* is being increasingly used by scientists who work in this field. The greatest reason, therefore, why people smoke is because they simply cannot stop. They are hooked on nicotine. As stated by former Surgeon General Luther Terry, "Ninety five per cent of smokers know the dangers of their habit and seventy five per cent of them want to quit, but can't."[11] Research has been initiated to find ways of withdrawing people from addictive smoking. The medical record for reversing addictions, however, is not encouraging.

THE EFFECTS OF SMOKING ON THE BODY

Many physiological changes take place when one lights up a cigarette. One of the offending substances resulting from cigarette combustion is nicotine, "a poisonous volatile alkaloid ($C_{10}H_{14}N_2$) derived from tobacco and responsible for many of the effects of tobacco."[12] In small amounts nicotine acts as a stimulant, but in larger doses it serves as a depressant. Hence, smoking will cause an increase in the heart rate of an individual, a temporary rise in the blood pressure, and a slight elevation of blood sugar level. Smoking reduces the blood flow in the coronary arteries of the heart similar to that seen in heart disease. Those individuals already suffering from narrowed coronary arteries as a result of atherosclerosis may often experience anginal pain pointing to the further narrowing of the arteries by nicotine-induced spasms. There is a narrowing of the blood vessels, causing a lowering of body temperature in the fingers and toes. In subzero temperatures, the possibility of frostbite of the fingers and toes is greater in the smoking individual.

In individuals with an *unusual* sensitivity to nicotine, severe spasms of the small arteries of the fingers, toes, cheeks, nose, and ears will result in a slowing down or stopping of the blood flow. Blood clots forming here will eventually result in gangrene of the extremity. This condition, Buerger's disease (thromboangiitis obliterans), is seldom fatal, but is most painful and handicapping because the amputation of fingers, toes, and other parts is usually necessitated.

[11] National Clearinghouse for Smoking and Health, *Newsweek,* September 27, 1971.

[12] Definition of nicotine in *Stedman's Medical Dictionary* (Williams and Wilkins Co., 1965).

DON'T SMOKE...
MEDICAL RESEARCH
THE LUNG YOU SAVE MAY BE YOUR OWN

HAPPINESS – IS THAT GOOD FEELING – WHEN YOU STOP SMOKING

FOR HEAVEN'S SAKE
STOP SMOKING NOW!

AFTER THE LIFT
COMES THE LETDOWN
R.I.P.

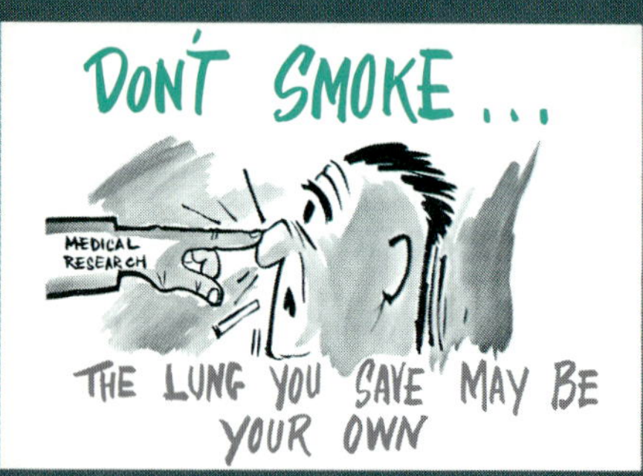

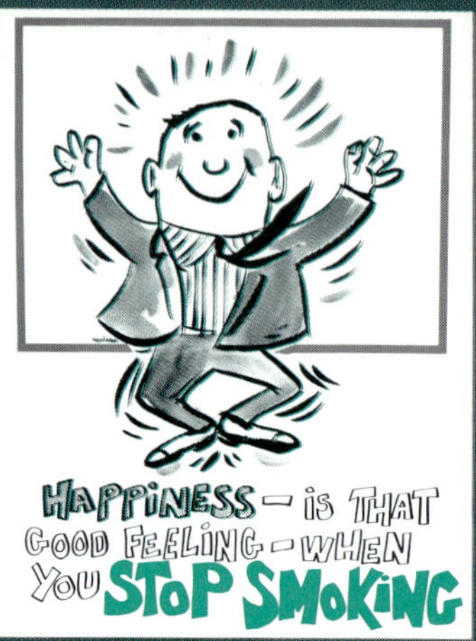

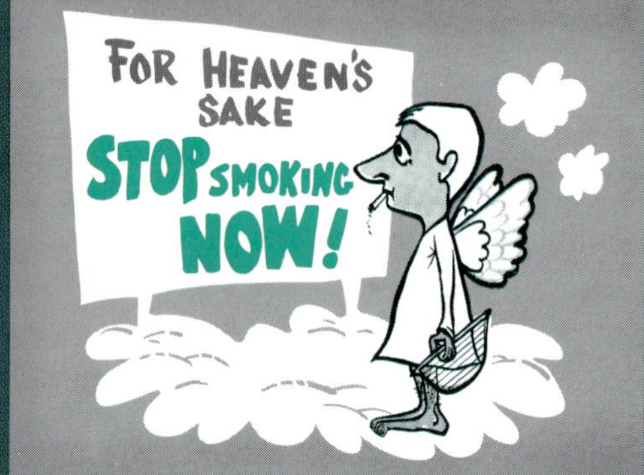

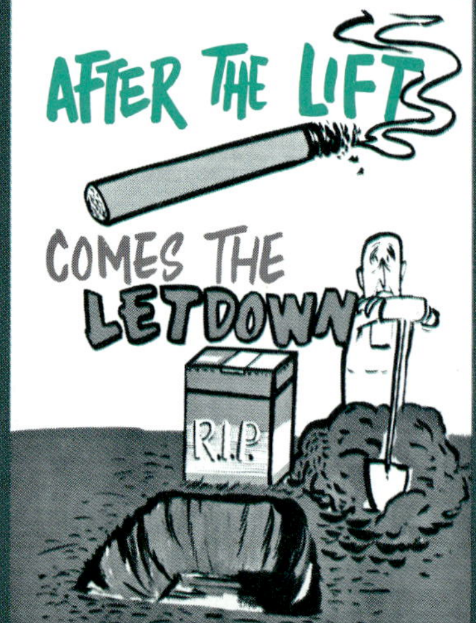

Figure 7–5

A series of posters developed by the Roswell Park Memorial Institute.

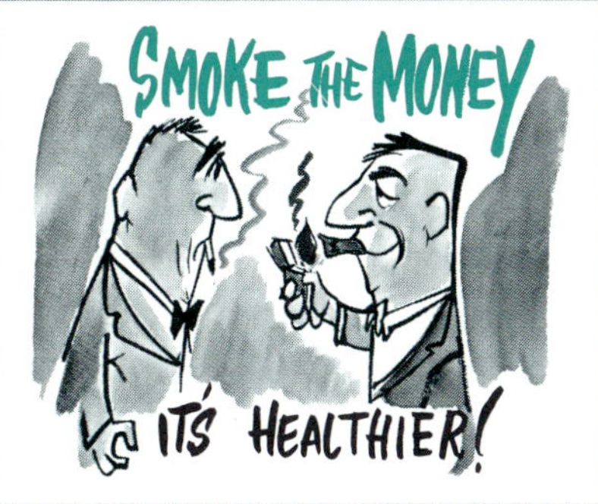
SMOKE THE MONEY
IT'S HEALTHIER!

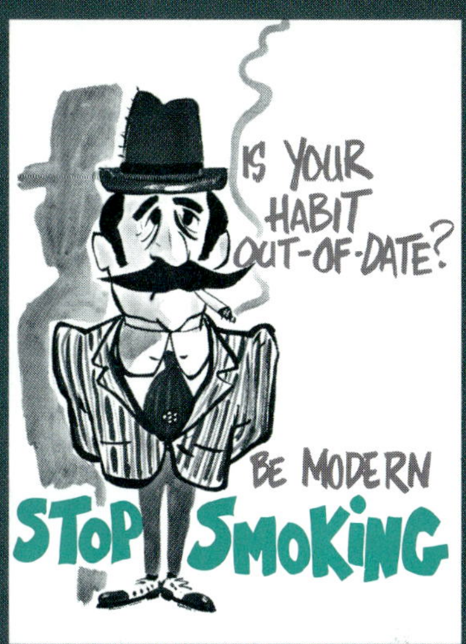
IS YOUR HABIT OUT-OF-DATE?
BE MODERN
STOP SMOKING

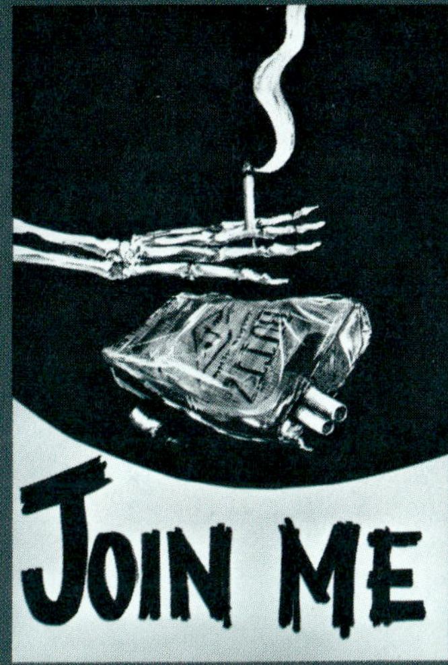
JOIN ME

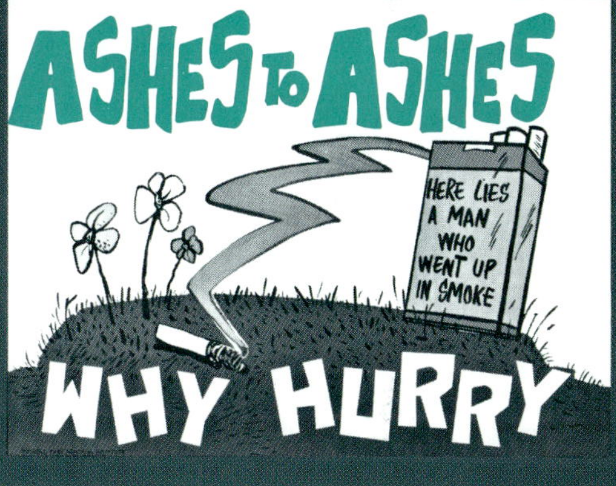
ASHES TO ASHES
HERE LIES A MAN WHO WENT UP IN SMOKE
WHY HURRY

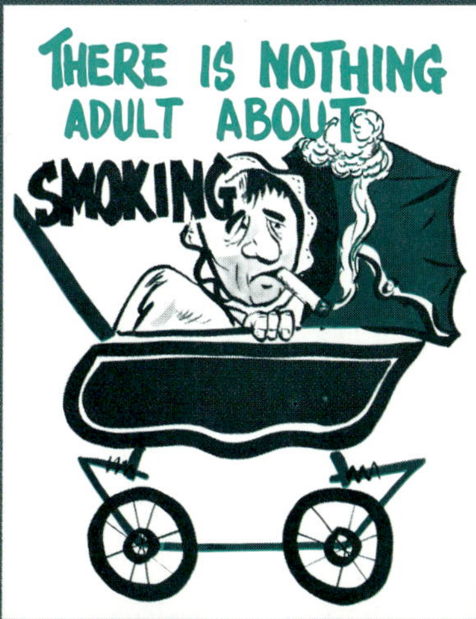
THERE IS NOTHING ADULT ABOUT
SMOKING

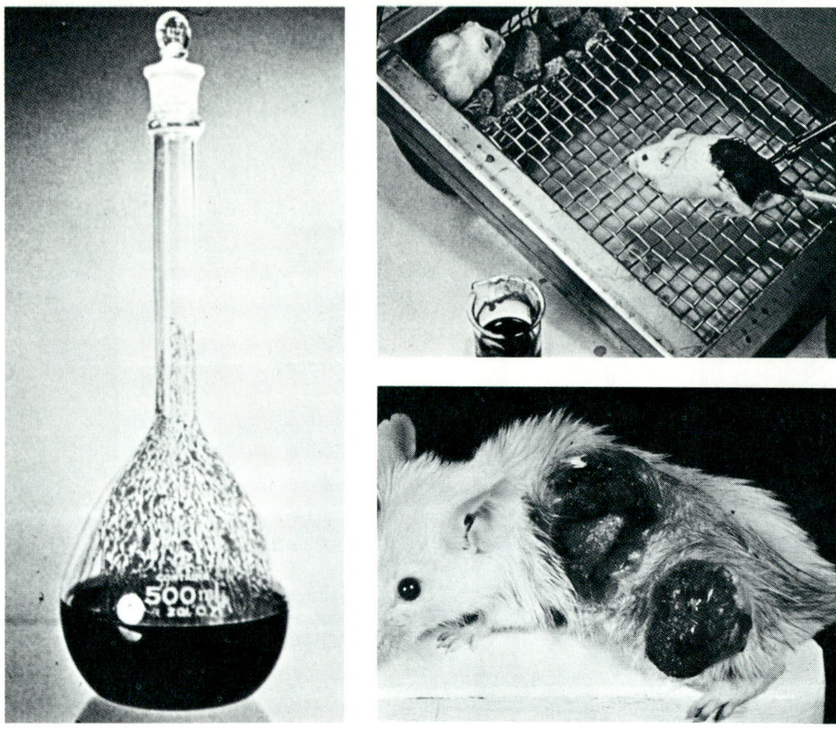

Figure 7–6

A, left: This collection of tar can be analyzed and is used in biological experimentation. B, top right: If tar is taken from just a few packages of cigarettes and a dilute solution is made, the application of this solution to the skin of small animals will cause 60 percent of these animals to have tumors of the skin within a year. C, bottom right: This can be done repeatedly and consistently under laboratory conditions.

(Roswell Park Memorial Institute)

The disease is terminated when smoking stops; however, in the individual addicted to smoking a return to the habit precipitates a resumption of the disease. "It is a startling fact indeed that some patients who have already lost their toes, and who have been warned that they will lose their legs next, nevertheless have continued to smoke."[13]

Nicotine is only one of the many offending compounds found in smoke. Other substances include hydrocarbons, alcohols, esters, sterols, aldehydes, acids, phenols, arsenic, potassium, and some metals. Though these substances are

[13] *The Consumers Union Report on Smoking and the Public Interest* (Mount Vernon, N.Y.: Consumers Union, 1963), p. 88.

found in minute amounts, several have been proved to be cancer-producing. Upon the inhalation of smoke, the lining of the trachea and bronchial tubes are bathed with the smoke condensate or tar. In the lining of the trachea and bronchi, the production of mucus and the whiplike action of the cilia normally catch and then sweep upward any foreign particles that may be inhaled. However, the inhalation of cigarette smoke slows down and may completely paralyze the ciliary action while it stimulates an increase in the production of mucus. The result is a persistent cough which endeavors to expel the accumulated, excess mucus. This is referred to as a "cigarette cough" or more correctly a chronic bronchitis (inflammation of the bronchi). As the mucus accumulates in the bronchioles, there is a tendency for these tubes to close shut, often trapping air in the alveoli (air sacs). Over a period of years this trapped air can stretch the alveoli to large blisters, or bullae. When a person coughs, the increased pressure exerted on the delicate walls of the alveoli is enough to rupture them, thereby eventually cutting down the lung capacity of the individual. This is essentially what occurs in emphysema, with the person constantly short of breath because so much of his lung tissue has been destroyed in this fashion.

Emphysema can have a negative effect on the heart because it tends to cause a decrease in the amount of oxygen that may be taken in by the lungs. The effect is that it increases the work load of the heart to pick up the same amount of oxygen. A further strain on the heart is caused by the fact that emphysema reduces the number of channels through which blood can pass through the lungs. Cardiac failure is often associated with advanced cases of emphysema.

Polonium 210, a radioactive substance, is dispatched into the mainstream smoke, and some researchers believe that this substance is at least one of the causative agents of lung cancer. Several autopsy studies have shown that the bronchial epithelium of smokers contains significantly more Polonium 210 than that of nonsmokers. Though research with Polonium is inconclusive, study continues to pinpoint relationships between specific carcinogenic substances in cigarette smoke and the development of lung cancer.

CIGARETTE ADVERTISING

From its early beginning, the tobacco industry in this country was a highly competitive one, requiring the use of varied promotional techniques and schemes. The advertising appeals were of a positive nature, with opera stars stating that certain brands of cigarettes would help to "save" their voices. Athletes were quoted on how a particular brand of cigarette helped them to "stay in shape."

In the early 1950s, the American Cancer Society presented a research report indicating a possible relationship between smoking and cancer. The immediate reaction to the report was a decline in the sale of cigarettes. The reaction of the tobacco industry was to increase advertising expenditures and to develop the filter-tip cigarette. The report also stimulated the "tar derby," in which each manufacturer made the attempt to convince the public that his cigarette was lowest in tar content. Though the filters that were placed on cigarettes were not very effective in filtering out tars, they did serve to satisfy the customer that he was now "safe from cancer." In 1954 the total cigarette sales in the United States had slumped to under 369 billion. By increasing its advertising costs by 134 per cent in the next six years, the industry caused an upswing in cigarette consumption so that by 1961 cigarette sales soared to 490 billion cigarettes. There were those who hailed this turnabout as one of the supreme achievements of marketing strategy! In 1964 the report of the Surgeon General's Advisory Committee indicting cigarette smoking as a cause of lung cancer and relating it to the high incidence of cardiovascular disease, emphysema, and a number of other conditions, again caused a dip in cigarette sales. In response to this challenge the tobacco industry once again increased its advertising expenditures. In 1965 this expenditure reached the total of 250 million dollars. This added effort reclaimed initial losses in sales due to the Surgeon General's report.

Since the publication of the report, advertising techniques have changed so that the mention of health factors in cigarette commercials is rare indeed. The tobacco industry has sensed that the average teenager has not been frightened by medical reports indicating the relationship between smoking and disease. It is difficult for a young person to be concerned about the possible developments of disease that might occur twenty years later. The result is that the teenager has been made an advertising target of the industry. Cigarette advertisements relate the use of cigarettes to athletic prowess, popularity, and datability.

Attempts to Control Cigarette Advertising

From 1955 to 1960 the Federal Trade Commission sought to control the many false claims made by manufacturers about the effectiveness of their filters, and the tar and nicotine content of their cigarettes. The FTC finally persuaded the tobacco industry to discontinue the tar derby because of this federal agancy's inability to properly supervise claims being made in this area. In 1962, Italy banned all tobacco advertising. In Finland, as of July 1962, television advertising of cigarettes ended. In February of 1965, the British Labor Government said that it would ban all cigarette advertising from television and was considering a similar ban on newspaper and poster ads. The United States government, which had been slow to act in this area, finally approved a health hazard warning which began appearing on all cigarette packages in January 1966. Some people have implied that the United States government has not acted forcefully against the tobacco industry because it is one of the giant industries of this country, with an annual output worth approximately $4 billion. It is one that has large areas of agriculture dependent solely upon it. Because this country is also the largest exporter of tobacco products, the crippling of this industry would hurt the country financially.

On January 2, 1971, cigarette commercials were banned from television. While some viewed this action as a victory for the consumer over the tobacco industry, it has proven to be a reversal. A few years prior to the 1971 ban of the cigarette TV commercials, the Federal Communications Commission (FCC) declared that significant (if not equal) time could be given to anticigarette commercials. Health organizations such as the American Cancer Society, the American Heart Association, and the National TB and Respiratory Disease Association developed anticigarette commercials that began to have an effect on cigarette sales. As indicated in the *Wall Street Journal,*

> It now seems clear that the continuing falloff is attributable to the antismoking campaign, but the rate of year-to-year decline should begin to level off in 1971 for the somewhat ironic reason that Congress has banned all cigarette commercials on radio and TV after January 1, giving stations less incentive to run antismoking commercials.[14]

As the tobacco industry shifted its advertising to magazines, newspapers, and billboards, it moved into media that the health organizations could not follow without enormous sums of money (which they do not have). The health organizations could not receive "public service space" in these media as it did public service time on the airways. The tobacco industry thus shifted its advertising from media where their messages relating cigarette smoking to enhanced masculinity, femininity, Women's Liberation, spring, and independence could not be counteracted by messages relating cigarette smoking to lung cancer, emphysema, heart attacks, and premature death.

THE DECADE SINCE THE SURGEON GENERAL'S REPORT

In 1964 the ten members of the Surgeon General's Advisory Committee, all outstanding physicians and scientists of this country, evaluated three kinds of scientific evidence: (1) animal experiments, (2) clinical or autopsy studies, (3) population studies. In animal experimentation, animals were exposed to tobacco smoke, tars, and the various chemical compounds they contained. Seven of these compounds have been established as being cancer-producing (carcinogenic) in nature.

[14] *Proceedings of the N.Y. State Conference, Smokeless 70's Independently or Interdependently?* N.Y. State Interagency Committee on Hazards of Smoking, April 1970.

Clinical and autopsy studies among smokers showed that many kinds of damage to body functions and organs, cells, and tissues occurred more frequently and severely in smokers.

Population studies showed that cigarette smokers had a proportionately higher incidence of lung cancer than nonsmokers. The prevalence of specific signs and symptoms such as chronic cough, sputum production, breathlessness, chest illness, and decreased lung functioning were found consistently in much higher incidence among smokers.

In 1972 the Surgeon General's Report had been updated and further substantiated through the years by additional research studies. Recent findings not only confirmed a relationship between cigarette smoking and coronary heart disease but further indicated its relationship to the sudden, fatal form of heart attack. There is evidence that cigarette smoking accelerates the pathology of preexisting heart disease, thereby contributing to the individual's sudden and unexpected death. Further experimental studies on animals and autopsy studies have indicated that smoking contributes to the development of atherosclerosis of the aorta and coronary arteries.

Cigarette smoking has been established as the most important cause of chronic obstructive bronchopulmonary disease (COPD) and far outranks atmospheric pollution as a causative factor. Respiratory disease as well as mortality is higher in smokers as compared to nonsmokers. The updated report further indicated that the hazards of cigarette smoking may fall on the smoker and *nonsmoker* alike—though not in equal amounts. He stated, "We cannot overlook the fact that exposure to these concentrations of carbon monoxide may be especially hazardous for those who are suffering from heart disease or chronic bronchopulmonary disease."[15]

The new information relative to lung cancer was quite specific. Whereas the 1964 report said that cigarette smoking *was causally related to lung cancer,* the 1972 report, "confirms the conclusion that cigarette smoking is the main cause of lung cancer in men."[16] There no longer seems to be an honest disagreement among medical scientists concerning the hazards of cigarette smoking. The incidence of oral cancer, as well as cancer of the larynx and esophagus, is clearly greater in smokers than in nonsmokers. An alcohol and tobacco interaction has been indicated as a lethal combination associated with especially high rates of cancer of the esophagus.

In summing up developments concerning cigarette smoking since the original Surgeon General's report of 1964, former Surgeon General Dr. Steinfeld said there would probably have been many more millions smoking cigarettes had the government not campaigned against the habit. With all this evidence one wonders how long the offering of a cigarette will continue to be viewed as a friendly, social grace instead of the threat it really is.

[15] National Clearing House for Smoking and Health, January 18, 1972.

[16] *The Health Consequences of Smoking,* A Report of the Surgeon General, 1972, p. 11.

PREVENTION

Inevitably the question is being asked, what can be done to prevent or at least slow down this developing catastrophic situation? A number of suggestions have been made and in many instances actions taken in an attempt to implement them.

Many feel that the development of an effective filter would significantly reduce tar and nicotine content in cigarette smoke. Current filters, however, are not highly effective. The most optimistic estimate is that current filters reduce the risk of lung cancer by 30 per cent over nonfiltered cigarettes. Other estimates are more pessimistic. A related factor is the tar and nicotine content of the tobacco in front of the filter. In some cigarettes, stronger tobacco is used to compensate for whatever filtering action the filter may effect. Dr. Ernest Wynder, President of the American Health Foundation, has suggested that we put "a maximum level (of tar and nicotine) on all American cigarettes and set it at 20 milligrams for tar and 1.2 milligrams of nicotine. I picked that level because 50 percent of all American cigarettes meet that level. That suggestion was violently opposed by the tobacco industry."[17] It is felt that it is easier for a smoker to break away from the cigarette habit if he is using cigarettes of low nicotine content. The University of Kentucky Agricultural Experiment Station is currently attempting to produce a low-nicotine burley tobacco breeding line in order that cigarettes with a low-nicotine content may be produced. In addition, of course, lowered tar content would protect the smoker to some extent from lung cancer and other tobacco-related diseases. Other efforts to create a nontobacco cigarette has not yet been fruitful. Until such time as a safe cigarette can be produced, people who feel a need to smoke are still urged to switch to pipes and cigars.

As indicated by the Surgeon General, 75 per cent of those people who smoke would like to stop but cannot, and further do not know where to go for help. Smoking withdrawal clinics have been experimented with over the past ten years. It would seem that it is time to routinely establish such clinics in hospitals (for patients and staff), schools (for students, faculty and parents), and industrial plants. These clinics have had varying success in terms of the percentage of participants who can kick the nicotine habit. However, even those who fail can learn to smoke more safely by means of low-tar and low-nicotine cigarettes, switching to pipes or cigars, smoking a cigarette only halfway down the butt, and so forth. The constant availability of such clinics makes it possible for a person to try to break the habit a second and third time should he fail on the first attempt. Such clinics may also serve to comfort

[17] *Smoking and Health Newsletter,* National Interagency Council on Smoking and Health, Vol. 8, No. 1 (January–March 1972).

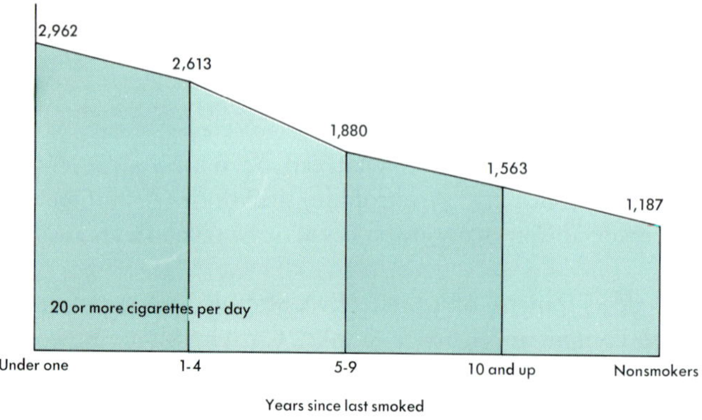

Figure 7–7

Death rates fall when smoking stops (males age 55–64, rates per 100,000 person-years).

(Roswell Park Memorial Institute)

those who feel trapped in a dangerous habit. It has been suggested that smoking withdrawal clinics be subsidized by health insurance companies as a preventive activity. Since the treatment of tobacco-related diseases represents the greatest expenditure of health insurance monies, this kind of preventive activity would seem justified because it would save lives as well as money. It would also have the effect of shifting health professionals from a purely *treatment* context to one involving *prevention*—a long overdue shift!

Increasing numbers of schools around the country have become involved in education programs in an effort to discourage people from taking up the smoking habit in the first place. Where schools have used knowledgeable teachers who know how to approach this kind of social health problem, the results have been laudatory. Too often, however, the educational program is attempted by teachers who are ill informed and convey the notion that it is all right for adults to smoke, but not for young people to do so. The latter does nothing more than to reinforce tobacco industry advertisements that have already planted the idea that smoking is associated with sophistication, adulthood, and independence. It amounts to throwing a gallon of gasoline on the fire. The growing demands by high school students for smoking rooms reflect the failure of these programs. Certainly the demand for smoking rooms in our present state of knowledge cannot be classified as an informed one.

Instructional programs related to smoking and health have been most successful when they are started at the elementary level (before a decision on tobacco use has been made) with the students actively involved in the study of this health issue backed by well-informed teachers who see no place for propagandistic approaches in the classroom. Many of these programs have their students active in the community taking surveys of various kinds, assisting in the conduction of smoking withdrawal clinics, seeking out legislators to discuss possible legislation, and serving as a speaker's bureau to report the findings of their studies.

A fifth grade boy who was a part of an activist-oriented education program

Figure 7–8

Shock Tactic: This poster of a child smoking is part of the antismoking drive of the British Health Education Council urging parents and other adults not to endanger their children's wellbeing or set a bad example by smoking.

(The Health Education Council)

How many cigarettes a day does your child smoke?
When a child breathes air filled with cigarette smoke
it can be as bad as if he actually smoked the cigarette himself.
Don't smoke when there are children present.

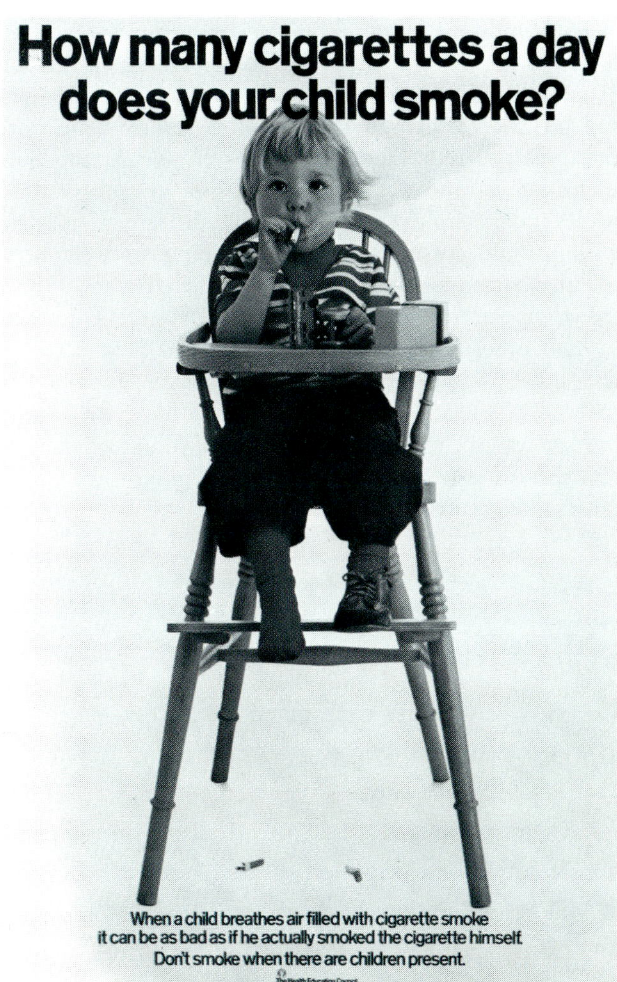

pursued his studies at home by badgering his cigarette-smoking, psychiatrist father. He clearly outlined for his father the various health risks his smoking habit exposed him to and that he was in the process of shortening his life expectancy by some eight years. The fifth grader asked, "Who is going to take care of me? Who will provide for my college education? Are you trying to tell me you don't love me any more?" The father indicated that the only way he could avoid the badgering was to duck into the clothes closet everytime he felt the need to have a cigarette. He soon admitted that being a psychiatrist, he realized that hiding in the closet was rather peculiar behavior. He ultimately resolved the conflict by breaking his smoking habit. There was a time when children used to be afraid to smoke in front of their parents. Where good education programs are instituted in schools, it is the parent who is afraid to smoke in the presence of his children.

Following the pronouncement from the Surgeon General's Office with regard to the harmful effects of tobacco smoke on the nonsmoker, a new band of militants has arisen with a nonsmoker's Bill of Rights. Airlines, railroads, and bus lines began to take action by establishing nonsmoking sections in their vehicles. All the action was not due to the Surgeon General alone. Increasing numbers of nonsmokers have complained to transportation companies and to smokers who pollute the air. A number of airlines were threatened with lawsuits by nonsmokers who felt they were being forced to breathe polluted air that posed a danger to their health. Typical was an altercation that took place on a commuter train. Two men entered the train and sat next to each other. One lit up a cigarette and blew a ball of smoke. The other responded, "Would you mind not blowing your smoke over me?" The smoker retorted, "Where do you expect me to blow it?" The response of the nonsmoker was such that it precipitated a round of fisticuffs exemplifying how sensitive the issue has become. The 164 million Americans who do not smoke can no longer be classified as the *silent* majority!

REVIEW QUESTIONS

1. How have drugs contributed to man's welfare?
2. A prescription drug is a personal thing. Explain.
3. Why are side effects in reaction to drugs a common response?
4. Why is it important to read the label on nonprescription drugs?
5. What is your definition of drug abuse?
6. What are the psychosocial implications of marihuana use?
7. What appear to be some of the limitations of methadone maintenance as a solution to heroin addiction?

8 Drug abuse is a social-health problem, not a moral-legal one. Explain.

9 Barbiturate addiction may be the most widespread form of addiction in this country. What have been the underlying reasons for the extensiveness of this problem?

10 What procedures would you propose for the control of the drug abuse problem?

11 Discuss the relative dangers of the nonaddicting drugs as compared to the addictive drugs as societal problems.

12 Describe the various physiological effects of alcohol on the body.

13 Review the various reasons why people drink or do not drink alcoholic beverages. Support a point of view, pro or con.

14 What appear to be the underlying causes of alcoholism? Explain the susceptibility of alcoholics to habituation to other drugs.

15 What have been the contributions of Alcoholics Anonymous in the rehabilitation of the alcoholic?

16 Explain the futility of jailing the alcoholic.

17 One of every ten of the American work force have serious drinking problems. The United States Public Health Service describes the disorder as having reached epidemic proportions. To what extent do you feel remedial actions are in order?

18 How has cigarette advertising influenced the development of a gigantic tobacco industry?

19 To what extent has the Federal Trade Commission managed to control cigarette advertising?

20 What are the relationships of smoking and health as related in the Surgeon General's report?

21 Identify the offending substances in cigarette smoke. Explain their effects on the body tissues.

22 What are the preventive approaches that might be used to alleviate the numerous health problems related to cigarette smoking?

8. Man & His Environment

LUNAR TRAVEL has made man see his existence on earth from a different viewpoint. As we view pictures of earth taken from the moon we realize that the planet earth is all we have. It looks like an oasis that harbors life in a vast sea of celestial bodies that are beyond our reach and are hostile to life. The concern, therefore, for the preservation of our environment must be a primary one.

Our environmental health problems of water and air pollution, pesticide and radiation control are reflective of man's progress. Paradoxically, they also represent obstacles to his future development if not properly dealt with. The increasingly sophisticated technology developed by man means not only a better way of life and perhaps the elimination of more primitive threats to health, but also the development of new health problems with shorter fuses. Our ability as a society to respond quickly and effectively to these newer problems will determine our levels of well-being, in fact, of our very survival as a species.

AIR POLLUTION

While public health officials have been aware of air pollution problems for quite some time, it took a series of disasters before public awareness and interest in the problem was developed. The first of these to occur was in the 1930s in the Meuse Valley in Belgium. The valley is a highly industrialized area that is approximately 15 miles long and $1\frac{1}{2}$ miles wide. An acute air pollution condition resulted in 63 deaths and the illness of many persons. In 1948 a combination of air pollution and adverse weather conditions precipitated a similar disaster in Donora, Pennsylvania. Within a few days this condition caused the death of 20 people and the illness of 6,000 more. In 1952 London underwent a similar experience. Air pollution plus fog and an inversion condition that lasted for about a week resulted in 4,000 deaths and untold illness. London has been the site of a number of such episodes, the last occurring in the summer of 1962. New York City has had a chronic air pollution problem for a number of years, with one of its episodes ironically occurring during the Thanksgiving Day weekend of 1966. According to a recent study a high concentration of sulfur dioxide during a ten-day period in 1953 was responsible for a rise in the average death rate per day in that city from 170 to 260. Although specific disasters have the effect of dramatizing the situation, we should perhaps be more concerned with the chronic air pollution problem faced by our society and with the daily toll that it takes not only in lives and illness, but in terms of its effect on crops, animals, and property as well.

THE POLLUTANTS

The impurities found in the air are essentially the waste products of a highly industrialized community. In the past, air pollution concern revolved around the amount of smoke that was produced by a busy factory. However, as a result of our technological advances, air pollutants are now many and varied. They are generally classified in two basic groups. The first group consists of gases which are usually the result of fuel combustion. In this grouping we find the nitrogen oxides, the sulfur oxides, carbon monoxide, hydrocarbons, aldehydes, acids, and ozone. The aerosols represent the second group, which are suspensions of solid or liquid particles. Examples of these would be smoke, dust, mist, gas, and fog.

The Gases

Nitrogen oxides are formed by the combination of nitrogen with one or two molecules of oxygen. The exhaust gases of engines and the effluents of furnaces will contain this pollutant. It has the effect of causing irritations to the eye besides reducing visibility and causing vegetation damage.

Ozone is a gaseous pollutant that is poisonous as well as ill smelling. The action of the sun on nitrogen oxide causes it to lose a single atom of oxygen which unites then with an oxygen molecule to form ozone.

Sulfur oxides are formed by burning fuels containing sulfur, such as coal, gas, or fuel oil. These fuels are used not only for industrial purposes but for home heating as well.

Carbon monoxide is formed by the incomplete combustion of those materials containing carbon such as wood, charcoal, paper, coal, and oil. When it is present in high concentration in closed areas, it can prove to be fatal. The concentration level of carbon monoxide in a number of urban areas is being monitored and its effects on the population studied.

Hydrocarbons are composed of hydrogen and carbon atoms. The incompletely burned gasoline from the automobile exhaust represents a major source of hydrocarbon pollution.

Aldehydes are made up of hydrogen, carbon, and oxygen atoms, and they may be formed from the incomplete combustion of fuels or from the action of sunlight on hydrocarbons and nitrogen dioxide. The aldehydes are known to cause eye irritation.

Organic acids are found in smoke coming from wood fires and from the incomplete combustion of fuels.

Inorganic acids are generated by the burning of coal or petroleum. The inorganic acids are known to be particularly damaging to vegetation.

The Aerosols

Smoke is a product resulting from incomplete combustion of a material. As a result, it will contain fine solid and liquid particles which will create dirt as well as odor.

Fumes are made up essentially of solid particles. These often are by-products of various industrial processes in which paint, rubber, metals, or chemicals are being manufactured.

Dusts are solid particles which can be produced from various industrial processes that involve the making of cement, asphalt, soap, metals, rubber, and other products. They can be particularly damaging to vegetation.

Mists are liquid particles that are oftentimes released by spraying, coating, or impregnating processes. An additional source of organic mists can be the automobile exhaust, with mist being produced by the reaction of nitrogen oxides and hydrocarbons to sunlight.

Natural pollutants are supplied by nature in the form of ozone, bacteria, soil dust, water droplets that evaporate from the sea, nitrogen dioxide created by lightning, spores, pollen, volcanic dust, meteoric dust, sodium chloride from seawater, and ice or snow. These natural pollutants would exist in the atmosphere even without man.

Smog and the Temperature Inversion

It is interesting to note that there are really two types of smog: the London type and the Los Angeles type. The London type is made up of fog plus sulfur

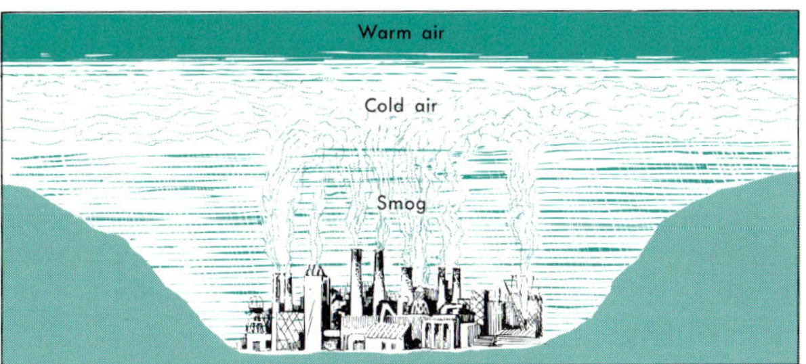

Figure 8–1

An inversion system is formed when atmospheric conditions permit a cold air mass to form under the warmer air. Under these circumstances the pollutants given off in an urban area are trapped over a city by the inversion system.

compounds developed from the burning of coal and fuel oil. The Los Angeles type is composed mainly of partially burned gasoline resulting from the extensive automobile use in that city. We also know that these hydrocarbons, when released into the atmosphere, can be converted by sunlight into more damaging and more reactive substances. Any city with a substantial amount of vehicular traffic will experience a certain amount of the Los Angeles smog.

The London-type fog, or famous "pea-souper," is almost something of the past. In 1956 the Clean Air Act was passed as a result of the 1952 smog catastrophe that killed thousands. This Act created smoke control areas where only authorized fuels could be burned (thus prohibiting the use of soft coal). In 1968 the Clean Air Act was amended to make its application even more effective. The results of these legislative measures is that the number of sunny days in London have increased by 80 per cent and the quality of the atmosphere has improved significantly. In addition, the number of deaths from chronic bronchitis in the large urban areas has decreased.

An atmospheric condition known as temperature inversion is one that contributes to critical periods of air pollution. During an inversion, warm air makes up the upper level of the atmosphere, keeping the cold air closest to the ground. This combination results in air pollutants being held down by the cold air. Because of their inability to escape into the upper atmosphere, pollutants increase in concentration over a city. It was during inversion periods of this type that the disasters of Meuse Valley, London, and Donora occurred. Where industrial areas are located in valleys with high hills on either side, they are particularly prone to periods of temperature inversion. It has been shown that inversion periods occur about one hundred days each year in Los Angeles. This city is particularly prone to this kind of condition because the cool sea air moves in under the warm desert air and an inversion layer is produced. It is only when the warm air rises high enough to permit the cool air to escape that the inversion period is broken.

THE EFFECTS OF AIR POLLUTION

Numerous studies have demonstrated a relationship between air pollutants and various disease conditions in man. Air pollution is a causal factor in the incidence of respiratory disease. Bronchitis-emphysema is found to be much more common among city dwellers, where air pollution rates are higher, than among their country cousins. The incidence of chronic bronchitis in Britain is found to be higher than in any other country in the world. This condition and its complications are now the leading cause of death in men over 45 years of age and the fourth leading cause of death for the entire population in that country. Scientists studying the problem of chronic bronchitis-emphysema are having difficulty separating out the effects of cigarette smoking, which in essence is a form of self-pollution, as compared with environmental pollution. While both appear to be definite factors in the increased incidence of this disease, results so far show that cigarette smoking probably has five times the effect of a polluted environmental area. Studies have also shown that there is a relationship between lung cancer and air pollution. The lung cancer death rate is approximately twice as high in cities, where air pollution is a problem, as compared to the death rates in rural areas. Cancer of the prostate in men has also been found to increase because of high levels of particulate matter in the atmosphere.

Carbon monoxide poisoning of the driver in heavy traffic is a developing problem in this country. While the carbon monoxide level in heavy traffic conditions is not high enough to cause asphyxiation, it can affect one's driving ability and be a contributing cause of an accident.

In addition to affecting man and his health, air pollution can also cause damage to crops and cattle. It has been found that it became impossible to grow vegetables commercially in certain areas because of high levels of air pollution. There have also been incidents in which cattle have become ill for the same reason. The pollutants found in air will oftentimes cause premature rusting of metals, and they have been known to discolor and deteriorate house paint. They have the effect of soiling clothes and can mar and even decompose public buildings and monuments. Current national estimates with regard to the widespread economic damage caused by air pollution range anywhere from 4 to 11 billion dollars annually.

INDUSTRY AND AIR POLLUTION

Industries all make their contributions to the state of air pollution in varying ways and amounts. The steel industries, chemical plants, oil refineries, and the power industry, to name a few, emit waste products into the air peculiar to their particular industrial activities. Industry has already embarked on a program of air pollution control. While the program has a long way to go, it does reflect an awareness of a public health problem. New plants are now being constructed with air pollution control in mind, not only in terms of equipment, but also in terms of plant location. The geography of the area is considered as well as its topography. Old industrial plants are being retooled in order to minimize their contributions to air pollution.

It has long been suggested that national standards be developed for permissible emission of pollutants of every industrial process. The uniform enforcement of such standards would then guarantee the country a strong measure of control over industrial pollutants.

CONTROLLING AIR POLLUTION

At the present time, the automobile is the country's number one air polluter. In a study recently conducted in a Los Angeles area it was found that 1,000 operating automobiles contribute the following amounts and types of air pollutants a day:

1. 3.2 tons of carbon monoxide.
2. 400 to 800 pounds of organic vapors (hydrocarbons).
3. 100 to 200 pounds of nitrous oxides.
4. Plus added amounts of sulfur and other chemicals.

Additional studies are needed to determine to what extent pulverized rubber from automobile tires and particles of asphalt are further contributors to air pollution. It is estimated that the automobile contributes more than the four-fifths of the 85 million tons of pollutants given off by all forms of transportation vehicles that include trucks, buses, railroads, and airlines.

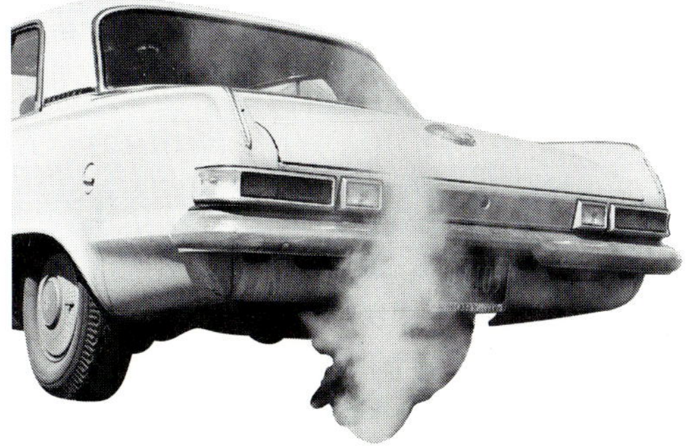

Figure 8–2

The automobile has become the country's number one polluter. Should the gasoline-burning car become a thing of the past?

(New York State Department of Environmental Conservation)

Attempts to control the emissions of the internal combustion engine have not proved to be overly successful. While emission-control devices reduce the amounts of some pollutants, the increases each year in the number of cars wipes out the gain. The emission-control devices actually increased the amounts of nitrogen oxides given off by pre-1973 cars. The effects of the nitrogen oxides were initially underestimated, but are now found to be a factor in the development of emphysema. In Los Angeles, on occasion, automobile-caused smog has even resulted in the cancellation of physical education classes at school to protect the respiratory health of the children.

In addition to smelly, dangerous exhausts, 60 per cent of urban land is given over to roadways, parking areas, and other facilities needed by the automobile. The overpopulation of the cities with cars is inversely related to the small amounts of money invested in badly needed mass transit systems. One or two persons in every car is hardly an efficient way of transporting large numbers of people in and out of a small geographic area, particularly during rush hours. The 1970 Urban Mass Transportation Assistance Act has made some federal money available to begin the improvement of now archaic mass transit systems. Some demonstration projects trying out new transit systems are under way. They include lightweight, rubber-tired vehicles that are computer controlled. They are propelled electrically and neither make noise nor pollute the atmosphere. Since they do not need operators, they can be run economically with continuous service at all hours.

The energy crisis that surfaced in 1973 dramatized the need to develop modern systems of mass transit. The big question with mass transit systems is when will we go from the pilot project stage to nationwide application? The infusion of large amounts of federal money is necessary to initiate the development of the needed change.

The Clean Air Act of 1970 proclaimed that:

1. Standards for emissions be established by the federal government for facilities that currently emit pollutants as well as establish standards for new facilities.
2. a pollution-free automobile be produced within 5 years.
3. a federal authority could seek court action against those facilities not meeting pollution standards.
4. failure to meet established air quality standards be made subject to fines of up to $10,000 per day.

Air pollution levels are continually monitored by automatic instruments that measure sulfur dioxide, carbon monoxide, and smoke shade. Should the air pollution index rise to a dangerous level because of a thermal inversion system, the population is alerted to this fact to take appropriate control measures. These might include the shuting down of factories, limited use of automobiles, and the prohibition of incinerator use.

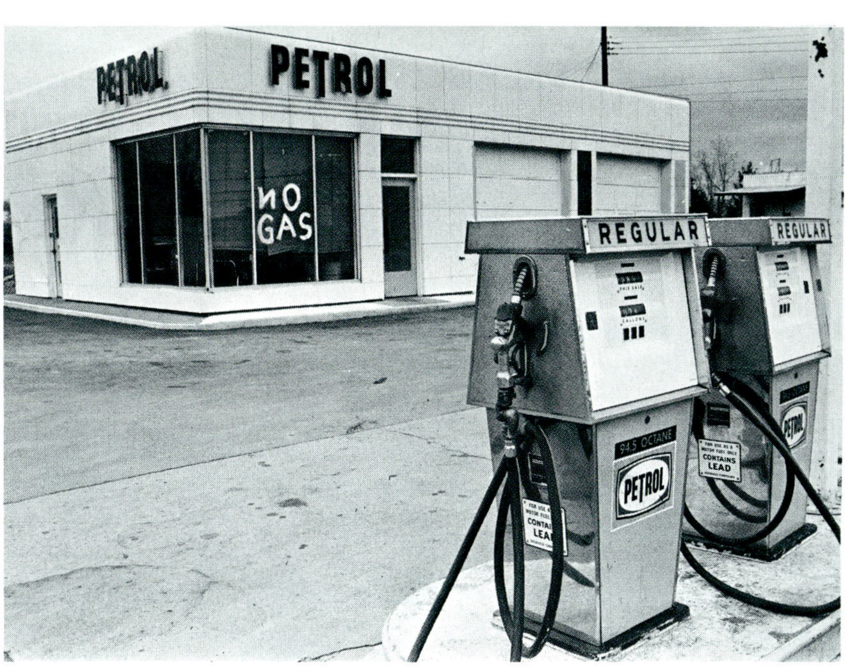

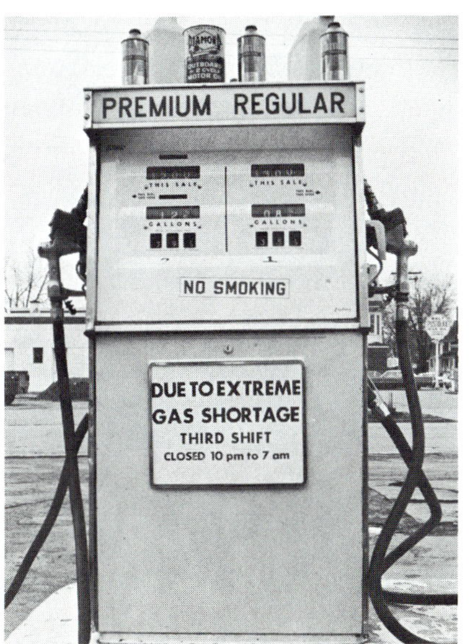

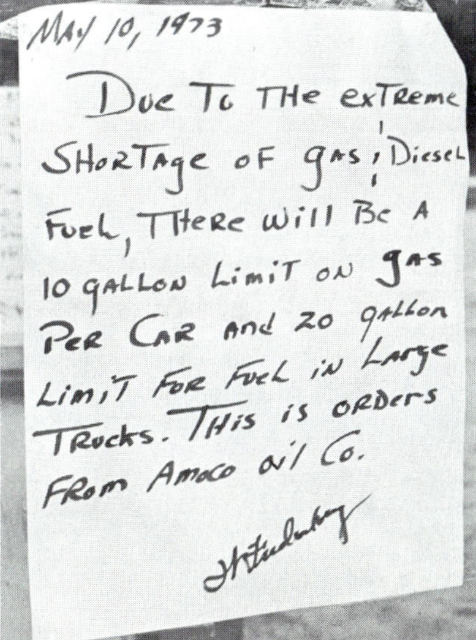

Figure 8–3

Some loud arguments for mass transit.

(Capital Newspapers, Albany, N.Y.)

WATER POLLUTION

We have been blithely looking the other way while our extensive problem of water pollution reached such proportions that it could no longer be ignored. We now have the choice of cleaning up the mess or stagnating with it as a community.

In the past, we have used our waterways as open sewers and as reservoirs for industrial wastes. There was a time when this could be done without its having great impact on our civilization. However, with the growth in our population and our industrial complex, we find that the wastes are now almost six times what they were sixty years ago in our rivers, lakes, and streams. These conditions have had a number of unfortunate effects. There has been the outbreak of disease, particularly when shellfish were taken from polluted waters. Detergent foam has become a more and more familiar sight floating on the surface of rivers and streams and in the drinking water of some communities. Large areas for fishing and swimming have been rendered useless by industrial wastes and other pollutants. Each year more bathing beaches and boating areas have been closed down because the water is unsafe. Some of the newer chemical substances such as pesticides that are finding their way into our waterways in increasing quantities represent a new facet of the pollution problem. Probably the greatest danger presented by water pollution is that it contaminates our sources of water. Three-fourths of our water needed for industrial, agricultural,

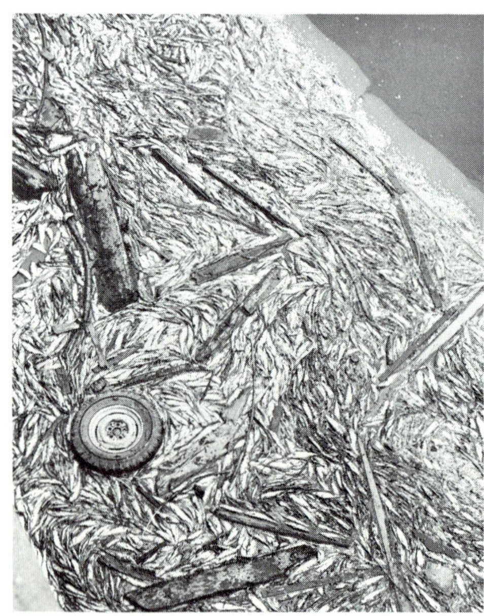

Figure 8–4

A massive fish kill due to polluted water.

(New York State Department of Environmental Conservation)

and municipal use comes from the rivers, lakes, and streams that we have been busy polluting. With our continued population growth as well as industrial and agricultural growth, the demands for water will surely increase. The challenge of producing enough usable water for the next few decades must be met. Water is without a doubt the number one raw material used by industry.

Agriculture, because of increased use of irrigation, has many times multiplied the amount of water it uses. Fortunately, water is a material that can be cleaned and its impurities removed. There just will not be enough new water to meet the needs of our communities. The answer to the maintenance of an adequate water supply is to use water over and over again. This means that ways must be found to remove the impurities as well as to prevent them from getting into the water in the first place.

Nuclear energy has begun to be used as a source of power. At the present time little more than 1 per cent of the country's power is developed by nuclear reactors. The great majority of the power plants burn fossil fuels (coal, oil, and natural gas). However, by 1980, 35 per cent of the country's power will be produced by nuclear reactors and by the year 2000, more than half the country's power needs are expected to come from this source. Nuclear plants are located by bodies of water because water is used as a coolant in the process. The heated waters emitted from the nuclear power plant can have detrimental effects on aquatic plants because of reduced levels of oxygen. When nuclear plants are placed by large bodies of water such as an ocean rather than a river or lake the thermal effects could have a positive effect by stimulating desirable biological growth. The pollutant potentials of nuclear plants need to be weighed against the kinds of pollution now being caused by power plants using fossil fuels.

CONTROLLING WATER POLLUTION

There is a great need for modern sewage plants that would properly treat sewage and release it into the nearest waterway only when it is completely safe. In a modern sewage treatment plant both primary and secondary treatment is given. Sewage treatment plants have difficulty removing industrial waste materials, particularly some of the new substances such as plastics, detergents, pesticides, nylons, or radioactive materials. These are best prevented from entering the waterways at their source. The biggest difficulty with sewage treatment plants is that there are not enough of them. There is no question that these are expensive facilities, their costs ranging from $50,000 to several million, dependent on their size. However, no community is properly assuming its responsibilities if it does not adequately treat its sewage but merely sends it downstream for the next community to deal with.

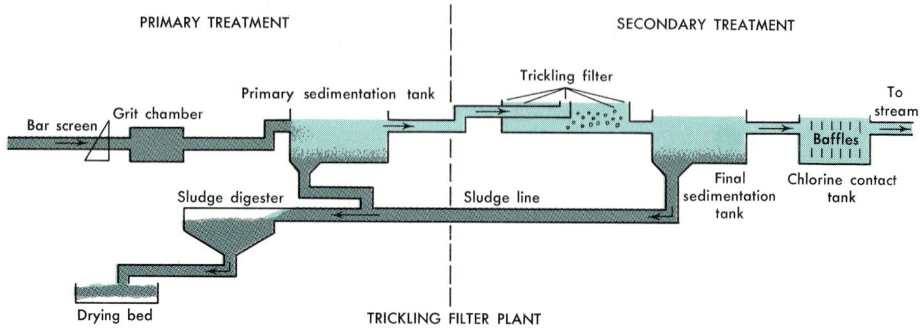

Figure 8–5

Diagram of sewage treatment. During *primary treatment* the water or sewage passes through a bar screen which catches large objects. The water next flows into a grit chamber that allows small objects like sand and gravel to settle out. It is then sent into a large settling tank where solid materials in the water will either settle to the bottom or rise to the top. The water between these two layers is drained off and sent to that part of the sewage plant that gives secondary treatment. In *secondary treatment* water is sprinkled over a bed of stones and permitted to trickle through. Bacteria grow on these stones and their function is to dissolve organic matter from the water. The water then goes through a final sedimentation tank and from there to a chlorine tank. The treated water is then discharged into a river or a stream. The solid wastes that are removed from the sewage are deposited in a sludge digester and from there they move out to a sludge drying bed. This treated sludge can be used for land fill or fertilizer.

Industry has a vital interest in conserving the country's water supply. Some industrial plants use more water than the entire city they are located in. By 1980 it is estimated that industry will be using two-thirds of the nation's water supply. Many industries have started water conservation programs. Changes in production procedure have curtailed the amount of water needed initially and have reduced the amount and nature of industrial wastes emitted. Most major industry is currently conducting research designed to curtail its waste output further. Industry has been reacting more quickly to the pollution problem, for while it is the major consumer of water it contributes less than half the pollution. The ability and the willingness of industry to move toward completely effective waste control programs will continue to be vital.

The federal government likewise is making a concerted effort to halt pollution and revitalize those areas which are already polluted. The Water Pollution Control Act of 1948 was enacted as temporary legislation so that it could be reviewed and revised after a five-year trial period. After a three-year renewal of the rather limited 1948 act, Congress in 1956 passed the Federal Water Pollution Control Act. This legislation was more extensive than its predecessor. It assisted 2,750 cities to build sewage treatment plants as well as to clean up some of our waterways. Before this legislation was passed, our municipalities and industries were spending less than half of what was needed to keep up with the enlarging pollution problem. Though the 1956 Act was a stimulant for increased pollution control, it was not strong enough to turn the tide. In 1961, in response to President Kennedy's appeal for stronger legislation, Congress amended the 1956 Act. The amendments made provision for the following:

1. Increased Federal support for the construction of municipal waste treatment facilities.
2. Broadened and strengthened the Federal Government's enforcement powers.
3. Called for an intensified program of research looking toward more effective methods of pollution control, with special emphasis on regional variations.
4. Authorized increased federal support of state and interstate pollution control programs.
5. Established in law the principle of water storage in planning and building federal reservoirs to maintain water quality during periods of low flow.[1]

The Water Quality Act of 1965 called for water quality standards for interstate water and for satisfactory state plans to meet these objectives. This legislation was supplemented by the Clean Rivers Restoration Act of 1966 which authorized $3.4 billion for the building of sewage treatment plants. However, there are usually great gaps between the amounts of money authorized and those actually spent. In some areas states have come together as regional compacts such as the Ohio River Valley Water Sanitation Commission involving eight states. This has resulted in coordinated and more effective ways of dealing with the problems of water supply and the prevention of water pollution. The federal government has enforcement powers provided through the Water Quality Act of 1965. Enforcement power was given the Secretary of the Interior who can bring suit against violators.

State laws will usually empower a control agency to make rules and regulations and to enforce them. They provide that a permit be sought from the control agency before any new or increased waste discharges are permitted. In June 1973, 15 states and 54 cities banned the sale of detergents with levels of phosphates above 8.7 percent. Some communities banned the use of detergents containing *any* phosphates. How effective a state's control agency is will be determined by the quality and number of its staff.

The international implications of pollution are being increasingly recognized.

[1] "Protecting Our Water Resources" (Washington, D.C.: U.S. Dept. of Health, Education, and Welfare, Public Health Service, 1962), p. 6.

The International Joint Committee that involves the United States and Canada, and the International Boundary and Water Commission involving the United States and Mexico have been established to investigate water pollution as it affects the respective countries and to develop remedial procedures.

Community Interest Stimulates Action

The emergence of some isolated instances of success in the fight against pollution is now being seen. A remarkable example can be found in the greater Seattle area in the state of Washington. This metropolitan area is located between the salt waters of Puget Sound and the fresh waters of Lake Washington. The quality of water in the area was in the process of being destroyed by 70,000,000 gallons of raw sewage which was dumped into Puget Sound. Lake Washington suffered from bacterial pollution that closed down its beaches as well as from an overgrowth of algae. The latter's growth was stimulated by the effluents being discharged from existing sewage treatment plants. The effluents from these sewage treatment plants were serving as fertilizer for the algae. The lake was in essence being killed by overfertilization. The water transparency declined from 12 feet in 1950 to $2\frac{1}{2}$ feet in 1962.

An enormous citizen effort then went into action. A municipal government was set up with the single function of sewage disposal for the city of Seattle and the surrounding counties. A comprehensive ten-year plan was developed for the rehabilitation of Puget Sound and Lake Washington. It required $125,000,000 worth of new sewage treatment facilities. The project progressed in many instances ahead of schedule. It was initiated in 1961 and by 1970 all effluent discharges into Lake Washington had ceased as well as the flow of raw sewage into Puget Sound. The waters were returned to their esthetic best as well as to varied recreational uses. Only 4 per cent of the cost of the project was subsidized by state or federal funds, an outstanding example of self-determination exemplifying what can be done when a community vigorously pursues a worthwhile objective.

Increasingly, various groups are showing interest and concern for the conservation of the nation's water. They range from Junior Chambers of Commerce and Leagues of Women Voters, to the Outboard Boating Club of America and the National Wildlife Federation, among many others. As an interested and responsible citizen of your community, how many of the following questions can you answer?

Are Wastes Treated?

Does your community have a sewage plant?
What kind of treatment is provided—primary or secondary?

Do Wastes Escape?

In normal dry weather, is some sewage bypassed into the stream?
In wet weather, when pipes and plants may be taxed by stormflow, is some sewage bypassed? What percentage? How often does this occur?

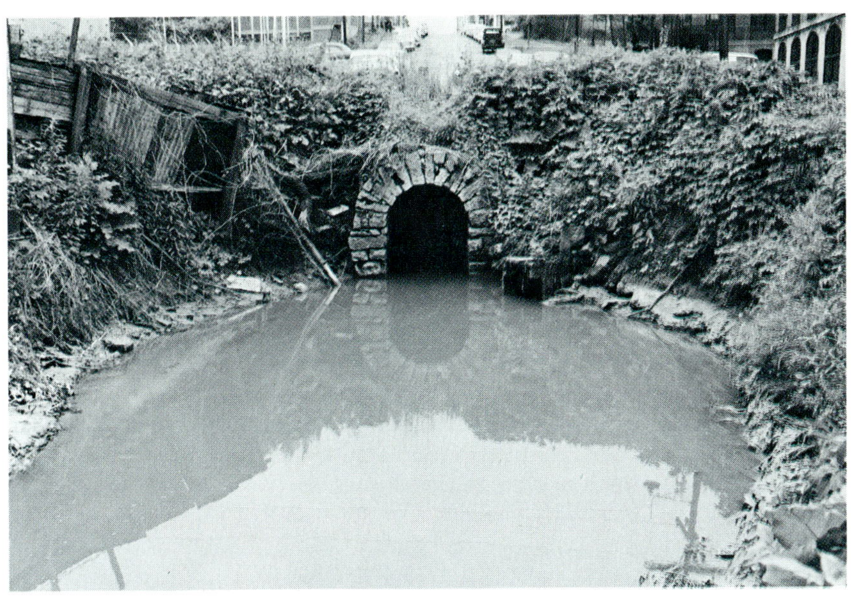

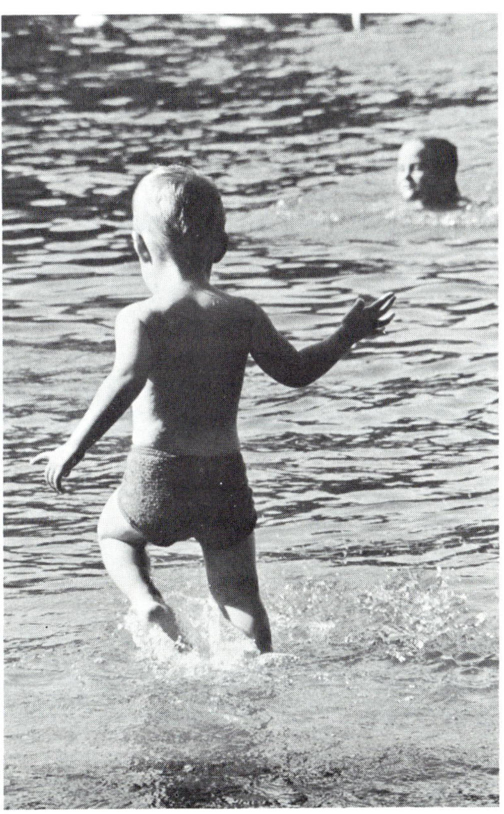

Figure 8–6A

How shall we use our waterways? . . . as a place to dump sewage. . . .

(New York State Department of Environmental Conservation)

Figure 8–6B

. . . or as a place for recreation?

(New York State Department of Environmental Conservation)

Adequate Staff?

Does your waste treatment plant have enough employees to operate it efficiently on a 24-hour, 365-day basis?

Proper Training?

Does your State provide training programs for plant operators?

Does your plant (if it's large enough) provide in-plant training? If so, are the programs utilized?

Does your community pick up the tab for such training courses?

Staff Certified?

Does your State or other agency have certification requirements for plant operators?

Does your community live up to these requirements?

Adequate Plants and Sewers?

How many homes are not connected with sewer pipes?

How many sewer pipes are not connected with a waste treatment plant?

Is the plant itself modern and up to date?

Does your community prohibit connection with roof and other storm water drains?

Future Needs?

Has your community drafted a plan to build new sewers and new plants as its area grows?[2]

LAND POLLUTION

The third phase of pollution which has been ignored far longer than either air or water pollution is land pollution. Through the years, the only progress made in garbage or trash removal was the hiring of persons to "take it away." Where they took it was of no concern to the suburban or urban dweller. With the establishment of air and water controls the elimination of many of the solid or semisolid wastes which were heretofore burned or dumped in riverways was prohibited.

> The land, therefore, inherits not only the solid wastes of our urban society, but also the unwanted solid and liquid wastes resulting from water and air pollution control.
>
> It is increasingly being recognized that the third dimension—the land, must be protected from pollution by urban, commercial, industrial and agricultural solid wastes. The land is the ultimate depository for the unwanted solid wastes from our society.[3]

[2] "Focus on Clean Water" (Washington, D.C.: U.S. Dept. of Health, Education and Welfare, Public Health Service Publication No. 1184), p. 8.

[3] Joseph A. Salvato, "The Third Dimension: Land Pollution," *Health News*, Vol. 44, No. 2 (February 1967), p. 13. N.Y. State Dept. of Health.

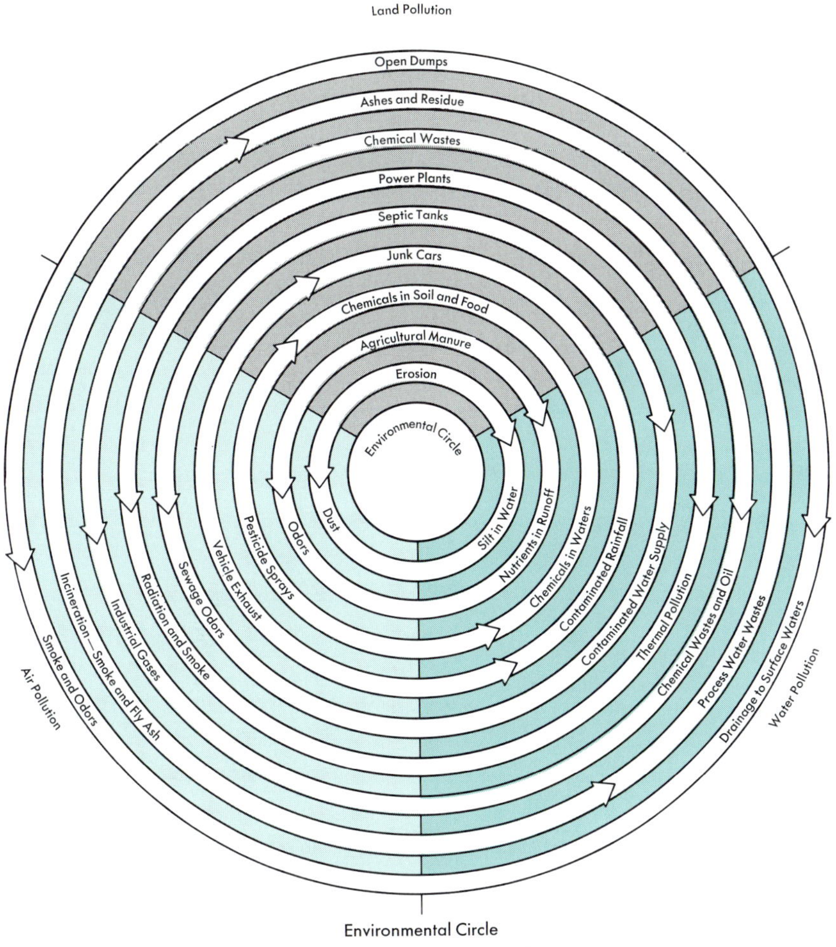

Figure 8–7

Environmental circle, showing many kinds of pollution and the effect on the total environment.

(New York State Department of Health)

Because of advanced technology and production we are now faced with the problem of getting rid of 500 billion pounds of solid waste each year, 4 billion pounds of which are plastic wrappings alone. For the most part, three-fourths of this solid waste is being delivered and periodically burned in open dumps. This primitive and unsatisfactory method is being replaced in some forward-thinking communities by sanitary landfill operations. This is a controlled method of disposal whereby refuse dumped in a trench or lower

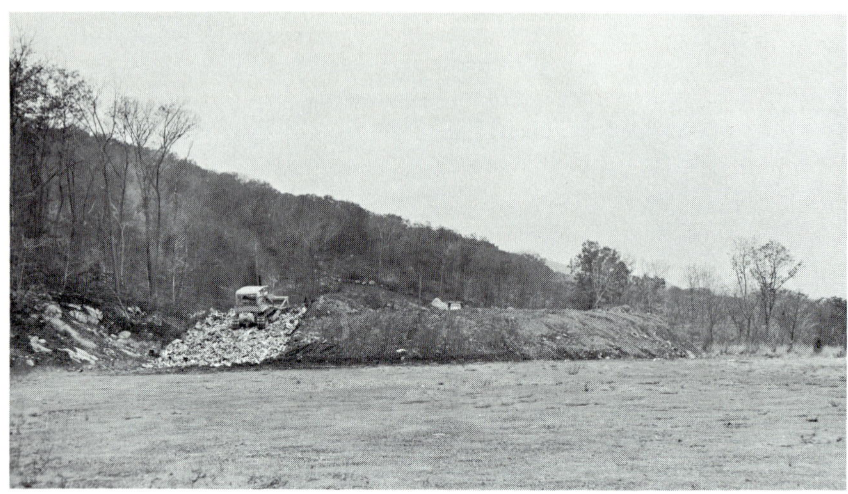

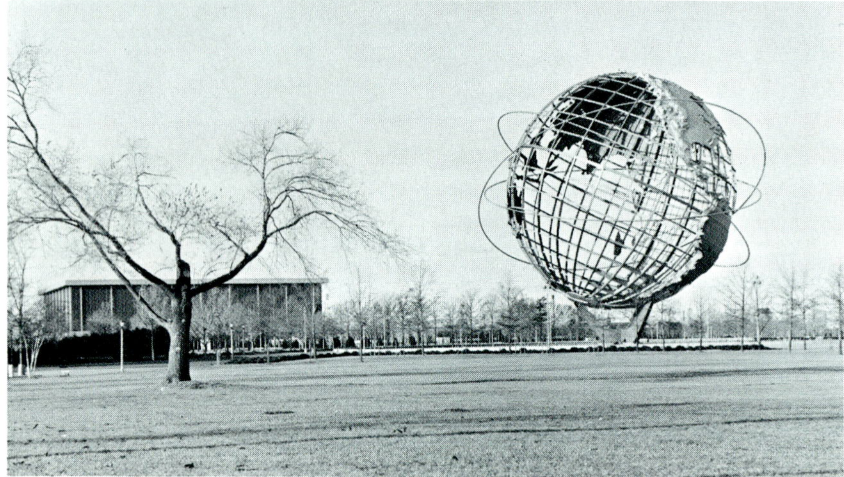

Figure 8–8

A, top- Sanitary landfills are replacing ugly, open dumps. B, bottom: When the sanitary landfill project is completed, the land can be put to a variety of good uses.

(New York State Department of Environmental Conservation)

valley area is covered by dirt at the end of each day. It is a carefully engineered project that eliminates the smoke, insects, rodents, odor, and ugliness of the open dump. When the sanitary landfill project is complete, the area can be slavaged for use as parks, golf courses, or structures not requiring excavation for basements.

With the increased awareness that the disposal of solid wastes is an important problem, cities and states have set up special agencies to arrive at a solution. The federal government has passed a Solid Waste Disposal Act which has been appropriating funds for demonstration projects. Though legislative mandates are by no means the complete solution to a problem—it is a start. Franklin, Ohio, is one community whose ingenuity, coupled with federal funds in the form of a grant, has come up with a promising solution to the problem.

> Here's how the complex works: A disposal plant reclaims reusable fibers from waste paper and separates and salvages metals and glass through centrifuge action.
>
> Adjacent to this plant is a sewage treatment facility. Sludge from this facility is mixed with the pulp residue from the disposal plant. This mixture is burned in a "fluid bed reactor"—a new kind of incinerator that burns trash more completely, thereby reducing the amount of residue.
>
> The treated effluent from the sewage plant is used to supply the water requirements of the disposal plant paper-pulping process. The fine ash from the fluid bed incinerator is piped to the sewage treatment plant and used in *that* process.
>
> After all this processing, there remains only about five percent of the original volume in the form of a clean, inorganic powder, which is placed in a nearby sanitary landfill.
>
> But this favorable disposal ratio is only part of the story. Initial operations of the complex indicate that it will salvage daily nine tons of reusable paper fiber, with a market value of $25 a ton; three tons of glass cullet, worth $15 a ton; three tons of ferrous metals, worth $10 to $15 a ton; and one-half ton of aluminum, worth $175 a ton. Thus Franklin's new waste disposal facility will help to pay for itself.[4]

Two counties in Wisconsin and Florida are pulverizing garbage, and elsewhere a new method compresses waste into 4-foot-cubed bales which seem excellent for landfill projects. In California wastes are burned in a

> high pressure incinerator to produce hot gases used to power a gas turbine. The turbine, in turn, drives a 15,000-watt electric generator. The projection is that not only will waste be burned up, but that the income from the production of electric power will offset the cost of operating the plant.[5]

The solutions of our land pollution problems will come from the creative professionals who can use the disposal process to fulfill other community needs and thus produce a constant productive cycle. The overenthusiastic, amateurish attempts at solid waste management that sporadically organizes community groups to collect bottles, cans, and newspapers are not effective in all instances.

[4] Richard D. Vaughan, "What to Do with Your Six Pounds of Garbage Every Day," *Today's Health* (June 1972), p. 47.

[5] Ibid.

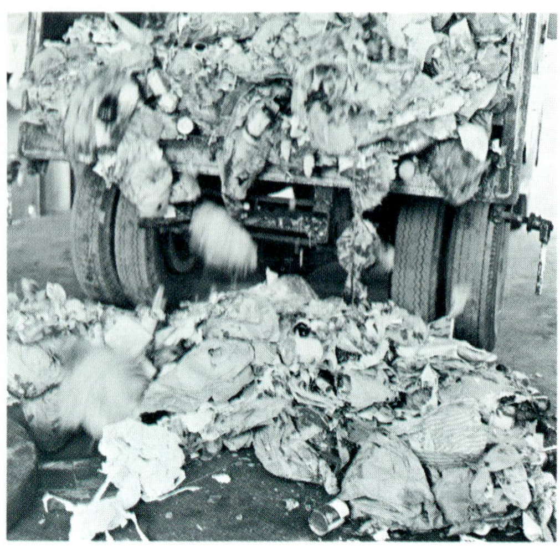

Figure 8–9

As the amount of garbage increases, its proper disposal becomes more important.

(New York State Department of Environmental Conservation)

The collections are usually carried off to the town's open dump to add to the problem because arrangements were not made with recycling units (where they exist). Instead, community groups should arm themselves with knowledgeable professionals and evaluate their community's waste disposal system, then move to effect the changes needed.

PESTICIDE USE AND EXPOSURE

The widespread use of these chemicals and how they find their way back to man are worth considering. Pesticides can enter the human body in three ways. They can be ingested as part of pesticide residue that may remain on food or contaminated dishes and utensils. They can also be inhaled when used as a spray, or they may be absorbed through the skin. The latter is a type of pesticide contact that is generally overlooked. Pesticides can be quite insidious, because we are often unaware that we have had contact with them. Pesticide poisoning frequently occurs without the persons' even considering pesticides as a source of his difficulty.

There has been an expanded use of pesticides in the last two decades. They are widely used in the protection of food crops. Carpet manufacturers use them in their products to discourage the presence of carpet beetles. In those areas where termites are a factor, termite poisoning is placed by the builder in the foundation of the home as well as in the soil around it. The dust from the soil could serve as a contaminant if inhaled. Some dry cleaning establishments impregnate clothes with pesticides, which can come in contact with the skin.

When fields are sprayed to eliminate certain kinds of pests, the insecticides are eaten along with the grass by animals. The insecticide can then return to the dinner table via game shot by the hunter. Insect sprays of various types are used to get rid of mosquitoes and flies in the home. Many people use insect sprays in the home as gayly and as indiscriminately as demonstrated on television commercials, ignoring the fact that these are poisonous materials. The result is the subsequent contamination of utensils, dishes, table tops, food, and human bodies. Also to be considered is the greater ability to inhale the spray as well as absorb it through the skin in an enclosed area. A number of pesticides are used in the garden in the form of powders, liquids, and sprays. The gardener who stands downwind from an insecticide is giving the insects all the advantage.

About 150 deaths a year are attributed to pesticide poisoning. Most of these occur among young children who ingest the poisonous chemicals. The incidence of pesticide poisoning that proves to be nonfatal can only be guessed at and some estimates run as high as 50,000. Some authorities believe it is probably even higher than this, because the symptoms produced by pesticide poisoning are similar to those of many common illnesses and are often not properly diagnosed. One of the real concerns in this whole area is the gap in our information with respect to the consequences of long-term exposure to pesticides. There just has not been enough research done in this area to give us clear-cut answers as to the significance of cumulative effects over periods of years. In one limited study, people who had a 35 milligram intake of DDT each day showed no ill effects from the exposure. However, it was found that there were 270 parts per million of DDT in their fatty tissues. This is more than twenty times the average level found in adults in the country. What continued exposure to DDT will mean to these people is unknown.

It has also been noted that there is an increased rate of pesticide poisoning among agricultural workers. What long-term exposure will mean to people in this occupation is yet to be determined. There is also little known about the effects of undue accumulation of more than one pesticide in the body. There is no question that there has been some improper use of pesticides. It has been noted that where these poisons have been used too casually there have been high fatalities among fish, birds, and other wildlife. Even when pesticide programs are carried out as planned, wildlife can be seriously affected. As reported by the President's Science Advisory Committee, mortality among birds approached 80 per cent in those areas where DDT was used for Dutch elm disease control. When DDT gets to bodies of water it can have a devastating effect on fish. In terms of sensitivity, it has been noted that fish are more sensitive to these substances than birds, and birds more so than mammals. One of the difficulties in controlling pesticide poisoning of animals is that wild animal populations roam freely and cannot be kept from treated areas. Birds, for instance, may fly into an area that has just been sprayed and eat worms that are now a source of poison and death to them.

BENEFITS OF PESTICIDES

It has been estimated that the production of apples, cotton, citrus fruits, and potatoes would be reduced by some 50 per cent without the use of pesticides, and the production of meat, milk, and wool would be reduced by 25 per cent. Many people feel that they have now become essential for the adequate production of food in this country. They unquestionably have contributed a great deal to the economic strength of the country and the nutritional well-being of the American people.

Insecticides also serve to control disease incidence. In an effort to control an outbreak of encephalitis in Dallas, Texas, in 1966, an insecticide was used to spray the city as a way of destroying mosquitoes and controlling the spread of this dread malady. Worldwide control of such diseases as malaria, yellow fever, bubonic plague, cholera, and typhus is being successfully pursued by the spraying of DDT. The incidence of malaria in India, for instance, has been reduced from 70 million cases a year to 5 million. The cry against the use of DDT that has arisen from Western Europe and North America has restricted its use in some of these areas. For example, as a result of premature cessation of spraying in Ceylon, their malaria rate went from 110 cases in 1961 (after a 15-year campaign against malaria) to 2.5 million in 1968–1969. The dilemma of DDT as an environmental threat on the one hand, and as the protector of human life on the other hand, will continue. In the meantime, a good deal of research is going on in a quest for alternative means of controlling pests other than through the use of pesticides. Pesticides, like many other potentially dangerous aspects of our environment, need to be used properly so that we may reap the benefits they afford and avoid needless undesirable consequences.

CONTROLLING PESTICIDES

When Rachel Carson's *Silent Spring*[6] was first published, there were mixed reactions to the book. Some indicated that the writing was emotional and exaggerated. Others felt that the book was most timely and one that would stimulate public interest in the subject as well as better controls in pesticide use. Perhaps Dr. W. B. Bean said it best in his editorial entitled "The Noise of Silent Spring," when he referred to the book as, "a call to attention rather than a call to arms."[7] Rachel Carson's publication set in motion a reexamina-

[6] Rachel Carson, *Silent Spring* (New York: Fawcett, 1962).

[7] "The Noise of *Silent Spring*," Editorial, W. B. Bean, Archives of Internal Medicine, AMA Publication 112:62, 1963.

tion of legislation and public practices and some soul searching with regard to the manner and the extent to which pesticides had been used. In the minds of many, the objectives of the writing were thus achieved.

The Federal Insecticide, Fungicide and Rodenticide Act is one of the federal laws controlling pesticide use. The administration and enforcement of this law is assigned to the United States Department of Agriculture (USDA). When new pesticides are developed by an industry, application must be made to the USDA requesting permission for its use. Recent legislation now requires that the FDA, the Public Health Service, and the Department of the Interior also review these applications to ensure the safety of the pesticide. When a pesticide is going to be used on food crops, the application must indicate which crop it is to be applied to, along with necessary data regarding its effectiveness and relative toxicity. If the pesticide leaves a residue and it is to be used on food crops, then a given residue tolerance (or a level of residue that may remain on the food when it reaches market) is tested for by the Food and Drug Administration.

Consumers Union, in its publication *Consumer Reports,* expressed some concern with regard to the permissiveness of current USDA pesticide labeling regulations. The USDA apparently classifies pesticides in four groups according to the danger presented by the chemical used. A mere taste of chemicals of the first group would prove fatal to a human. On the label of these appear a skull and crossbones and the words "POISON" and "WARNING." On all containers for these pesticides will appear a prescription for an antidote to be used in case of poisoning. In the second grouping the word "WARNING" must appear on the label. A mere teaspoon of these pesticides could kill a child, yet no antidote need appear on the label, nor need the word "POISON" be placed on the label, either. In the third grouping the word "CAUTION" must appear on the label, although this is not necessary for the fourth group. In fact, on the labels of the fourth group are occasionally found the words "SAFE and NON-TOXIC" even though it is a known fact that all pesticides, at least those presently known, are poisonous. The small print usually adds "if used as directed." Since some manufacturers are honest enough to put the word "CAUTION" on even their fourth grouping of pesticides, the result is a confused situation as far as the consumer is concerned.

The Federal Hazardous Substances Act under the jurisdiction of the FDA also plays a role in protecting the consumer from poisonous substances. The law requires that substances that are poisonous if swallowed be labeled "POISON" (with skull and crossbones). The label will also include instructions for special handling or storage, the chemical name of the hazardous substance, first-aid instructions, the statement "Call a physician immediately," and a warning statement, "Keep out of reach of children."

PROPER PERSONAL USE OF PESTICIDES

Where pesticides are to be used by the individual in the home or in the garden, the United States Public Health Service recommends that the following precautions be taken:

> READ THE LABEL each time you use a pesticide—no matter how often you have used it and no matter how well you think you know the instructions—and FOLLOW THE LABEL DIRECTIONS EXACTLY. KEEP PESTICIDES AWAY FROM CHILDREN AND CHILDREN AWAY FROM PESTICIDES.
>
> Other precautions are:
>
> 1. Use a pesticide only when you are sure it is needed. Use the one best suited to your needs. The label on the product explains the proper uses.
> 2. Keep the pesticide in a plainly labeled container, preferably the one in which it was bought. NEVER transfer pesticides to unlabeled or mislabeled containers.
> 3. Store pesticides under lock and key, away from food items and OUT OF THE REACH OF CHILDREN, pets, and people who might not be able to understand their danger.
> 4. When handling, mixing, or applying pesticides, avoid inhaling dust and fumes and avoid getting materials on the skin.
> 5. Check the label of the product BEFORE USING, so that you know what to do quickly if there is an accident. In case of an accident, call a doctor or get the patient to a hospital immediately.
> 6. The very few people who suspect they may have a special sensitivity to pesticides should consult an allergist, and if necessary, take steps to avoid any exposure to the offending agent.
> 7. Wash hands thoroughly after using pesticides and before eating or smoking.
> 8. Get rid of used pesticide containers in a way that will not leave the package of leftover contents as a hazard to people—particularly children—or to animals or plants.
> 9. Work in a well-ventilated area, to avoid inhalation of fumes.
> 10. Do not spray into the wind.
> 11. When so directed by the label, wear protective clothing, such as goggles, gloves, aprons, respirators, and masks.
> 12. When mixing or using inflammable chemicals, be especially careful to avoid the fire hazards caused by smoking, defective wiring, and open flames.

13. Cover food and water containers when using pesticides around livestock and pet areas.
14. Do not spray or treat plants or animals or animal feeding areas with pesticides unless you are certain such treatment is safe for that use.[8]

RADIATION

The atomic age has brought with it great hopes for the future as well as some concerns. The detonation of nuclear bombs and the ensuing fallouts have been watched and tested very carefully by scientists. We are seeing greater use of nuclear power in industry and consequently greater amounts of radiation wastes that need to be disposed of carefully. The question that must be answered is, What is the significance of this radiation exposure when added to the natural radiation that we receive from the sun and to that from medical and dental X rays?

The greatest source of natural radiation is, of course, cosmic radiation that originates in outer space with the sun as its source. The amount of cosmic radiation that one would be exposed to would multiply as the person left the surface of the earth and moved toward the upper atmosphere. It is estimated that cosmic radiation is three times as high at a level of 3,000 meters above the earth than it is at sea level. The amount of radiation on various parts of the earth will vary depending on different types of soil and rock, each having a varying ability to carry radioactivity. There will be certain deposits, of course, like uranium and thorium, whose radioactive content is quite high and can serve as a source of radiation. Man thus has been in contact with natural radiation from his very beginnings. What the effect of this natural low-level radiation has been on man is open to conjecture at this stage of our knowledge.

THE NATURE AND EFFECTS OF RADIATION

Radioactive chemicals have the tendency to disintegrate or decay. It is as a result of this disintegration that they give off various kinds of radiation, as exemplified by gamma rays or X rays. The rate at which this decay takes place varies considerably among these materials. Cesium 137, for instance, would require something like 250 years to decay to less than 1 per cent of its original level. Strontium 90 would require 150 years for a similar amount

[8] *Pesticides* (Washington, D.C.: U.S. Dept. of Health, Education and Welfare, Public Health Service Publication #1081).

of decay or disintegration. The great majority of radioactive materials, however, decay within a few days or a few weeks. A basic characteristic of all radiation is that it serves to carry energy from one point to another.

Radiation is measured by a unit of measurement called a roentgen. A thirty-year exposure of fallouts amounts to .1 roentgen, more or less, with medical radiation amounting to 2 to 5 roentgens. A chest X ray is rated at about .3 roentgen.

Studies have shown that radiologists and others occupationally exposed to increased doses of radiation are more likely to develop leukemia. Studies of the people of Hiroshima and Nagasaki exposed to radiation from the first atomic bombs confirm that a single high-dosage exposure produces a higher leukemia rate.

Another effect of radiation is that it tends to shorten the life expectancy of the exposed. Specifically why this occurs is not understood, but it has been noted.

Geneticists warn that doses of radiation considered to be below threshold level for somatic (bodily) effects can have potential for genetic harm. Early experiments by Dr. Muller with the drosophila (fruit fly) indicated that mutations increase with the amount of radiation received. Dr. Muller's studies and others also demonstrated that the vast majority of the mutations prove harmful to the species. Geneticists feel that the number of mutations that will occur in humans is in direct proportion to the amount of radiation reaching the reproductive cells. According to this principle, any amount of radiation is harmful, and therefore the less radiation we expose ourselves to, the better.

SOURCES OF MAN-MADE RADIATION

Fallout from nuclear bomb testing has been a source of man-made radiation that has stirred up vehement controversy, with some outcries against it bordering on hysteria. When a "small" nuclear device is exploded, most of the radioactive debris falls to earth within a few days or a few weeks. With larger devices, the radioactive materials are sent up into the stratosphere and take longer periods of time to descend back onto the earth. It is estimated that in these instances it takes ten years for 50 per cent of the radioactive material to descend. During this time, it becomes rather evenly distributed around the globe. Most of the radioactive particles will have disintegrated during this period, except for the more persistent ones like strontium 90 and cesium 137.

Radiation can enter the body by penetrating it directly. It can enter the body indirectly via radioactive materials taken in with food and water, or by inhalation. With fallout, the most common route of bodily entry would be by means of the food supply. The radioactive material may be deposited on food crops or may become a part of the soil and be absorbed by the plant. It may be deposited on grass that is eaten by the cow and thus is found in trace amounts in milk. Some estimates indicate that the amount of radiation we are exposed to via fallout is about 5 per cent of what we receive by natural radiation. It is difficult to make clear-cut assessments of this type, however, because different areas receive varying amounts of fallout. It has also been found that children will have larger amounts of strontium 90 in their bones because of its presence in milk and its ability to act like calcium in the body. Indications are that the amounts of these materials are minute and do not constitute dangers to health at these levels. The virtual elimination in recent years of atmospheric nuclear testing has brought this source of contamination under control.

Television sets give off what are referred to as soft X rays. They are not nearly as penetrating as radiation produced by X-ray machines and are shielded by the sides of the tube as well as the cabinet and outer glass covering on the set. Radiation exposure from this source is normally not considered significant.

Luminous radium-painted dials on watches and clocks give up small amounts of radiation. Their principal danger would be to young children who might remove the glass from the timepiece and either inhale or eat the flakes of paint. It is interesting to note that the sale of radium-dial pocket watches has been restricted in New York City. These watches are usually carried face inward below the waistline, and concern developed with regard to unnecessary exposure to radiation of the reproductive organs and the possible genetic effects.

Medical and Dental Radiation

The X ray and other forms of radiation are used for treatment purposes in cases of cancer. Cancer cells are more susceptible to the effects of radiation than normal cells and can thus be destroyed.

The utilization of X rays by physicians and dentists for diagnostic reasons has become more conservative in recent years. The principle adhered to is that X rays are unquestionably to be employed when necessary for a diagnosis—but only when necessary.

Some obstetricians at one time would X-ray the unborn child to check its size and position. Studies have since shown that children X-rayed prenatally suffered a higher incidence of leukemia. Mass chest X-ray programs have also been reduced in number. Only specific groups with high tuberculosis incidence in the community are being screened. Broadscale X-raying of all groups in a community is now considered unwise.

A good deal of progress has also been made in reducing the amount of radiation given off by X-ray apparatus. Work along these lines continues to further reduce radiation exposure from this source.

Industry

Lack of experience or instruction, and carelessness have been the bases of those few industrial accidents that involved radioactive materials. However, with the increasing production of these materials, more complex problems

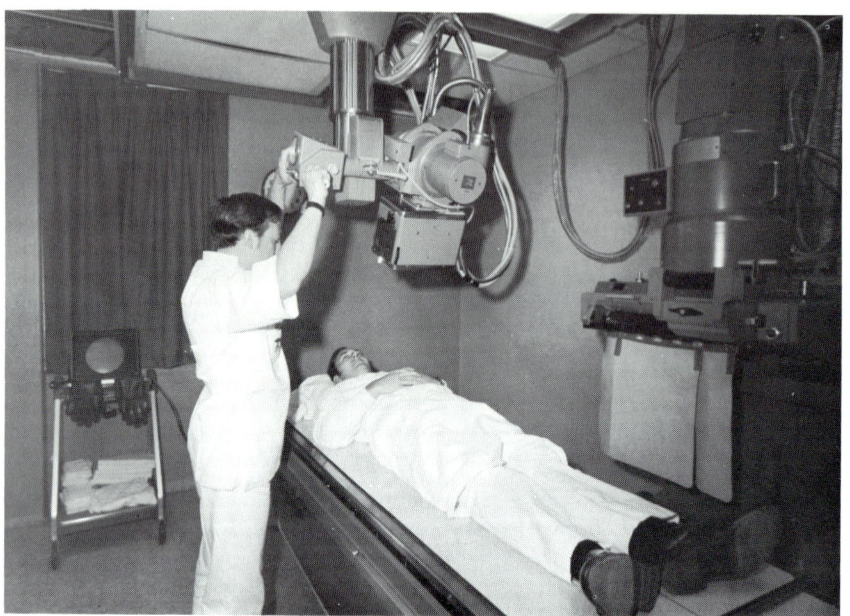

Figure 8–10

New Standards require improved diagnostic X-ray equipment.

(*FDA Consumer,* October 1972)

related to their handling and transportation will arise. Where an accident such as a fire occurs in a plant producing radioactive materials, other problems present themselves. Firemen need to know how to handle the situation lest they unduly expose themselves to radiation or inadvertently contaminate other areas with the radioactive materials that they have been in contact with. Smoke from such a fire may also contain radioactive contaminants and serve to spread them in the adjoining community. A truck carrying radioactive cargo involved in an accident presents problems peculiar to its load, relating again to radiation and contamination dangers. Accidents such as these are covered by very carefully worked-out plans of assistance by federal and state agencies prepared to take immediate action.

A source of concern and controversy has been the rapid increase in the number of nuclear-powered electric plants in the country. In 1972, 22 such plants were in operation, with 55 under construction and 49 more being planned. A major concern of some scientists is that the radiation released by these plants into the atmosphere could reach dangerous levels.

> Target of much of the criticism is the Atomic Energy Commission (AEC), which is responsible for promoting the peaceful use of atomic energy and

> for protecting the public from atomic danger. Critics maintain that these responsibilities conflict; they accuse the AEC of working harder to promote atomic energy than to protect the nation from it. . . . Dr. Gofman and other scientists have been producing studies since 1963 which indicate that the incidence of radiation-caused cancer and genetic disorders is 20 times greater than the AEC claims. The AEC maintains these studies are not scientifically accurate, but the commission did set new standards in June 1971, which reduce by 100 times the level of permissible radiation emission.[9]

While controversy revolves around the relative safety of nuclear power plants, power companies are caught in the middle needing to construct additional plants as the electric power needs of the country doubles every ten years. They also recognize that the sources of coal, oil, and natural gas are rapidly being depleted.

Several concerned citizen groups have managed to delay the construction of some nuclear plants. One U.S. senator has proposed legislation making the electric companies rather than the federal government (AEC) liable for radiation damage caused by nuclear plants. This is aimed at dampening their enthusiasm for nuclear power. Some companies have begun to consider the possibility of solar (use of the sun's energy) plants or geothermal (use of the heat from the earth's core) plants which would be pollution free. Planned expansive use of nuclear power plants in the meanwhile persists. Continued public surveillance of this controversy is necessary so that future plans best represent the public interest.

> Our civilization in this nuclear age has a staggering responsibility to the future. The costs to coming generations of our mistakes are almost beyond the power to imagine. Our technologists must be nothing less than infallible. Accordingly, everything must be done to increase our chances of being right when we finally decide what to do.[10]

REVIEW QUESTIONS

1 Why are our current environmental health problems actually reflective of man's progress?

2 What is the nature of the pollutants found in the air of our urban communities?

3 Describe a temperature inversion and its relationship to air pollution.

[9] "Do Nuclear Plants Make Deadly Neighbors?" *Today's Health,* February 1972.

[10] Peter H. Metzger, "Dear Sir: Your House Is Built on Radioactive Uranium Waste," *New York Times Magazine Section,* October 31, 1971.

4 What have been the effects of air pollution on health and property?

5 What forms of air pollution control are being developed for the automobile, industry, and municipalities?

6 How extensive is our water pollution problem? What are the causes of this environmental problem?

7 Describe primary and secondary treatment of sewage. What are the limitations of modern sewage treatment plants in handling some of the newer chemical industrial wastes?

8 Why does industry have a vital interest in conserving the country's water supply?

9 What role has the federal government played in water pollution-control programs?

10 How can a community go about evaluating how well it is succeeding or failing in the area of water conservation?

11 What has been the contribution of Rachel Carson's book, *The Silent Spring,* to the more discriminate use of pesticides?

12 What are the means whereby pesticides can enter the human body? What can be their effects?

13 What effects can the careless use of pesticides have on wildlife?

14 How has recent legislation given greater protection to the consumer from the harmful effects of pesticides?

15 What are the sources of man-made radiation? To what extent have controls been developed to limit human exposure?

16 What are the potentials of radiation for bodily and genetic harm?

9. Living Safely

THE ACCIDENT has become the neglected epidemic of our modern society. It is now the leading cause of death in the first half of the life-span. The time has come to dispel the notion that the accident is inevitable and beyond our control and to initiate some positive action.

The dramatic decline in the death rate due to infectious disease has left the accidental death rate standing like a tall oak in a leveled forest. The death rate due to accidents has actually gone down in some age groups; however, as compared to other problems, we have not made significant progress in this field. It can now be said that the accident is the leading cause of death in the age group 1 to 37, and that in the age group 1 to 14, accidents claim more lives than the next five leading causes of death combined. In the 15 to 24 age group, accidents are responsible for more lives lost than *all* other causes combined, with the automobile accident as the predominant cause of death.

For too long we have accepted the accident as an unavoidable aspect of our environment. The result has been that as a society we have developed a tolerance for accidental death that we would not have for death caused by disease. If a plague were to hit this country and cause over 100,000 deaths, all kinds of emergency actions would be initiated and great concern would be evident. Yet we have this very situation caused by the accident with very little reaction or concern being shown. Death, as we know, is not the only means of measuring the seriousness of a problem. Accidents result in a loss of approximately 18 billion dollars in medical and hospital expenses, wage loss, property destruction, and damage. They also cause over 10½ million injuries, with 400,000 of these resulting in permanent, partial, or total disability.

While the accident represents an environmental problem that is not as well recognized by society as it should be, better-informed elements of the community have been at work. Increasingly, professionals from the areas of preventive medicine and public health are being involved in the study of safety problems. It is felt that the methods used by these groups to control the communicable diseases can have application in the field of accident prevention. Newer and more comprehensive research methodology is needed for more complete understanding of this environmental hazard. Even the definition of the accident has come under closer scrutiny. Generally, accidents have been described as unplanned or uncontrolled events that have resulted in injury or damage of some kind. Current thinking is that for purposes of research broader definitions of the accident are more appropriate.

EPIDEMIOLOGY IN SAFETY RESEARCH

Epidemiology is the scientific study of those processes and factors that influence the health of people. The epidemiological study of an accident involves the study of the interactions between the *host* (the person), the *agent* (those things that inflict injury—glass, fire, poison, explosives), and the *environment* (lack of visibility at night, nonskid rugs, highway design). Studying the accident from this rather broad approach usually leads to the conclusion that it takes a combination of factors to cause an accident.

An epidemiologic approach was used in the study of off-duty motor vehicle accidents in the armed services. The motor vehicle accident ranked ahead of diseases and other types of accidents as a cause of death and disability. Study revealed that the accidents were not related to long-distance weekend driving, but to driving short distances around the army base, usually during late evening or early morning hours. It was found that 70 per cent of the accidents occurred within 10 miles of the base, and 90 per cent within a 50-mile radius. The high-rate accident group was identified as the young, unmarried, enlisted man who was in search of recreational activity which usually included drinking. A high proportion of the accidents also occurred on a few particular sections of the highway. As a result of the study recommendations, the military police patrolled the high-incident sections of the highway. They took into custody those who appeared excessively fatigued or under the influence of alcohol. Countermeasures that were put in effect resulted in a 42 per cent decrease in the accident rate.

Epidemiologic principles in accident prevention revolve around (1) *Making the "host" less susceptible to accidents.* This could involve such things as increasing the person's skill (driver education), or developing positive attitudes and safer practices. (2) *Making the "agent" less hazardous.* For example, safety lenses in eyeglasses, safety devices on machinery, shatterproof glass on cars. (3) *Modifying the environment to make it more accident-free.* Dual highways, guardrails, proper lighting to prevent falls—these would be but a few examples of this principle.

In the study of the host or human being, researchers have become concerned with determining the keenness of the person's senses (vision, hearing, and others) and therefore the ability of the individual to react to his environment. In addition, motor ability as measured by reaction time, coordination, and habit patterns are considered important. The physical condition of the body is also noted, with age, sex, strength, body build, and general physical fitness taken into account. The person's social attitudes and feelings of responsibility for himself and others are also reviewed. The driver in the flow of traffic is essentially in a social situation. Driving that would reflect the individual's lack of regard for others invariably would be more conducive to a higher incidence of accidents. Nothing the person may do to affect his physical and mental abilities can be overlooked. The keenest of senses and the highest level of coordination can be blunted by the use of drugs and alcohol. Patterns of behavior that lead to the habitual misuse of these substances can quickly negate other positive qualities the person may have and reduce them to a level that would make the person accident-prone. Safety knowledge and intelligence are also considered in evaluating the "host."

The environmental approach in the prevention of accidents has been influenced most by safety engineering and related disciplines. Various types of safety equipment that have made contributions here include machine guards, safety belts, and better door locks. There has also been developed greater control of atmospheric pollutants through engineering, although we still have a long way to go in this field. In the past, studies of accidents have attempted to relate a single factor or "cause" to the accident. It is comparable to pulling a factor out of context. For example, suppose a driver is momentarily distracted by a bird that flies into his windshield. As a result, the car swerves enough to cause the two right wheels to leave the pavement. In many such instances the driver might slow down and then return to the road. If, however, the shoulders of the road are soft or muddy, we have an environmental factor that might complicate the situation. The driver might find that he does not have the strength to control his vehicle on the soft shoulder (a physical factor). He may also have been exceeding the speed limit (a judgment factor). If he was driving a car with the engine in the rear, when leaving the pavement the added weight in the back of the car might have caused the vehicle to fishtail, resulting in the car's overturning (a vehicular factor). The driver might also react to the situation by slamming on the brakes, resulting in a loss of control of the vehicle (driver skill factor). So although a misguided bird may have initiated a potential accident, a number of factors such as the environment, driver strength, obeying the speed laws, vehicular construction, and driving skill could all come into the picture for consideration.

The attempts to develop accident prevention programs by modifying human behavior, though helpful, are not as rapid as effecting environmental changes. Things in the environment can be modified, rearranged, and added to with relative ease. The rearrangement of human behavior, however, does not take place as easily. Nevertheless, a full program of accident prevention will aim at effecting changes in the human (host), the agent, and the environment.

TRAFFIC SAFETY

The automobile has become an inherent part of American life. In addition to providing a major means of transportation, it has also become a status symbol, a living room on wheels, a major source of air pollution, and a means of committing suicide and murder. The automobile, in becoming a part of our culture, has made major social and economic contributions to it. At the same time, it is exacting a price that makes us pause to question why the automobile must kill approximately 50,000 Americans a year and injure millions. At the present rate, more than one out of every two Americans can be expected to be killed or injured in an automobile accident. Is the carnage on the American highways a necessary price for the "luxury" of a car?

The automobile manufacturers have responded to this question by supporting driver education courses, the implication being that the driver is basically at fault in the accident. Properly train the driver and you reduce the accident rate. The government has responded to the situation by subsidizing the construction of new and safer highways. The publication of the book *Unsafe at Any Speed,* in 1966, by Ralph Nader, opened up a third facet, the heretofore untouched issue of the unsafe construction of the automobile.

THE AUTOMOBILE AS AN ACCIDENT FACTOR

Mr. Nader's thesis is that for too long we have focused on the driver as the basic cause of all accidents. Law-enforcement personnel, in investigating accidents, look first for the presence of alcohol and, failing to find that, generally place the accident in the realm of reckless driving. In essence, the philosophy has prevailed that the accident can result only from the violation of a law and if laws are obeyed you cannot possibly have accidents. This foolproof, if illogical viewpoint, does not take into account the accelerator that got stuck, the brakes that locked or failed, the tire that blew out, or the windshield wiper that reflected sunlight into the driver's eyes at the time of the accident.

Mr. Nader used the following example to make his point. He indicated that in order to make shaving safer, we progressed from a very crude cutting device to a straight razor, to the safety razor, and finally to the electric razor (or shaver). He pointed out that advising people to have a steady hand, not to be temperamental while they are shaving, and to keep their eye on the mirror would not significantly reduce slashed faces if they were using a crude razor. The redesigning of the instrument in the form of an electric razor, for instance, would permit the individual to make an operational slip without slashing his throat. The obvious conclusion drawn, then, is that we can significantly reduce injury and death by making the car safer. Because one out of every two cars produced will be involved in either a death or injury-producing accident, examination of the vehicle seems logical.

Mr. Nader has further contended that the stylist for the automobile industry has been acting as a quack engineer, designing the car for its outward appearances rather than for its functional excellence or crashworthiness. The publicity generated by Mr. Nader's attacks on the automobile industry and a Senate subcommittee hearing on the subject led to the conclusion that the imprudently built car, just like the imprudent driver, represents a social menace.

In September 1966 the National Traffic and Motor Vehicle Safety Act was passed. This legislation provided for the establishment of a National Agency to carry out its provisions. One of the first actions of this agency was to recommend 23 safety features that would apply to 1968 automobiles, both domestic and imported.

Recent research has sought to ascertain how well the structure of the average car will protect its occupants in a crash. Unfortunately, cars constructed with what must be described as *basic* safety features are still the exception rather than the rule. Tests conducted on the crashworthiness of the conventional car indicate the need for the following basic changes:

1. The frame of the automobile needs to be redesigned to increase its energy-absorbing capability for the front end and the sides of the car.
2. The engine of the car should be mounted in such a manner that in a head-on collision it is deflected toward the ground rather than into the passenger compartment.
3. All cars should have roll-bar construction to prevent the roof from caving in on its passengers in a roll-over accident.

The bumpers on cars have been completely inadequate. Starting with the 1973 models, cars had to be equipped with bumpers that would not result in damage to such equipment as headlights, cooling systems, trunk doors or tail lights in low-speed impacts (5 mph going forward, $2\frac{1}{2}$ mph in reverse).

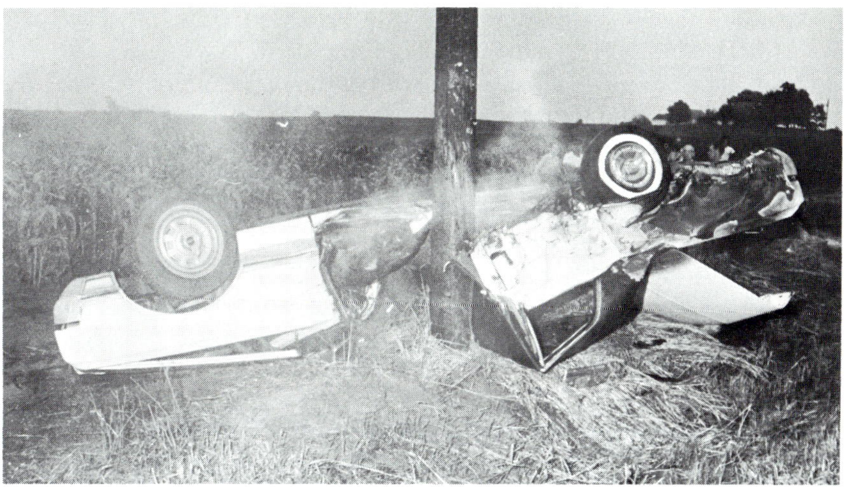

Figure 9–1

All cars should have roll-bar construction to prevent the roof from caving in on its passengers.

(Capital Newspapers, Albany, N.Y.)

This will reduce repair costs for parking lot mishaps. What are now needed are bumpers that are effective where cars were intended to be used, namely, on the highway.

In recent years the recalling of cars by the automobile industry for the correction of structural defects has become a common practice. In the period between 1966 and 1971, 25 million American and foreign-made vehicles were recalled. This represents 40 per cent of all cars and trucks sold in this country. In 1971 General Motors set a new record by recalling 6.7 million cars and trucks for possible faulty engine mounts. It offered to install straps to hold possibly faulty engine mounts in place. While an official of General Motors described the failure of motor mounts as no more serious than a flat tire, motorists who went through the experience described it as terrifying.

In 1972 the Ford Motor Company recalled over 400,000 Torinos and Mercury Montegos to guard against bearing failures causing the rear end to fall to the pavement. Ford offered to place an extra set of retainer plates on the rear axles of the cars. In case of bearing failure these retainer plates would cause a loud screeching noise warning the motorist to head for his nearest Ford dealer before it was too late. How's that for a better idea! If the motorist made it to the Ford dealer, the bearings would be replaced without charge. The trauma is also free. Ultimately the Ford Company consented to replace the entire axle unit. The screeching that precipitated this action did not come from retainer plates but from consumer groups, including Ralph Nader.

Recalls generally come about when the National Highway Traffic Safety Administration (NHTSA) or an automobile manufacturer suspects that a safety defect may be present in a vehicle. The recall, however, can only be ordered by the company. The NHTSA can only recommend a recall. Ralph Nader has contended that in the interests of public safety the government should have the power to order such recalls and advocates the need for new legislation to effect this.

The Air Bag

At the present time approximately 30 per cent of the nation's motorists use the safety belts (shoulder straps and lap belts) which were mandated for all cars. It is estimated that about 5,000 lives a year are saved as a result of the current level of use of safety belts. If all motorists could be convinced to use them, it is estimated that an additional 10,000 lives a year would be saved. An objective has been to get more motorists to wear their safety belts. People are still not using their seat belts even though belt systems are connected to the ignition system and require the motorist to buckle up in order to start the car. The result of all this has been serious thought about a passive restraint that operates automatically. The air bag has been proposed as the solution. On impact, the air bag would inflate inside the car cushioning

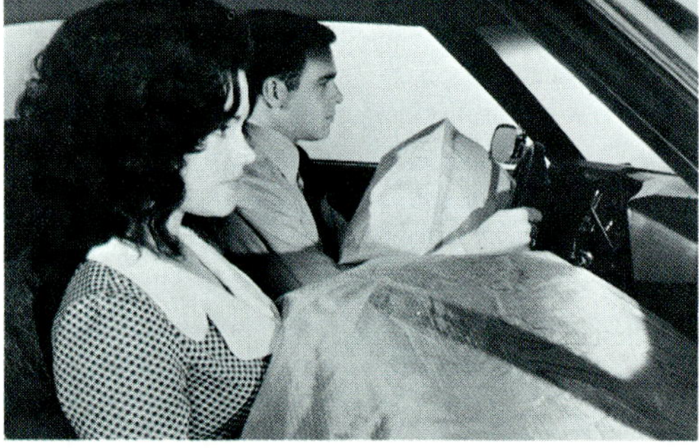

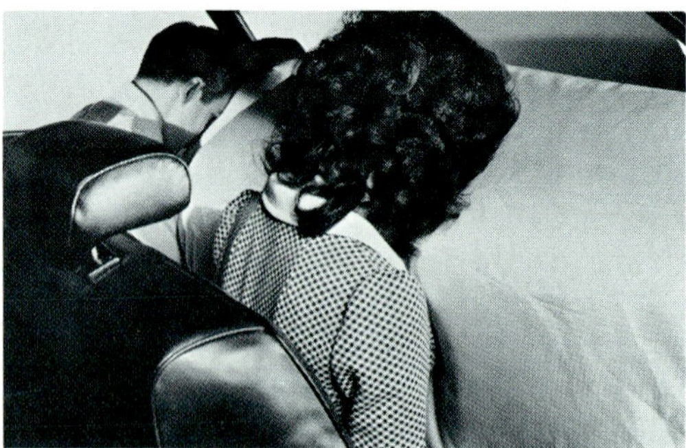

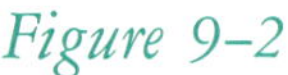

Figure 9–2

Air bags add a new dimension to protecting automobile passengers from injury.

(Fisher Body, Division, General Motors)

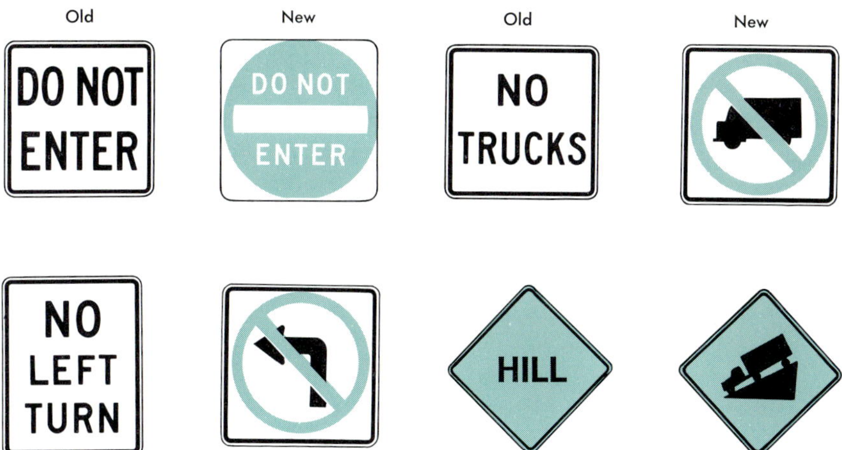

Figure 9–3

In order to cut down the accident rate on our highways further, a new international system of road signs is being implemented. The new symbol signs are more effective than words where reaction time and understanding are important. By adapting these signs on a nationwide level the differences in state-to-state travel signs will be minimized.

its passengers from the shock of impact. Standards call for the air bag to protect the occupants of a car when hitting a parked car at 60 mph. Federal safety standards are requiring the installation of air bags for all cars sold in the United States as of 1976.

Some serious questions about air bags have been raised. Since the air bag deflates in one second, it gives little protection to the motorist in a roll-over accident in which he may be bounced about the vehicle. The bags would also not protect the occupants of a car against a second collision, as might happen in a chain series of accidents on a highway. They also provide little protection in side impacts. At this stage in its development, the air bag would seem to be an excellent supplement to seat belts and head rests. It would thus make the American car safer in time of accident.

THE INTERSTATE HIGHWAY SYSTEM

Travel on the nation's developing interstate highway system is safer than on other kinds of roadways. The mileage death rate on the interstate system has been 2.2 per 100,000,000 miles of travel. This compares favorably with the 6.4 rate for all other roadways. The continued development of the interstate system will provide an extended environment for safer highway travel.

However, some controversy has arisen because the preponderance of transportation funds are going to the development of superhighways, with other means of transportation being ignored. Road builders and administrators are being charged with indifference to the other transportation needs of the people, to say nothing of their human and environmental needs.

> Pared down to its core, this final argument says, "The trust funds have paid for the superhighways, and also have kept the gas and rubber and truck weight and parts sales taxes from being used for any other purpose except building those highways." Agreed: The Trust Fund concept, thus described, has been a whopping success. Because of it the United States today can claim the most impressive system of superhighways the world has ever known—along with a collection of run-down railroads, limping urban transit services, and archaic local streets and roads that have been starved of public funding support by the Trust Fund's "new highways only" preoccupation.[1]

THE DRIVER

The safest vehicle and the safest highways can be negated by the driver who for one reason or another cannot perform in a responsible manner. A study by the Department of Police Administration at Indiana University indicates that where the alcohol level in the blood of the driver reaches .15 per cent the chances of that driver's having an accident increase 25 times.

The increase in the use of drugs has also resulted in larger numbers of people driving while under drug influence. Prescription as well as self-prescribed proprietary drugs can have side effects that can seriously affect a driver's performance. A number of drugs produce drowsiness, some affect vision and equilibrium, while others produce a dangerous overconfidence.

It has been standard procedure for the Interstate Commerce Commission to require medical examinations of commercial drivers involved in interstate travel. Operators of private vehicles who do most of the nation's driving are not subjected to the same scrutiny. There is apparently a need to establish some national norms to be used as guidelines indicating kinds of physical conditions that would prevent a person from acquiring a drivers' license. Though some states have set standards, the nationwide picture is rather spotty. In many communities, people drive when they should not, simply because there is no other means of transportation readily available in the community. Some taxi companies have recognized this need and have offered monthly rates (that reduce the cost per ride) to senior citizens and the chronically ill. The savings in yearly depreciation and insurance costs of a car can take care of a good many taxi fares.

[1] Ben Kelley, *The Pavers and the Paved* (New York: Donald W. Brown, 1971), p. 36.

The relationship of emotional stress to accident causation is another matter of concern. A person's driving can be affected by his emotional state. Careful research studies in this area are unfortunately lacking. There are no data on the number of highway fatalities that were actually successful suicide attempts. Nor is there any real attempt made to determine if risk-taking drivers have unconscious motivations to commit suicide. When such drivers are "caught," they are usually fined and then released. "A study relating to accidents in California states that 61.9 per cent of the teenage drivers are at fault. Speeding was considered the prime factor, followed in order by failure to grant right-of-way, improper turning, and driving on the wrong side of the road. These are all violations of the type to be associated with risk-taking, or unsafe practices."[2] Physical performance being at a peak during these teen years, other reasons must be responsible for the high accident rate. Inexperience as well as attitudes reflecting emotional immaturity and risk-taking appear to be related factors.

The need to conserve fuel because of the energy crisis has made an unexpected contribution to highway safety. The traffic accident rate was lowered as a result of reduced speed limits. In essence the driver was induced to modify his driving habits to conform to the legal, lowered speed limits.

THE EXPANDED USE OF THE MOTORBIKE AND SNOWMOBILE

The number of motorcycles (including motor scooters and motorized bicycles) has been increasing at a rapid rate in the United States since 1960. In the ten-year period between 1960 and 1970, there has been a marked increase in this type of vehicle. There has also been noted a sharp increase in the incidence of rider deaths associated with the motorcycle, out of all proportion to the increase in the number of these vehicles. The rider death rate for these vehicles during 1972 is estimated to be 17 deaths per 100,000,000 vehicle miles traveled. The death rate for all motor vehicles, including pedestrians and occupants, was 4.5 deaths (per 100,000,000 vehicle miles).

The reason for the increased death rate appears to be related to the increased number of inexperienced and improperly equipped riders. The most common cause of death to the cyclist is the head injury. Upon impact, the rider is projected forward, head first. The pavement, another vehicle, or a variety of other objects may be struck. An adequate helmet, then, is a must for the cyclist. Leather clothing also has a protective function in case of an accident. The cyclist riding with bare arms or legs is inviting serious injury.

[2] Frank Freeman, Charles E. Goshen, and Barry G. King, *The Role of Human Factors in Accident Prevention* (Washington, D.C.: U.S. Dept. of Health, Education and Welfare, 1960), p. 39.

The motorbike is also found to be a precarious vehicle when ridden on wet pavement. The more stable four-wheeled vehicles need to be driven with more care in wet conditions. The two-wheeled vehicles under these conditions can be outright menaces, particularly in the hands of the unskilled driver.

"If you can't beat 'em, join 'em." This has basically been the philosophy of the portion of our population who live where winter means snow. Instead of complaining about the weather, thousands have now joined in using the snowmobile as the vehicle for communing with nature or destroying it—depending on its use or abuse.

In order to ensure that snowmobiling is the fun it was intended to be, it is important to dress warmly for the occasion. Dress should include a one-piece insulated snowsuit, snowboots, goggles, heavy leather gloves, and helmet. On a cold night the wind-chill factor on a fast-moving snowmobile can cause frostbite for the inadequately dressed.

It is also important to snowmobile in familiar territory, preferably on well-marked trails. To scout out new trails, particularly at night, can be

Figure 9–4

With the more extensive use of bicycles in the last decade the rate of accidents involving bicycles has also increased. The number of deaths related to bicycle use increased from 1962 to 1972 by 120 percent. The increase from 1971 to 1972 was an alarming 25 percent. The bicycle in this picture is equipped with reflectorized tires and rims so it can be more easily seen at night.

(Capital Newspapers, Albany, N.Y.)

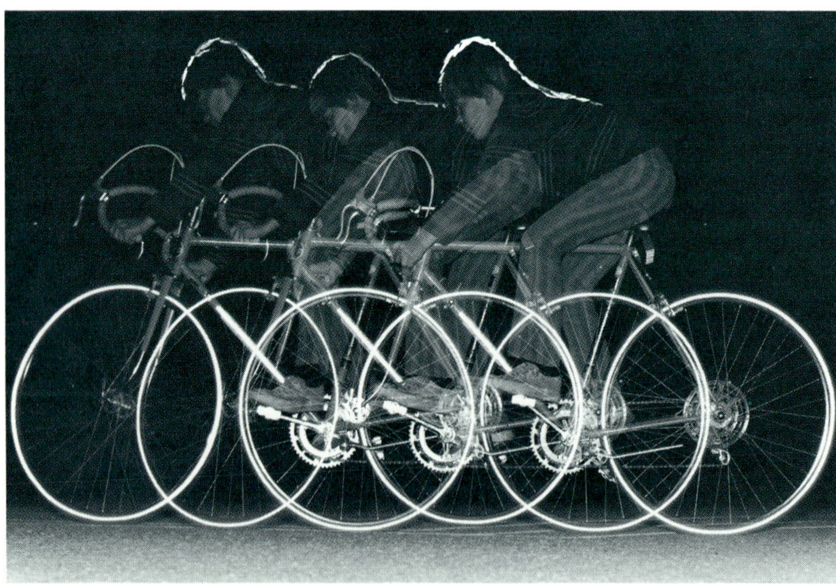

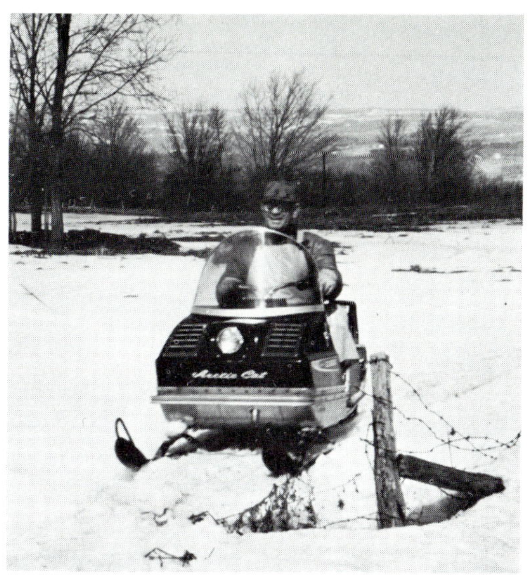

Figure 9–5

It is important to know the countryside when traveling by snowmobile. Barbed wire, tree stumps, and snow-covered bodies of water can all serve as unsuspected hazards.

(New York State Department of Environmental Conservation)

dangerous. The number of accidents involving snowmobiles running into barbed wire fences has been increasing. Permission to travel through someone's farmland is essential. It is only the abuses of the activity that have angered so many of the naturalists and farmers.

HOME ACCIDENTS AND THE CHILD

Home accidents in 1972 accounted for 27,000 deaths and 4,200,000 disabling injuries. The accident threat to the lives and limbs of our children under five is far greater than the threat of disease. The high accident rate stems basically from the child's lack of experience and knowledge, which leads to his inability to recognize danger. In infancy, the human factors of the guardian, rather than the infant, are of greatest concern, for while the infant is this young, the guardian has the greater responsibility for accident prevention. When a child can crawl, he has access to only limited hazards; as he learns to walk and climb, the possibilities for trouble are limitless. Because safety must be learned, the parent must acknowledge that most of the learning of a preschooler is through imitation. The parents who are unconscious or careless of the need for safety spawn youngsters that are "accident-prone."

Our data indicate that fires cause the greatest number of preschool deaths. Children, whether awake or asleep, should never be left unattended at home for even short periods of time. Children trapped in a burning building are gripped with panic and do not even try to escape. More often than not they will attempt to hide under beds or in closets, waiting for rescue. The child who has been trained through fire drills is at a definite advantage here. Though the responsibility for the escape of the preschooler from a burning home is usually left with an older child or parent, the cooperation of the young child may be ensured if the child has been properly prepared for such an emergency.

In 1972, death from suffocation both ingested and mechanical, claimed the lives of 1,250 children under the age of five. Ingested suffocation refers to death resulting from some particles of food or other object the child has inhaled instead of swallowed. The parent or babysitter must know the level of development of a child and never offer hard candy or carrots to the young toddler incapable of handling these kinds of foods.

The child who finds an old refrigerator to "play" in, only to find the latch cannot be opened from the inside, is bound to be a victim of mechanical suffocation. The removal of doors or latches on any discarded refrigerator or freezer is essential. Likewise, children playing "space man" with plastic bags over their heads are prime candidates to become accident statistics. Because of plastic bags' extreme thinness, static electricity is generated through friction, causing the plastic to adhere to the skin. If brought in contact with the nose

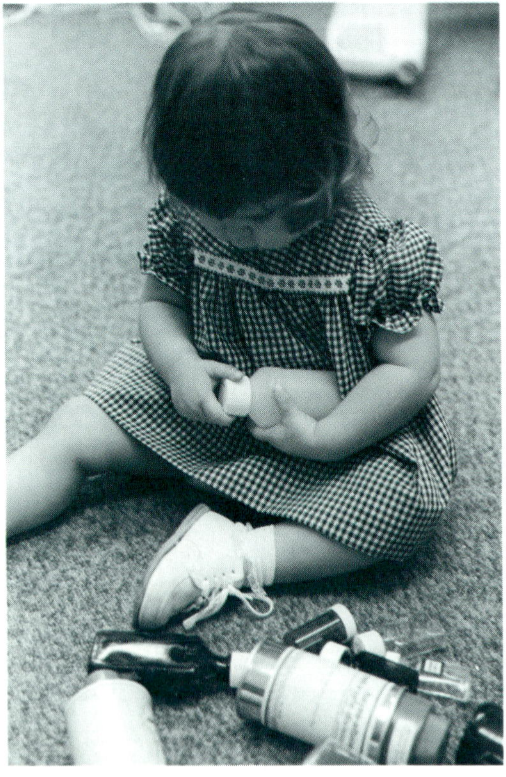

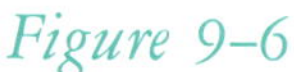

Figure 9–6

Bottles with multicolored pills hold a special and sometimes deadly fascination for children.

(*FDA Consumer,* March 1973)

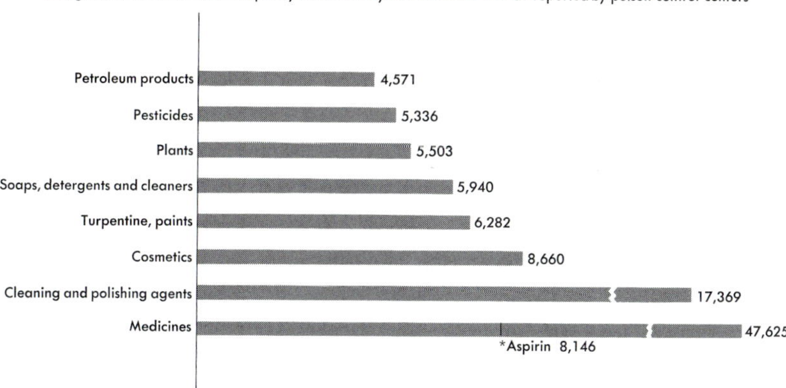

Figure 9–7

The graph indicates the amount of work that still needs to be done to make the home safe from poisoning of young children.

National Clearing House for Poison Control Centers, Bureau of Drugs, Food and Drug Administration (May–June 1973)

and mouth, the air is cut off and the struggling child will suffocate. Legislation has mandated that all thin plastic garment bags be labeled with regard to their potential danger.

The ingestion of poisons and potential poisons has become a significant medical problem. There are a great variety of substances that a preschooler will experiment with. Medicines, cleaning agents, and pesticides, if left under the sink or in unlocked medicine cabinets, are fair game for the curious and imitative youngster. Authorities indicate that tranquilizers have dramatically increased as agents of juvenile death. In this age of increased drug use it is important that medicines be locked up or out of children's reach. This is particularly true of aspirin, which is the substance most frequently involved in children's poisonings. Parents must make a concerted effort to impress children with the fact that this is medicine, not candy, and that medicine must only be taken under parent's supervision. It is wise not to have children watch parents who must regularly take pills—the urge to imitate is strong in the preschooler.

It might be worth the time and effort to learn if your community hospital has a poison treatment center as part of its emergency room facilities. Since 1953 poison control centers and poison information centers have been established. The purpose of the information center is to collect and disseminate all information concerned with poisoning. Thus, in case of a poisoning, a physician may call for information about the poisoning agent and learn the level of toxicity as well as the specific toxic agent in the substance. If a nonmedical person seeks information, he is given first-aid instruction and advised to call a physician immediately. Poison information centers operate on a 24-hour basis and are usually located in large health departments or university medical or pharmacy schools.

Certainly any accredited hospital will have facilities for a gastric lavage (stomach pumping), which is usually the emergency treatment prescribed by the physician when a toxic substance has been swallowed. It is wise to bring the container of the substance swallowed to the physician or hospital so that there is no question as to the identity of the poison.

Most home pool drownings happen to children under 5, with the peak incidence being for 2-year olds (7 out of 10 are males). The chief causes of drowning are the temporary lack of qualified adult supervision and the absence of environmental protection. Because most children under 5 are not able to float or swim, the bulk of the responsibility for accident prevention in this area rests primarily with the parent. Secondarily, prevention must rest upon the child-proofing of the backyard pool. This should include proper fencing that children cannot climb over or dig under.

HOME ACCIDENTS AND THE ADULT

A basic problem in home safety is that in the home the person deals with a wide variety of tools, appliances, and substances that he or she is only casually familar with. In industry, a worker is often responsible for one kind of job and one machine. He becomes thoroughly familiar with the one piece of equipment and the specific function he is to perform. In addition, a safety engineer on the premises is constantly seeking ways of making the work safer. These advantages are not to be found in the home. The worker, upon arriving at home, in his attempt to be a jack-of-all-trades is often transformed from a skilled professional to an outrageously performing amateur.

The National Safety Council states that in the 25–to–64 age group 2,100 deaths represented the yearly death toll attributed to fires. In this age group, the frequent causes of fires are falling asleep while smoking, starting fires with inflammable liquids, using defective heating and cooking equipment, overloading electrical circuits, and using fuel oils, paints, or gasolines improperly. Becoming familiar with the materials and equipment one is using is an important first step. Inflammable materials are often well labeled and directions for their use described. Directions for the proper use and maintenance of the variety of appliances now found in households are usually available with the purchase of this equipment. The casual attitude that one does not need to read instructions or directions related to such items is fraught with danger.

The comparatively new idea of family fire drills is being urged by the

National Safety Council. Disorganization and panic at a time when precise and planned actions are imperative can only lead to tragedy and disaster.

The kitchen is often the place where fires start; the strategic placement of a fire blanket (preferably wool) in this room would seem logical. The installation of fire extinguishers throughout the home should be mandatory, along with the knowledge of their proper use.

An area of fire safety that has heretofore been ignored is the flammability of most camping tents. It has been demonstrated that tents can become ignited momentarily because of the paraffin-impregnated fabric they are often made of. Many tents are also made so that the sides come down and extend as a floor covering. These seamless "walls" make escape almost impossible if the fire starts at the tent opening. Very often the only escape is to go through the wall of fire. When using candles or heaters inside a tent, the potential for a fire should not be overlooked. It is essential that in buying a tent a person purchase one made of fire resistant material.

In this age group (25 to 64) poisoning is a common occurrence, and ironically it is most often caused by medication. Household preparations such as bleaches, lye, and pesticides also caused death in the adult group. Many of these tragedies could have been avoided if some precautions had been taken. Medicines that have been prescribed for a specific ailment should be discarded at the termination of the illness. Medicines may alter in composition while standing for months in the medicine cabinet and what was once a beneficial substance may now be harmful. Taking medicines in a dimly lit bathroom in the middle of the night may also be an invitation to disaster, particularly if medications for internal use are stored haphazardly with externally used compounds and disinfectants. To be sure, one must read and *reread* a label of the medication to be used, as well as clean out and organize the medicine cabinet. It is also recommended that medication not be left on the night table to be administered in the middle of the night; in addition to the hazard of poisoning oneself with an overdose, the medication on the night table is too accessible to the young child.

Poisons or possibly hazardous substances should never be placed in cups, glasses, soda bottles, or similar receptacles. The temporary pouring of caustic disinfectants into a soda bottle is bound to mean trouble.

Insect and rodent poison should always be used with great caution, particularly in or near the kitchen. Likewise, the use of pesticides in the garden must be done with care. Because certain toxic substances can be absorbed through the skin, the body should be well covered and upon completion of the spraying thorough washing should be encouraged.

There has been an increase in carbon monoxide poisonings as a result of the improper use of hibachis and charcoal grills. It is extremely hazardous to bring glowing charcoal briquets inside a trailer, camper, or poorly ventilated lodging to warm the interior. Several carbon monoxide deaths have been attributed to this practice, and the FDA with full cooperation from the briquet industry has published regulations for a warning label that reads: "Warning—Do not use for indoor heating or cooking unless ventilation is provided for exhausting fumes to outside. Toxic fumes may accumulate and cause death."

The Spray-Can Menace. Hair sprays, shaving creams, toothpaste, deodorants, pesticides, paints, de-icers, and polishes are now all available in pressurized cans which spray or spurt their contents in a most convenient way. However, with their misuse have come many tragic accidents.

One most obvious problem is disposing of the empty can. Though the can no longer dispenses its product, the vapor left inside can reach explosive proportions when heated. It becomes important, then, to dispose of the can without exposing it to any form of heat. The inhalations of toxic fumes from spray cans can also be a hazard as exemplified by the recent discovery that vinyl chloride gas that was used to expel the contents of some spray cans, was linked to liver cancer. Extensive spraying should be done in well-ventilated areas and not in the presence of a lighted cigarette or any other flammatory source.

HOME ACCIDENTS AND THE AGING

Our most vulnerable group in home accident fatalities are the elderly, 65 years and over. The majority of these accidents are due to falls. In a study by Sheldon,[3] he indicates that about a third of the falls are due to vertigo and another third are associated with the greater tendency of older people to trip. The slower reactions tend to result in an inability to recover when thrown off-balance, or to move quickly out of the path of a falling or moving object. Vision and hearing may become impaired at this age, lessening the acuteness of the individual's safety "alarm" system. With advancing age, the general brittleness of bones renders an individual most susceptible to fractures.

In order to prevent falling accidents among our elderly, it will be necessary to provide them with an environment that is free from hazards. This will include well-lighted stairways that are kept free of toys and other objects, and equipped with handrails; nonslippery floors and rugs that are well anchored; cellar stairs and porch steps that are kept in good repair. Housing specific for senior citizens includes, wherever feasible, ramps instead of steps, kitchen cabinets that are easily reached, and other facilities designed to prevent falls.

It will also be necessary to help the older person realize his physical limitations, the need to carry on former activities in a slower, more deliberate way, and the advisability of wearing properly fitted shoes to help avoid falls. This may be a difficult task after a lifetime of habit has already been established in the elderly.

[3] "The Role of Human Factors in Accident Prevention," op. cit., p. 50.

ELECTRICAL SAFETY

Though prevention is the ideal way of solving a major health problem, knowing what to do if the problem presents itself is next best. The Lightning Protection Institute indicates that although most lightning accidents occur outdoors, one-fourth do occur in the home. Lightning enters houses via chimneys, plumbing, wiring, TV antennas, or directly through the roof. The safest place in the home is usually in the center of a room, away from walls, fireplace, plumbing lines, electrical equipment, and metal objects such as the stove, sink, or tub. If one is caught outside the home, one should stay away from utility poles, trees, and wire fences. The camping enthusiast should be sure that his "home away from home" is not pitched on rocky ground in the open, because lightning shows some affinity for this type of location. Groups of people in the open also seem to attract lightning, so that it might be wise for individuals to scatter. If a storm is hitting so close that the lightning and thunder seem almost simultaneous and a strong odor of ozone prevails, it is best to "hit the ground!"

Although over 100 deaths due to lightning electrocution occur each year, a far greater number (over 1,000) of *accidental* electrocutions take place. In this era of electric gadgetry, which enables us to open cans, sandpaper walls, brush teeth, trim hedges, and wash dishes, the need for electrical safety education has become critical.

We have all at one time or another experienced an electric shock that is sometimes described as an unpleasant sensation, as a tingling, throbbing, or hot feeling. The rate of flow of current through the body is measured in milliamperes (1/1000 of an ampere). The human body is very sensitive to electric current and some few individuals can feel a current of only 2/10 of a milliampere. Most people, however, can feel a current approaching 1 milliampere. An electrical shock at this level is not dangerous in and of itself; however, a startled reaction could lead one to drop a power tool or jump back into a hazard. When the current exceeds 5 milliamperes, muscular contractions stimulated by the electric current are so severe that the individual cannot let go of the object (such as a metal handle of an electric drill). This continual shock could lead to fatigue, collapse, and finally death. A shock of 50 to 100 milliamperes (or 110 volts or less) could kill a person outright.

When an electrical appliance comes off the assembly line with insufficient insulation or poor circuit design, you have the potential for a leakage of electric current from the live interior of the appliance to the outer metal covers. Though the outer casing of this product may be alive with current, by touching the appliance alone you will not feel a shock. However, if some other part of your body is simultaneously touching a ground (an electricity-conducting

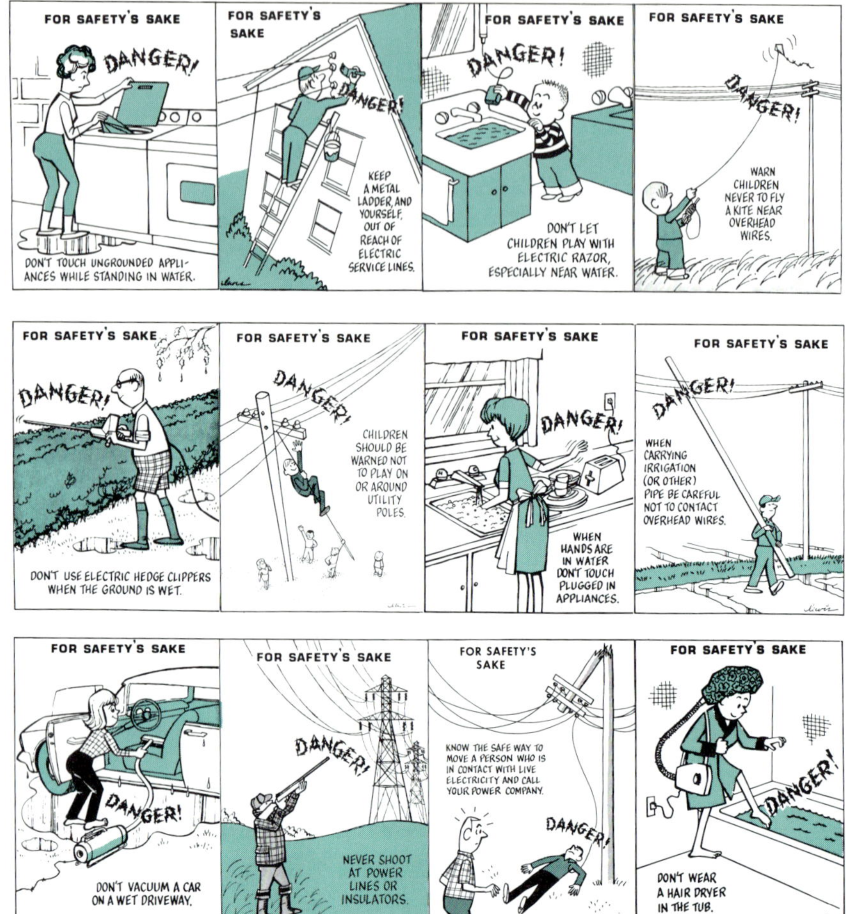

Figure 9–8

(Courtesy of Consumers Power Company)

material that at some point enters the earth or touches a conductor that in turn, enters the earth, e.g., metal sink, radiator, faucet, cold-water pipe, gas pipe, storm drain), you could receive a substantial electric shock. Most obvious grounds are moist earth, outside patios, and damp concrete basements. Persons may live with hazardous appliances for many years without experiencing any shocks, because they just never happened to touch a ground and the faulty appliance at the same time. This is a form of Russian roulette currently being played by thousands of people.

In order to minimize this possibility, electrical appliances and power tools should be properly grounded. This may involve the services of an electrician to convert outlet boxes to accept a three-prong receptacle and to be sure such boxes are correctly grounded. In some instances an adapter plug is utilized to enable one to use a three-prong plug into a two-prong receptacle. It is essential if an adapter plug is used that the small pigtail wire be secured by the screw holding the cover plate of the outlet. Using an adapter plug is considered a far less safe way to handle the situation, for very often adapter plugs are used without securing the pigtail wire to the outlet. Secondly, if the outlet is not properly grounded to begin with, even securing the wire of the adapter plug will not ground the appliance. It only gives one a false sense of security.

A safety device has been designed, which monitors the balance of current between the hot and neutral lines of a circuit. When the balance is off, as when current leaks to the ground because of a faulty electrical appliance, the

Figure 9–9

What this person does not know is that it is not even necessary to touch the high voltage lines or equipment to get hurt. Just getting close can cause an arc—blinding flash—which may inflict severe burns or cause a fall from a tower or pole.

(Niagara Mohawk Power Corporation, photo by Connie Moynihan)

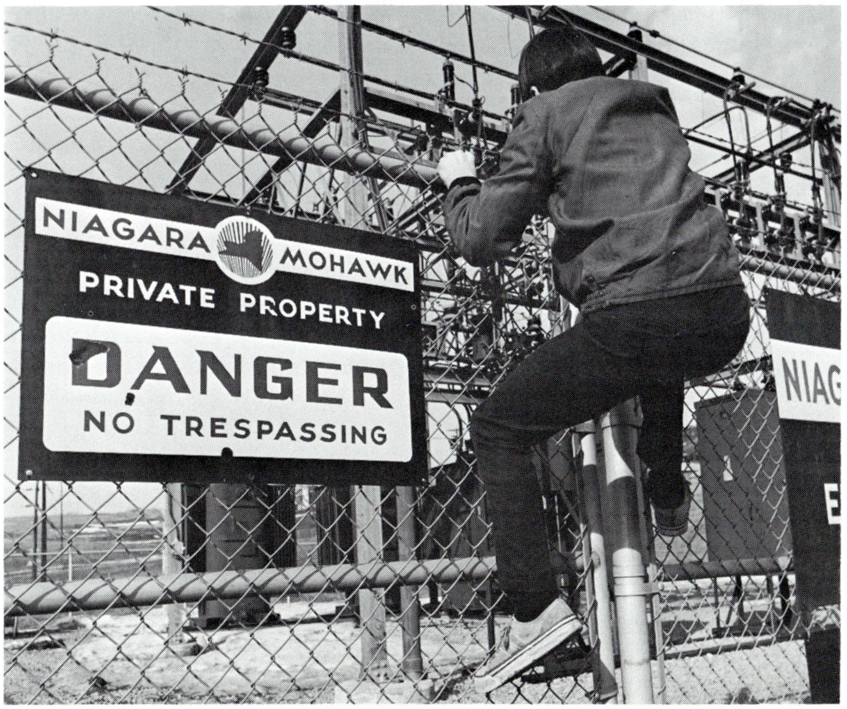

device activates a circuit breaker which shuts the power down. This *ground-fault interrupter* works fast enough so that a nasty shock is the result instead of a person's electrocution. A ground-fault interrupter in this day and age of electrical appliance use should be installed in the fuse box of every home.

Most people are unaware that many electric high voltage power lines are not insulated and that they pose a threat to the unsuspecting. The wet string of a kite can serve as a deadly conductor as can equipment such as a crane, or a well driller. In the summer, high school and college youths are often hired by tree-trimming companies and given little training with regard to the electrical dangers they may expose themselves to. A number of states have passed legislation to establish safety regulations for tree trimming. Certainly the tree trimmer whose job brings him close to power lines should have similar training as the employees of power companies who are taught to work cautiously and knowingly with these potential hazards. With the need for electrical power in our society doubling every ten years, the presence of power lines carrying thousands of volts of electricity will continue to be an environmental factor that we must learn to live with safely.

INDUSTRIAL SAFETY

The National Safety Council reports that since World War II the number of accidental deaths to workers on the job has *decreased* by 15 per cent. This, in spite of an increase in the number of workers. The rate of accidents resulting in death has actually been reduced by 13 per cent. It is also interesting to note that in 1970 three out of four deaths, and more than half the injuries suffered by workers, occurred *off the job.*

The reasons for the advances made in industrial safety revolve around the assumption by management of greater responsibility in this area. There are, of course, legal obligations that employers have had to meet that require reasonable standards of safety in the operation of their plants. They have also felt the social pressures of society reminding them of their obligations to their workers. Should management fail to meet these obligations, public opinion would then give support to increased government regulation in order to attain these goals. A key factor in the picture is that the employer has accepted responsibility for a portion of the financial loss involved in an accident. An accident invariably involves work stoppage and this in itself represents an economic loss to the company. In addition, accidents often involve expensive equipment or machinery that must be repaired or replaced. An accident often may result in machinery damage or loss without an employee's being hurt. The causes of these accidents are the same as those that produce employee injury or death. The point is that safety and production have become interwoven segments of the industrial pattern. Progressive managements have therefore recognized the need for accident prevention programs as part of the operation of a successful business.

Although the industrial safety problem has by no means been completely resolved, recent developments demonstrate the kinds of progress that can be made when some attention is given to the problem. It is at best ironic to note that death and injury rates run higher in the home than at places of work.

REVIEW QUESTIONS

1. Why have we as a society tolerated for so long the idea that the accident is an unavoidable aspect of our environment?
2. How does the human factor make its contribution to the accident picture? What are the effects of drugs, emotions, immaturity, disability, and old age on the driver?
3. How has the utilization of the epidemiological approach aided the study of accidents?
4. The development of accident prevention programs by modifying human behavior, while helpful, is not as rapid as effecting environmental changes. Explain.
5. What have been the contributions of Mr. Ralph Nader in calling attention to the automobile as an accident factor?
6. What are the functions of the National Traffic Agency?
7. To what extent has the expanded use of the motorbike aggravated the traffic safety problem?
8. Why does the home accident continue to reign as a leading cause of injury and death?
9. How can we better protect the preschool child from accidental injury and death?
10. What adaptations are being made to make homes safer for the aged?
11. What precautions should one take when caught in the open by a lightning storm?
12. How can the advances in industrial safety be explained?

10. Community Health

THE QUALITY of a society can be measured by how well it cares for its less fortunate. In our competitive society we have sometimes viewed the more fortunate as the "winners" and the less fortunate the "losers." We are rapidly learning that this attitude is inappropriate in the health area. Communicable diseases do not distinguish between rich and poor. Polluted air enters everyone's lungs. In essence, the health of our neighbor and the quality of our environment affects the health of all.

The individual oftentimes finds himself virtually helpless in trying to combat or avoid the effects of a broad-scale environmental health problem such as air pollution. The quality of his water supply, food, environmental sanitation, and medical facilities, to name a few, is beyond the control of the individual. He must rely on others to help ensure that elements of his surroundings are designed to support rather than hamper his existence. The ability to maintain levels of health is more and more becoming community based. Increasingly, how a community is organized and the effort it puts into the health area will determine the levels of individual health more surely than anything the individual can do.

The implications of this developing situation are quite clear. The person must first of all be familiar with those organizations in the community designed to protect his health. He needs to know how effectively they are working and to determine what he, as part of a citizen group, can do to support the effective functioning of these organizations.

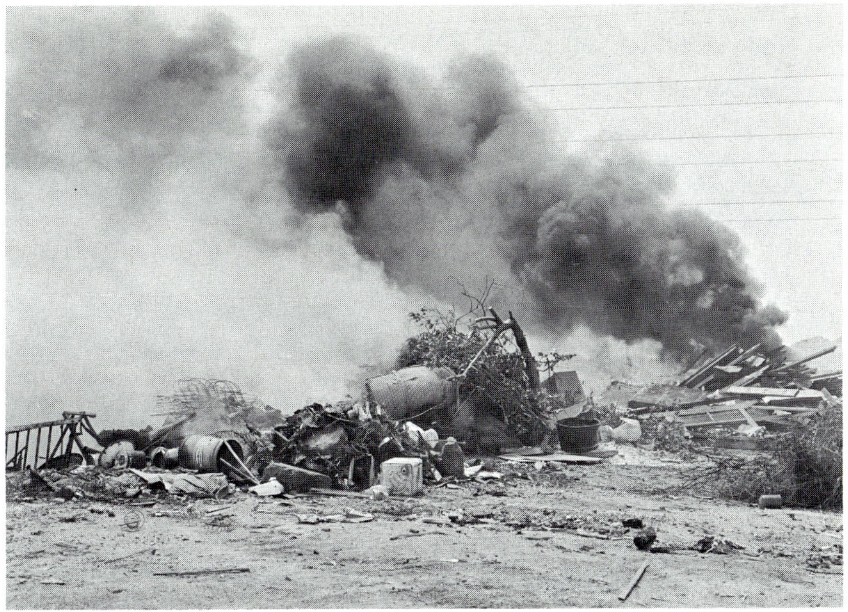

Figure 10–1

Polluted air enters everyone's lungs. In essence, the health of our neighbor and the quality of our environment affect the health of us all.

(New York State Department of Environmental Conservation)

THE OFFICIAL HEALTH AGENCY

The health department at the local level is a part of the community local government. The budget to support this organization comes from local tax moneys. Its basic purpose is the protection and further promotion of the community's health.

The health officer serves as the director of the local official health agency. He is usually an M.D. (medical doctor) who often possesses an M.P.H. (Masters Degree in Public Health). In some instances, the health officer is a nonmedical person with specific training in public health administration. This is similar to the definite trend of training nonmedical personnel to serve as hospital administrators. The latter degree would be obtained from one of the graduate schools of public health in the country and would specifically train a man for his responsibilities as a health officer. In this position he serves not only as the head of his department but as a coordinator for all community health activities that would involve a number of other community groups.

Functions of the Local health Department

Vital Statistics. Keeping a tally of such things as births, deaths, marriages, divorces, and incidence of reportable illness serves a basic public health purpose. Vital statistics act as a community barometer indicating how things are going. Sudden increases of a given disease forewarn the health officer and ultimately the community of an impending epidemic or of a breakdown in one of the preventive disease measures. Appropriate action can then be taken to correct the condition at an early stage of its development.

Vital statistics from local health units are sent on to state health departments, which chart a statewide picture of what is occurring. From there they are sent to the National Office of Vital Statistics, where conclusions are drawn with regard to the health status of the nation.

Environmental Sanitation. The health department plays a major role in maintaining the health of the community through its activities in the area of environmental sanitation. It maintains a constant check on the fitness of community water supplies. Health department sanitarians also serve to supervise the production and distribution of milk. Equipment used on dairy farms must meet optimum standards of cleanliness, with milk from diseased cows being barred from distribution. Sanitarians also supervise foods and food handlers in restaurants, and help set standards for cleanliness and food handling. These health workers will often have bacterial counts taken of waters from public swimming pools and beaches to determine their level of safety. Insect and rodent control is another key program in environmental health because insects and rodents often serve to transmit disease.

Communicable Disease Control. While the activities of the health department in the area of environmental health make a number of important contributions to the control of communicable disease, the department engages in a number of other specific activities in this area. Health departments often

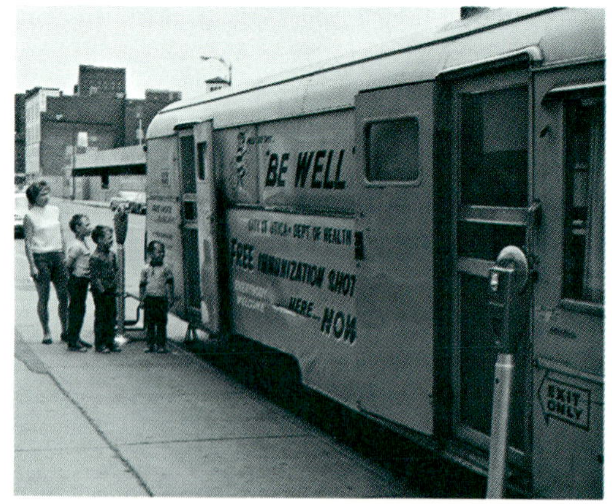

Figure 10–2

An immunization clinic goes to where the people are.

(New York State Department of Health)

conduct immunization drives as well as routine immunization clinics. The maintenance of high immunization levels in the community is considered a primary preventive objective. A number of health departments will operate special clinics, such as venereal disease or rabies clinics, where these particular communicable diseases pose special problems.

Maternal and Child Health. There is no other aspect of the public health program that is so broad and varied as that pertaining to mother and child. Probably every facet of public health, with its many programs and numerous personnel, touches this population group.

Maternal health programs start before marriage or conception. Educational programs, often in cooperation with the school, are conducted to prepare the person for parenthood. For expectant mothers, nursing service and educational programs are conducted and are designed to prepare the woman for childbirth. Classes for expectant parents often include fathers so that they too may become acquainted with the varied tasks and adjustments that come with having a family. Following childbirth, health departments will also provide nursing service on proper infant care (the bathing of the infant, how to prepare formula, and so forth), as well as on alertness to any postbirth complications in the mother or illness in the infant. The nurse can also pave the way for pediatric care for the baby. This care may be given by private physicians or well-baby clinics sponsored by the health department.

The health department is also concerned with the identification of the ill or handicapped child. These children are sought out so that they may be recipients of needed care.

Increasingly health departments are conducting birth control clinics. These clinics are designed to inform women of the various means of contraception and their effective use. The goal is to prevent the unwanted pregnancy.

The health department works closely with schools, assisting them in their health instructional program and often serving as the schools' source of health services. The objective is to provide the child with meaningful information that will lead to the development of positive health attitudes and practices. The health services are not only designed to assure well-being, but to make sure that the child is physically and psychologically prepared to learn. The child with a vision, hearing, or emotional problem can be insensitive to the best teaching in the world.

Health departments are also represented on school health councils whose function it is to identify and resolve health problems in the school environment.

Public Health Education. Many of the activities of the health department rely upon community understanding, support, and cooperation for their success. Essentially, every member of the department staff has an educational responsibility in his contacts with various groups in the community. In addition, health departments have on their staffs public health educators who use the mass media as well as community meetings. classes, and exhibits to get health information to the public. Understanding of the principles of disease prevention and the maintenance of health precede meaningful health activity. The best-equipped and -staffed immunization clinic, for instance, will go unattended unless there is public acceptance of its need. Recognition that public education is pivotal in determining the success or failure of a particular health program has led more health departments to utilize health educators to prepare their communities for health activities and programs.

Chronic Disease Control. Many public health programs are designed to facilitate the early detection of chronic diseases. Increasingly, health departments have been developing rehabilitation programs in this area, helping people to return to useful and productive lives. Educational efforts in that area are also being accelerated. As stated by Hanlon: "In the final analysis, it may well be that increased public education in these matters would represent the single most important service that may be rendered by public health agencies."[1]

Other Functions

Some local health departments will, in addition, conduct programs related to public health nutrition, dentistry, accident prevention, mental health, rehabilitation, medical care, and research. The activities of health departments have been expanding, making more and better services available to local communities. Closer liaison with state health departments also appears to be developing, with local departments participating in area-wide and even state-wide programs.

HEALTH ORGANIZATION AT THE STATE LEVEL

The role of state health departments has become an increasingly important one. Their initial functions were quite limited, with primary concerns centered on the recording of births and deaths. Through the years the responsibilities of this organization have been considerably expanded. Its programs now include activity in the broad area of environmental health, medical and laboratory services, research, preventive services, supervision of hospitals, nursing homes, and other medical care facilities.

The state health department plays a leadership role as far as the official (local) health agencies in the state are concerned. It generally serves in an advisory capacity and leaves the administration of direct health services to the local health department. It also works to establish full-time local units where they are nonexistent. Many times, it is instrumental in coordinating the efforts of several local health departments in the development of an area-wide program. Invariably, where broad-scale health problems (such as water and air pollution)

[1] John J. Hanlon, *Principles of Public Health Administration* (St. Louis: Mosby, 1964), p. 603.

occur the interactions of all the health agencies in a given region are required. The state health agency does in some instances act as a middle man between a Federal agency and a local one where federal assistance is given to local communities. The state health department will also coordinate its efforts with those of the voluntary state agencies when they share common health interests.

HEALTH ORGANIZATION AT THE FEDERAL LEVEL

The Department of Health, Education and Welfare

All of the agencies of the Department of Health, Education and Welfare (HEW) have some health-related responsibilities. The Social Security Administration manages the Old-Age and Survivors and Disability Insurance program as well as the Medicare program. The office of Education has a division for Drug and Health Education that seeks to stimulate the development of such programs in the schools of the United States. It also provides supportive services for handicapped and deprived children. The Public Health Service has through the years represented *the* federal health agency headed by the Surgeon General. In a reorganization of the Public Health Service in the late 1960s three major components of the Service were developed which consisted of the Health Services and Mental Health Administration, the National Institutes of Health, and the Food and Drug Administration.

THE HEALTH SERVICES AND MENTAL HEALTH ADMINISTRATION. This agency concerns itself with programs that involve comprehensive health planning and the development of comprehensive health services. It provides grants to states and to local recipients for these purposes. It also seeks to stimulate research designed to improve the quality and accessibility of health care for all segments of the population. Through the information provided by the National Health Survey it continually evaluates the health status of the nation.

NATIONAL INSTITUTES OF HEALTH. The NIH supports, through its many thousands of grants, medical research and training for research in over 700 of the nation's schools of medicine, universities, and other research centers, and provides grants for construction and equipping of health research facilities; it carries out an extensive program of direct research in laboratories and clinics at Maryland, and in the field. An added responsibility of the National Institutes of Health is the Bureau of Health Manpower, which promotes the quality and number of professional health personnel. It does this by providing training grants, student assistance, and funding for the construction of educational facilities.

The National Library of Medicine is also a component of the National Institutes of Health. This library has the largest collection of publications of its kind in the world, containing over a million volumes of medical literature.

It has combined a computerized storage and retrieval system with photo-duplication services as a means of making this giant store of medical information available to other medical libraries.

The Food and Drug Administration is fully described in Chapter 6, "Consumer Health."

Other Federal Agencies

The *Veterans Administration* is responsible for a medical care program through the utilization of its VA Hospitals and outpatient clinics. The program is basically designed to provide for veterans with illness or disability associated with military service. The VA, however, will also provide medical care for veterans with nonservice illness who cannot afford to pay for medical care.

The *Department of Defense* furnishes comprehensive medical care for members of the armed forces and their dependents. The Corps of Engineers also is actively involved in ensuing environmental sanitation in and around military posts.

The *Department of Housing and Urban Development* are responsible for the administration of grants for sewer and water facilities. In so doing, safeguards against the pollution of waterways is required. Grants are also made to finance health and recreation projects as well as other community services.

The *U.S. Department of Agriculture* has several health- (human) related programs. Its programs to eradicate tuberculosis, brucellosis, and other animal diseases also protects the human population. The department's meat inspection program is designed to protect the human population. It has also conducted a nutrition education program aimed at improving health and preventing nutritional deficiency diseases.

The *U.S. Department of the Interior* has within its structure several units with health-related functions. The Federal Water Pollution Control Administration has the powers to enforce federal water pollution laws. The Fish and Wildlife Service conducts programs related to animal-borne diseases. The Bureau of Mines conducts studies on accident prevention and the protection of the health of the miners.

The *Atomic Energy Commission* produces and distributes radioactive materials used in medical research. It has also supported and conducted such research itself.

The large number of federal agencies that have health responsibilities has caused the American Public Health Association to comment as follows:

> No important function of government has been more intentionally fragmented in recent years than has the health function. Federal fragmentation has made more and more difficult the maintenance of effective state and local health programs and departments. Each federal act should be, but rarely is, scrutinized for its effect on administration at the point of impact (usually state or local).

It then recommended,

> A unified health department, responsible and responsive to the entire population of a nation, a state, or a community, discharging agreed-upon governmental health functions, seems to be a reasonable, viable, and desirable proposition.[2]

THE VOLUNTARY HEALTH ORGANIZATION

The voluntary health agency is one that is supported by public donations raised in fund drives rather than by tax moneys. This kind of health organization is unique to the United States and not found in other countries. Its focus is usually delimited to a specific health problem, as exemplified by the American Cancer Society, the American Heart Association, or the United Cerebral Palsy Association. Voluntary agencies usually start with a few people who draw attention and interest to a particular health problem that might otherwise be overlooked. In the first organizations of this type, they were manned solely by volunteers. Though large numbers of volunteers are still used, these agencies now employ professionals as executive secretaries and in other key positions.

Education, service, and research are viewed as the major functions of voluntary health agencies. Many of their fund-raising activities revolve around making the public aware of a health problem, as well as community and personal actions that will help alleviate it. Year-round educational programs are usually constants with voluntary agencies.

These agencies often serve to supplement the efforts of the official health agencies of the community. Because they have greater flexibility with regard to their use of funds, they can pioneer in demonstration programs and try new approaches to old problems. Many times, when a voluntary organization demonstrates the worth of a new program, it will ask the official health agency to accept responsibility for its continuance. At times, the community's official health agency will lack funds to initiate a project alone. The voluntary health agency may then supplement the resources of the official health agency with its own funds and make the project possible.

These organizations are also active in the support of legislation that is in the interest of the public health.

Sizable portions of the voluntary agency's income are also contributed to needed research efforts. Noted researchers are often supported by funds from

[2] *The Nation's Health,* The Official Newspaper of the American Public Health Association, April 1972. Editorial by Thomas R. Hood.

these organizations and serve to supplement the work done by the National Institutes of Health and other research organizations.

Voluntary health organizations, like the official health agencies, have a state organization that advises and coordinates the efforts of its local agencies. Each local agency passes on a percentage of the proceeds of its fund drives to support the operation of the state organization. Every state organization then passes on a percentage of its income to support a national office. Educational materials such as printed materials, films, and other things are developed or purchased by the state office of the voluntary agency and passed on to its local units for use. The state office also sends field consultants to local units to advise the executive-secretary on the development of the local agency's program.

Many of our voluntary health organizations are strong, nationally organized groups making a significant, unique public health contribution. Some examples of these organizations follow:

ALCOHOLICS ANONYMOUS, P. O. Box 459, Grand Central Station, New York, New York 10017.

ALLERGY FOUNDATION OF AMERICA, 801 Second Ave., New York, New York 10017.

AMERICAN ASSOCIATION FOR MATERNAL AND INFANT HEALTH, 116 S. Michigan Avenue, Chicago, Illinois.

AMERICAN CANCER SOCIETY, INC., 219 East 42 Street, New York, New York 10017.

AMERICAN DIABETES ASSOCIATION, INC., 1 East 45th Street, New York, New York.

AMERICAN HEARING SOCIETY, 919 Eighteenth Street, N.W., Washington, D.C.

AMERICAN HEART ASSOCIATION, 44 East 23rd Street, New York, New York 10010.

AMERICAN INSTITUTE OF FAMILY RELATIONS, INC., 5287 Sunset Blvd., Los Angeles, California.

ARTHRITIS AND RHEUMATISM FOUNDATION, 10 Columbus Circle, New York, New York 10019.

EPILEPSY FOUNDATION OF AMERICA, 733 15 Street N.W., Washington, D.C. 20005.

MUSCULAR DYSTROPHY ASSOCIATION OF AMERICA, 1790 Broadway, New York, New York 10019.

NATIONAL ASSOCIATION FOR MENTAL HEALTH, 10 Columbus Circle, New York, New York 10019.

THE NATIONAL FOUNDATION, 1275 Mamaroneck Avenue, White Plains, New York 10605.

NATIONAL MULTIPLE SCLEROSIS SOCIETY, 257 Park Avenue South, New York, New York 10010.

NATIONAL SAFETY COUNCIL, 425 N. Michigan Avenue, Chicago, Illinois 60611.

PLANNED PARENTHOOD—WORLD POPULATION, 515 Madison Avenue, New York, New York 10022.

SEX INFORMATION AND EDUCATION COUNCIL OF THE UNITED STATES (SIECUS), 1855 Broadway, New York, New York 10023.

UNITED CEREBRAL PALSY ASSOCIATION, INC., 321 West 44th Street, New York, New York 10017.

THE HOSPITAL

The hospital is an integral part of the community's health organization. It has traditionally been viewed as a treatment center, though the activities of the hospital are to a greater extent becoming more concerned with services related to preventive medicine and the promotion of public health. Some hospitals have experimented with the use of the emergency ward as a springboard for preventive procedures. A person arriving with a badly cut hand may not only have the wound attended to, but have the readily available drops of blood tested for diabetes or anemia; the smoker may be advised to "kick the habit," and some vision testing may be thrown in for good measure before the patient is released. Two New York City hospitals routinely administered the Papanicolaou test (see Chapter 3) for cervical cancer to women admitted to the hospital for a variety of other reasons. In a matter of a few years, over 300 cases of cervical cancer were detected early enough to save the lives of the women involved.

A number of hospitals, as part of their new preventive role, are developing cooperative activities with school health education programs. The health professionals of the hospital participate in teacher training workshops. In addition, the hospitals have also provided field work experiences for the high school student. The student is involved in a variety of helpful roles, from reading to patients to conducting lead poisoning surveys in the community. These hospital-school interactions have not only added relevance to health education programs but have been helpful to the hospitals as well through the appropriate use of student manpower.

The United States Hospital and Medical Facilities Survey and Construction Act (Hill-Burton) of 1947 has stimulated construction toward the development of regional hospital systems. At the center of such a system is a hospital affiliated with a medical school. Smaller satellite hospitals service the outlying areas of the region. The purpose is to provide the most adequate medical care facilities possible in a given region.

This federal legislation is also subsidizing the remodernization of many of the older hospitals in the country located in the urban areas. Its initial efforts were directed toward the development of hospital facilities in rural areas where they were lacking. In addition, the Hill-Burton legislation provides funds for hospital research and demonstration programs. These activities are directed toward the development of improved patient care and more efficient hospital administration and operation.

THE SCHOOL

The school is not often thought of as a health organization. It can, however, make a substantial contribution in this area with its programs of health education. Any educational institution concerned with the study of man, his environment, and his interactions with it would be remiss to exclude so vital an area as the health sciences from its curriculum.

Because many patterns of health behavior are best initiated at an early age, the school has unusual opportunities to influence young peoples' health values at a most receptive time. The quality of school health education programs can determine the levels of health information in a community and its willingness to undertake needed public health measures. Public health programs can be best initiated with the consent and support of the citizenry in a democratic society. In order that such decisions be properly based, a health-informed public is essential. A cultural lag in this area can be literally incapacitating to a community.

Health education is more than the mere dissemination of knowledge. It also involves the development of values and even a life-style. Confining this kind of instruction within the four walls of a classroom immediately restricts its effectiveness. Intellectualizing about health information in a classroom accomplishes limited objectives. If we are to realize the real goals of health education we must increasingly make this form of education experientially based. Health education in schools ideally should become an inherent part of public health programs, with the student actively engaged in various field work experiences. If there is to be classroom discussion, let it consist of strategy meetings on what is to happen in the community and on how to effect the needed reforms in conducting our human health affairs.

Student involvement in the learning process should be all that phrase implies. Some high schools in the country are already planning public health field work experiences for their health education students instead of requiring a term paper. The reports they will be responsible for will be based on their actual experience. Students from a New York City school, for example, in

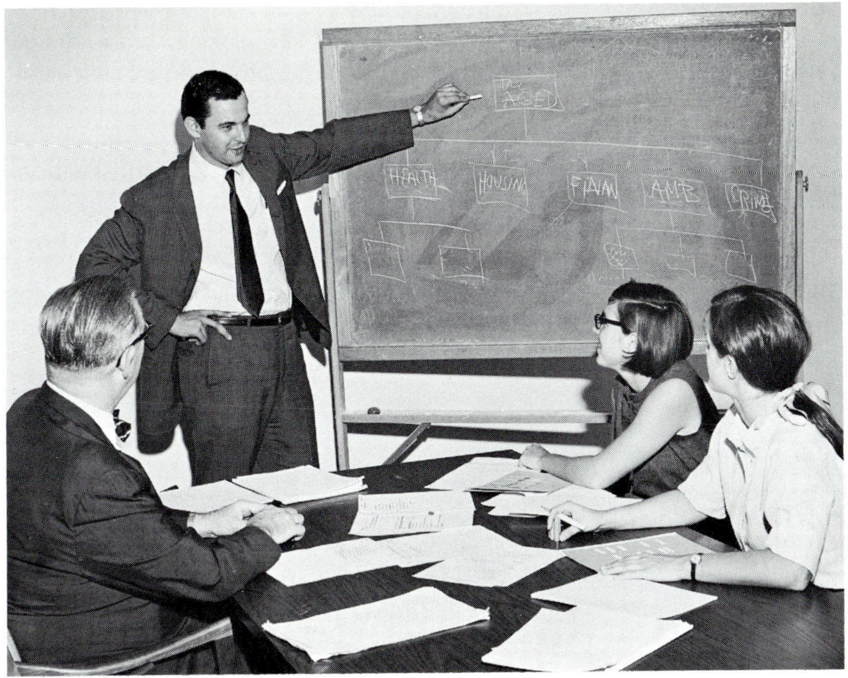

Figure 10–3

Health Education students gathering data at their local Health Department as part of their field work experience.

(New York State Department of Health)

cooperation with personnel from a local hospital, conducted a survey of 1,500 homes in an effort to detect cases of lead poisoning. The students *did* turn up 20 cases of lead poisoning, to the delight of their health colleagues at the hospital. The students in turn had the satisfaction of knowing that they helped to save 20 lives as well as to inform 1,500 families on the hazards of lead poisoning. (The latter is better than any letter grade a student can receive.) As part of their health education program in another high school, students are working in a program for mentally retarded patients in a nearby hospital. What better way for young people to understand the problems related to retardation and what better way of overcoming the unfortunate stigmas too often associated with these conditions. Many examples of school-community interaction are now evident as more complete approaches to our health problems and issues are sought. The community is the laboratory of the health sciences. If the education program of the school is to be effective, it needs to have access to that laboratory. It is also time that we ring an end to the "amateur hour" role of the school, by professionalizing its role in conducting our societal health affairs. This means that boards of education need to provide appropriate curriculum time and trained teacher personnel to carry out meaningful programs.

One important objective of a health education program is to bring some objectivity into the health classroom. We need to get away from the traditional format of the teacher *telling* the students the do's and don'ts of how to be healthy and lead the good life. Rather, the students need to be involved in the learning process, not only for the purpose of coming to his own conclusions and making his own decisions, but also to add his own constructive efforts to the resolution of societal health problems.

NURSING HOMES

The nursing home is rapidly becoming established as a necessary community health facility. It serves to care for people who do not need the elaborate services of the hospital, but are not quite ready to return home. These are often persons who have chronic diseases, are convalescing, or need long-term care for a variety of reasons. An advantage of the nursing home is that it provides the services needed for selected patients and is usually much less expensive than the hospital. Our nursing homes are populated mostly by the elderly, since the major chronic diseases affect them more heavily.

Though the caliber of the nursing home has been upgraded, the abuses, impatience, and despair prevalent in nursing homes has been well documented. The boom of the nursing home business brought with it many unscrupulous people. Privately owned, profit-making institutions were more often concerned with profit than the social, emotional, or physical welfare of its charges. In some cases they were being administered by businessmen whose training and qualifications were questionable. Legislation now requires the licensing of administrators of nursing homes, though owners of these institutions still need to meet no standards in education, training, or experience. The need for qualified personnel from the top administrator to the lowly aide has become critical. A beautiful new brick building "staffed by surly aides and minimally competent nurses is not much good."[3] An unprecedented effort to upgrade the services in some nursing homes must be attempted.

Pressure from consumer groups needs to be exerted to obtain funds for alternative services. The nursing home should not be the *only* answer in care for the elderly. The establishment of day care centers is desired for people needing only part time nursing or simply companionship; housekeeping services

[3] The Nader Report, *Old Age—The Last Segregation,* Claire Townsend, Project Director (New York: Grossman Publishers, 1971).

or home meals for those needing help with household chores; the payment of partial medicaid support for those families who want to take care of their own parents (these monies could be used for part time nurses' visits). A public health official in Michigan summed it up aptly when he urged that we spend some of our federal and state monies in keeping people *out* of institutions instead of spending all our money taking care of people *inside* institutions.

HEALTH CAREERS AND THE EXPANDING HEALTH INDUSTRY

The expanding activities of the public health professions have been necessitated by a number of factors. They have been attempting to find applications for pyramiding research findings, as well as to disseminate health information developed from these sources. In addition, they have been responding to changes and dangers affecting our environment (pollution, radiation, proliferate use of drugs) in our advancing technology. They have also heard the public demand for more and better health services by a growing population. The entire field of public health is in an era of rapid change and advancement. The expansion and development of its programs are to a great extent being delimited by the numbers of available health personnel. The current critical shortage of health professionals represents a major stumbling block to the attainment of desired public health goals.

To ease this personnel shortage, the United States Public Health Service has made available traineeships through Schools of Public Health. These public health traineeships will not only cover the educational costs of recipients but will provide a sizable monthly subsistence allowance as well. The program has been effective in attracting people to the public health professions. These have included students who had not as yet decided on a career, and personnel from other professions. There are over 200 possible health careers for individuals interested in providing services that will promote the health of peoples and communities. Financial remuneration in this developing health industry is also competitive.

HEALTH ORGANIZATION AT THE WORLD LEVEL

We are living in a rapidly shrinking world where air travel has made all parts of the world accessible within a matter of hours. Where there exist pockets of disease, such as smallpox and cholera, we now face the reality that these sources of infection are not in some inaccessible region of the world, but perhaps hours away. Our interests in world health, while many times sparked by humanitarian motivations, are increasingly being stimulated by the need to safeguard our own health.

The World Health Organization and Its Activities

In 1945, when the United Nations was located in San Francisco, Brazil and China made the joint proposal that an international health organization be formed. This was followed by an international health conference in which the constitution for the World Health Organization was drawn up. On April 7, 1948, the World Health Organization became one of eleven specialized agencies of the United Nations. Its stated objective is "the attainment by all peoples of the highest possible level of health." It operates as a fairly independent unit having its own constitution, budget, and administrative structure. Basic decisions for the World Health Organization (WHO) are made by the World Health Assembly. Delegates that represent each of the WHO member

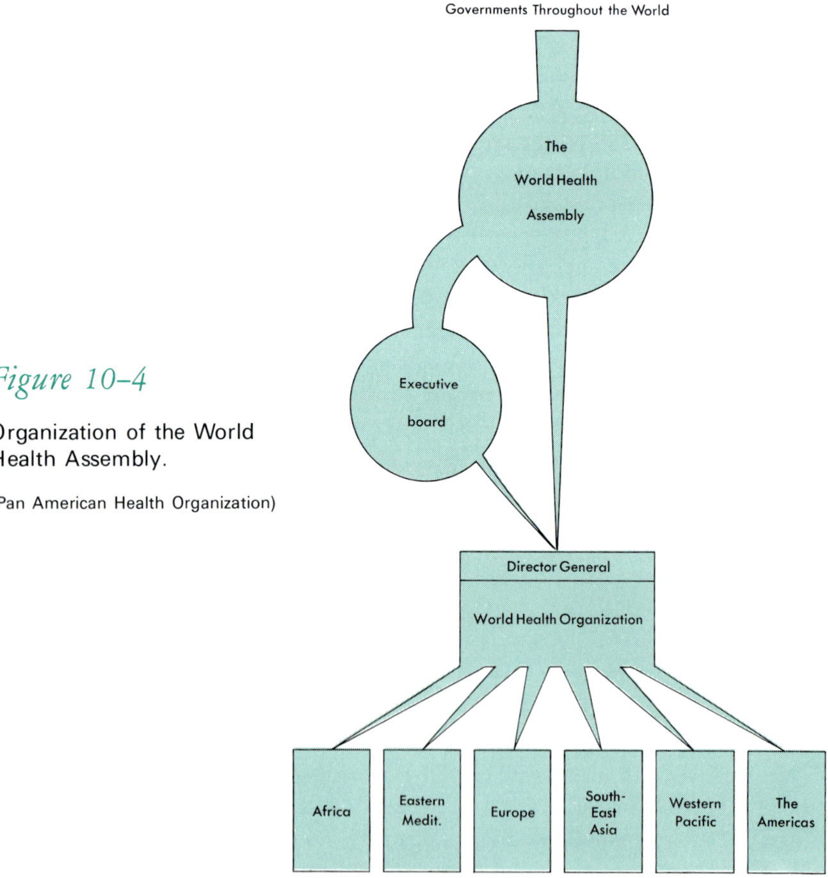

Figure 10–4

Organization of the World Health Assembly.

(Pan American Health Organization)

states make up the governing body. It is the World Health Assembly that determines policies, budget, and program. The Assembly meets annually, the meetings generally lasting three weeks.

The executive board of WHO is made up of 24 health specialists who serve three-year terms on this body. Eight are replaced each year, with the Health Assembly designating those countries entitled to choose persons to serve on this board. Members of the executive board are *not* there to represent their countries, but to make a contribution to the WHO.

In order to facilitate its operation, WHO has divided the world into six regions. The regional offices are located in Brazzaville (Republic of the Congo), for Africa; Washington, D.C., (United States), for the Americas; New Delhi (India), for Southeast Asia; Copenhagen (Denmark), for Europe; Alexandria (Egypt), for the Eastern Mediterranean; and Manila (Philippines), for the Western Pacific. Each of the regional offices is largely responsible for the development of projects within its area. In 1948, when the first World Health Assembly met, they chose Geneva, Switzerland, as the location for the organization's headquarters. The offices of the director General of WHO and his staff are located there.

International narcotics control is a responsibility the WHO inherited from the League of Nations. WHO has a committee, made up of international experts, that reviews various drugs considered likely to produce addiction. It then proceeds to place the addictive substances on the listing of controlled drugs. Biological standardization is another service rendered by WHO. WHO will provide samples of substances that have been internationally standardized such as vaccines, antibiotics, hormones, and other drugs. In this manner, laboratories have a standard of measurement and can compare the strength of their own products with that of WHO's standardized products. WHO also publishes the International Pharmacopoeia. It adopts internationally recognized names for pharmaceuticals which often have varying names in different countries. It also serves as a clearing house for new drugs and for information on dangerous side effects of drugs that may already be in use.

In order for it to obtain the best advice available on technical matters, WHO will many times set up expert panels made up of leading scientists and health administrators in the world. These experts are called together whenever a need arises. The services of these outstanding scientists are given free.

WHO maintains a watchdog service for the ever-present menace of epidemics of diseases like plague, cholera, smallpox, typhus, and yellow fever which still smoulder in our world environment. WHO also keeps nations informed about outbreaks of viral diseases like influenza. Before the WHO came into existence, there was little uniformity in quarantine regulations. There is now a uniform set of International Sanitary Regulations that give protection against the spread of disease. International health statistics have been made more accurate as the World Health Assembly makes provision for the uniform reporting of diseases and death.

The WHO also serves as a clearing house for health information. It has put out hundreds of technical publications on a variety of health topics and has stimulated and coordinated research activity, though it does not itself do research. Cooperative international research has obvious advantages in that it can focus the best talent and resources on a specific research problem.

The responsibilities of WHO will be rapidly increasing in the area of radiation control. The expanded industrial use of atomic energy will result in the need for international controls related to the transportation and use of radioactive products and the disposal of radioactive waste materials. It is assuring to know that WHO is anticipating these developments rather than waiting for them to mushroom into problems before taking remedial action.

UNICEF (The United Nations Children Fund)

The United Nations Children Fund represents the only branch of the United Nations whose activities are deveoted exclusively to the welfare of children. It was initially organized on December 11, 1946, as UNICEF (United Nations International Children's Emergency Fund). Its initial function was to help the children of war-torn countries. By 1950 UNICEF had completed its major tasks in Europe and in 1953 the General Assembly of the UN decided that UNICEF should continue under its changed name of United Nations Children Fund. Its purpose was designated as that of helping the millions of children, particularly in the underdeveloped countries, who were undergoing the hardships of hunger and illness. UNICEF has been working very closely with the WHO in its campaign against the major diseases of the world. UNICEF has provided various kinds of support for these campaigns. It has contributed supplies such as insecticides, sprayers, drugs, and health education materials. It has been busily at work helping to set up schools for the training of various health personnel. This organization has also made a major contribution by providing skim milk powder by the ton to alleviate nutritional problems. A drawback to the large-scale distribution of milk powder has been the discovery that some people cannot digest milk. They lack an enzyme (lactase) that is needed to break down milk sugar or lactose. The number of such people is more prevalent than has heretofore been realized. Even though lactase-deficient peoples can drink small to moderate amounts of milk and show no discomfort, there is a move toward supplying milk powder that is lactose-free so that intolerant populations can be provided milk—a major source of needed protein.

UNICEF has been at work with the FAO (Food and Agriculture Organization) and WHO in efforts to develop new high-protein foods. It has given assistance to communities in helping them increase their production of fruits, vegetables, and poultry. It has undertaken a program for the training of local workers to help overcome their many unscientific beliefs with regard to nutrition and health. At the same time it has instituted courses of study at the primary school level for the same purpose.

UNICEF is headed by an executive director who is appointed by the United Nations Secretary General. However, when it comes to budgetary matters, UNICEF is financed completely by voluntary contributions that come from governments and private groups of people from various countries. The United Nations does not provide money for the budget of UNICEF. Each year contributions that have been received from various governments have steadily increased, so that its budget now approaches that of the World Health Organization. Help from UNICEF is rendered only at the request of governments. Countries oftentimes will propose that various projects be carried out within their borders and make application to UNICEF for such programs. The requests are reviewed by UNICEF officers and upon approval are set into action. UNICEF activities are worked out very closely and cooperatively with the World Health Organization and other groups within the United Nations. The ultimate goal in any UNICEF program is the development within the country itself of *permanent* health, nutrition, education, and social welfare services that are supported entirely by the country's own efforts. Only in this way can the benefits to children be long-lasting.

Food and Agriculture Organization (FAO)

The food and Agriculture Organization is one of the specialized agencies of the United Nations. Its major purpose has been to relieve the hunger and inadequate nutrition that afflict half the world's population. It tackled the twin problems of overproduction and undernourishment and sought the best possible use of food surpluses for economic development of struggling countries. In 1963, after much study, the World Food Program (WFP) was created. It was conceived by the United Nations and Food and Agriculture Organization, and was concerned with economic and social development as well as nutrition and the production and distribution of food.

One of the two largest projects of the World Food Program is in India where the development of a dairy industry is under way. This involves increasing capacity and output of dairy processing facilities, switching raw milk suppliers to modern dairies, and bringing the cattle from the cities to the rural areas. The social, nutritional, and economic benefits of this project will be widespread. The health hazards caused by cattle in the city will be eliminated. There will be increased availability of wholesome milk, which is the most important source of animal protein in the Indian diet since a large proportion in the country are vegetarians. In addition the price for pure milk will be cheaper.

The World Food Program had also been engaged in settling people on new land, for example, many of those who had to leave the Aswan Dam area. Reclaiming and improving the land is done by the laborers who are paid with food (or rations) as part of their wages. Food aid is given to families until their land can support them. In 1974 there were approximately 40,000 new

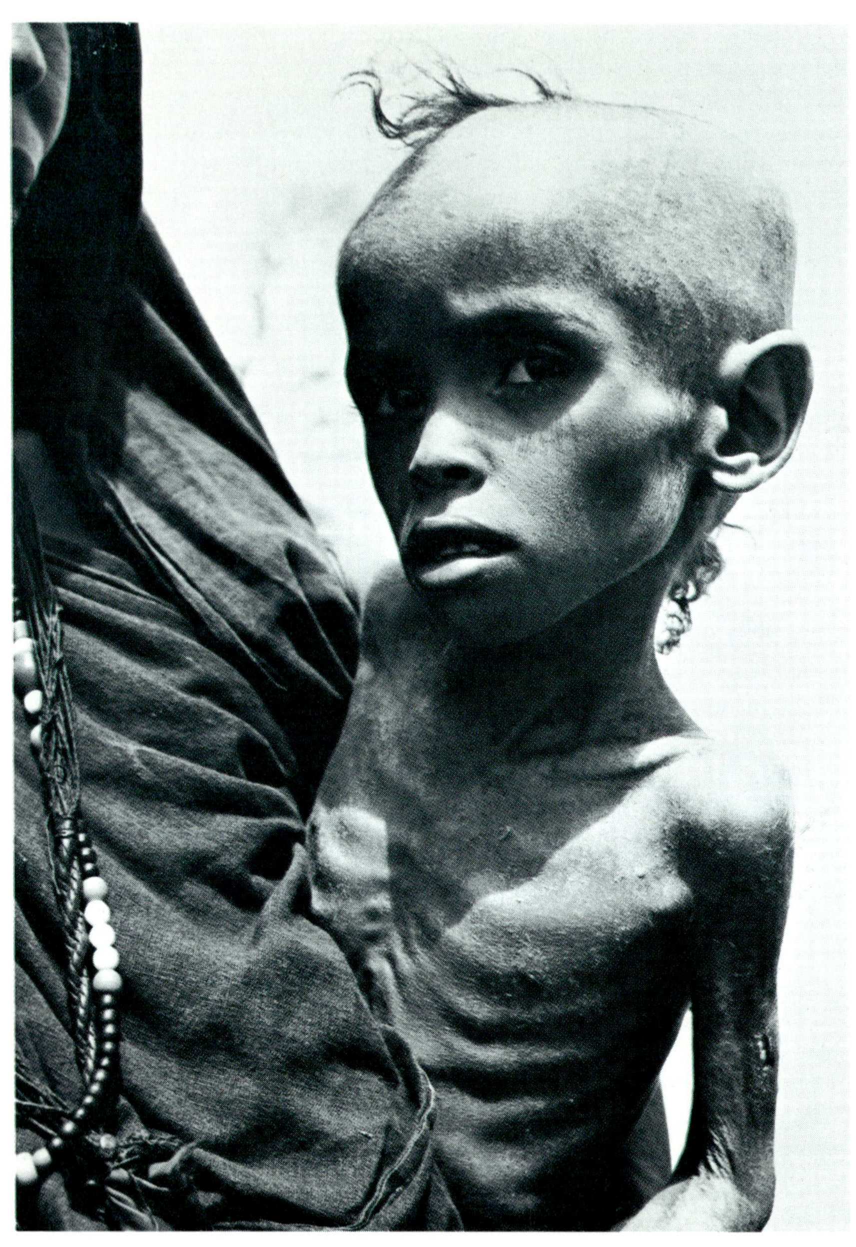

Figure 10–5

Inadequate nutrition and starvation are still prevalent world health problems.

(Photo: Jean-Marie Bertrand, Black Star)

settler families working with the program in this way. To meet the need for new and more abundant forests not only to provide timber but for erosion, control and general soil conservation, projects in forestry are now under way. Livestock projects are also an essential phase of the agricultural scene. Rangelands that are turning into deserts because of overgrazing of sheep and goats are being renovated.

CARE/MEDICO

The humanitarian work of Tom Dooley in the northern Laotian village of Nam Tha had far-reaching effects. He not only treated the disease-ridden people of that area, but taught and trained those Laotions who would follow him in running "their" hospital. With Dr. Commanduras, Tom Dooley appealed to the International Rescue Committee for the establishment of six medical teams to be sent to critical areas throughout the world. On February 4, 1958, he announced the founding of a new organization called MEDICO, which stands for Medical International Cooperation Organization. MEDICO was in no way a religious or political organization. Tom Dooley envisioned it as a person-to-person, heart-to-heart program in which therapeutic medicine could be practiced for sick people in areas that had little or no chance of receiving medical aid. "It will aid those who are sick and by that simple act it will win friendship for America."[4] Dr. Dooley died of cancer in 1961 at the age of 34. In 1964, MEDICO and CARE merged. In this alliance, CARE supplies the money and logistical support, and MEDICO supplies the doctors. Tom Dooley's work in the form of CARE/MEDICO and The Thomas A. Dooley Foundation, Inc., goes on, and his spirit lives on in those dedicated to helping their fellow men.

SS Hope

In 1960 the Project Hope (*H*ealth *O*pportunity for *P*eople *E*verywhere) was launched when an unused Navy hospital ship was refitted and renamed the SS *Hope.* Under the direction of its founder and medical director, Dr. William B. Walsh, the SS *Hope* traveled to South Viet Nam, Indonesia, Peru, Ecuador, Ceylon, and Nicaragua. Staffed by U.S. medical personnel, Hope participated in the development of emerging nations by elevating their health standards through education and by promoting international friendship and understanding. Though the ship is no longer being used, Project *Hope* still operates on the principle of helping people who wish to help themselves and goes only where it is invited. Its professional staff has trained over 5,100 physicians, nurses, dentists, and paramedical personnel in those countries. More recently, *Hope* has expanded its people-to-people health project to within the United States. A program with Mexican Americans in Laredo, Texas, and another with

[4] Thomas A. Dooley, *The Night They Burned the Mountain* (New York: Farrar, Straus and Giroux, 1960), p. 24.

the Indian Americans at Ganado, Arizona, have now been established. Project *Hope* has thus stimulated the development of medical services and facilities leaving some of its medical skills, texts, and dedicated zeal. In essence, it leaves a little hope.

Dr. Richard B. Stark, in his article "Medicine as a Force for Peace," stated:

> So, the Schweitzers, the Seagraves, the Dooleys, the Walshes, the Carlsons, the Commandurases, by reliving the parable of the Good Samaritan, have pointed the way. With planning and a continual supply of superbly trained humanitarian specialists, the medical export will grow. Administered with compassion as a gift of the giver, the parable of the samaritan need not be old hat, but may inject into our nervous, narcissistic, alcoholic, bored, rich, delinquent society, a sense of selflessness and indeed, of purpose itself.[5]

SOME WORLD HEALTH PROBLEMS

The health problems of the more developed countries of the world increasingly parallel those of the United States—heart disease, cancer, venereal diseases, problems of the aging, environmental pollution, automobile safety, and many others. It is not unusual to read of automobile pollution problems in Rome, or the traffic accident as a "man-made epidemic" in Buenos Aires. It is interesting to read of some solutions on aging from countries like England, Denmark, and Sweden. They are reportedly dealing with their aging population somewhat more successfully than we have done in the United States. These three countries emphasize preventive medicine and home care rather than institutionalizing or segregating old people in nursing homes.

"A backward nation to me is an area in which there are major sociological and cultural reasons which prevent the widest possible application of existing biological knowledge; New York City is a backward nation."[6] The failure to act because of ignorance is understandable. The failure to act in the health area in the presence of existing knowledge is tinged with immorality.

As political barriers began to fall in the early part of this decade, medical and health news from China and Russia began to be exchanged and explored. There developed widespread interest in acupuncture, a Chinese form of anesthesia. American physicians observed the technique of inserting long, sterile, stainless steel needles into parts of the body far removed from the site of surgery, and finally witnessed surgery under this method of acupuncture

[5] Richard G. Stark, M.D., "Medicine as a Force For Peace," *The Journal of the American Medical Association,* Vol. 195, No. 1 (January 3, 1966), p. 108.

[6] George James, M.D., M.P.H., *Human Potential in a Dynamic Environment,* School Health Education Study.

anesthesia. The increased interest in acupuncture precipitated a statement from the New York State Medical Board, which plays a key role in regulating (i.e. examining and licensing) the practice of medicine in New York. The statement read,

> The Board recognizes the need for, and desires to encourage, further research in the techniques, mechanisms of action, and uses of acupuncture. However, because acupuncture is considered at this time strictly as an investigational procedure, it should be performed only in medical centers and teaching hospitals having committees on human research, which will provide the necessary peer review of protocols and appropriate monitoring of such studies.[7]

Whether the use of needles will become a part of standard anesthetic practice in America remains to be seen. Considerable experimental data is being gathered so that a scientific judgment can be made. It is felt that if acupuncture is successful, it will be a panacea for those people in chronic pain who to date have no other means of treatment available. In addition, a great deal of surgery for older patients with cardiac and/or respiratory problems might be more safely carried out, since surgery for these patients presently is very risky with conventional anesthetic means.

The overall Chinese health care system has revealed that great strides have been made in some areas. For example:

- VD, which affected tens of millions, has been almost totally eliminated in most parts of China. In a few areas where sexual promiscuity is traditional, VD has been brought under control and is expected to disappear in the next generation;
- Drug addiction, rampant since the introduction of opium into China by foreign traders in the mid-19th century, has been wiped out. This was done in less than five years, by public education, stiff legal penalties for those selling drugs (but not for users), and medical care for the addicted;
- Childhood diseases, such as diphtheria, have come under control through inoculation programs. Immunization against poliomyelitis and measles is also universal, and the number of cases has become insignificant;
- Public education in sanitation, its implementation in city neighborhoods and on agricultural communes by "health activist" residents, guided by sanitarians, has resulted in a very substantial reduction in parasitic diseases that were endemic in the past. Schistosomiasis, which as late as 1955 still afflicted many millions in river delta and swampy areas, has largely been brought under control;

[7] "New York State Medical Board Adopts Position on Acupuncture," News Release, July 26, 1972.

- Emphasis has shifted from the curative aspect of medicine to the preventive. Checkups are on a regular basis, and people are urged to visit health clinics—located in the neighborhoods where they live, in factories, and on farms—as soon as they feel ill;
- Comprehensive care—medical, surgical, and dental, including hospitalization—has been instituted. It is either free or covered by cooperative plans that cost a few tenths of a per cent of an average income. Half the cost of drugs and hospitalization for nonworking members of the family must be paid, but it only costs about 50 cents a day.[8]

In Russia, cardiovascular disease research has been given high priority. At the S. L. Miasnikov Institute of Cardiology in Moscow, Russian scientists are exploring methods of prevention, diagnosis, and treatment of heart disease. The realization that education plays an important role in modifying the risk factors can be seen in Russia, where classes in exercise are encouraged; in Finland, where efforts to modify eating habits are in progress; and in England, where antismoking clinics are held. The risk factors have been identified, and the challenge to halt the coronary epidemic by modifying these factors is echoing the world over. The United States and Russia entered a Joint Agreement on Health Cooperation in 1972, which has resulted in a rich exchange of information, initially on heart disease and cancer but ultimately to extend to other areas of health as well.

DISEASES FOUND IN UNDERDEVELOPED COUNTRIES

The health problems of the underdeveloped nations of the world differ from those of the more highly technological societies. A review of the more prevalent disease conditions include the following.

Kwashiorkor is a disease caused by a lack of protein in the diet. The condition was studied in Africa by a group from the World Health Organization in 1914. Subsequent study showed the condition to be widespread in Asia and Central America as well.

Young children are particularly hard hit by the disease. They thrive well during their first year of life while they are being breast fed. Afterwards, they are given a diet rich in starch but lacking in protein. The child is particularly affected because he is in a period of rapid growth requiring a protein-rich diet. The adult is not as severely affected because he has attained full growth.

Characteristics of the disease include a swollen abdomen, thin arms and legs, stunted growth, streaks of patchy, reddish hair, and discolored patches of skin. General weakness and death often follow.

[8] *The Nation's Health,* June–July 1972.

Any protein-rich food can quickly correct the deficiency. Skim milk and peanuts are commonly used for this purpose. It is interesting to note that a liquid dietetic food that is rich in protein has been successfully used in correcting kwashiorkor. As stated by Dr. John Miller, a missionary physician directing medical work in Africa: "I wish the people who make Metrecal could only see what their product does for starving babies with kwashiorkor. Children who have long since lost all interest in food beg for it."[9] Educational programs are now being conducted to make mothers aware of the cause of the condition. Attempts are being made to teach these prople to grow protein-rich plant foods and to produce other sources of protein, such as cattle and milk. One of the real difficulties in reducing the incidence of kwashiorkor is that people like to cling to old, misconceived ideas about nutrition. In some areas, for instance, mothers refuse to give their children animal milk because they believe it is not good for them. In other places where fish, a good source of protein is plentiful, it is considered an acceptable adult food but unsuitable for children. The problem, therefore, is not always the lack of a source of proteins, but the difficult matter of changing old ways and ideas.

Malaria has been one of the deadly afflictions of man. At one time 300 million people a year were sick and 3 million people were dying of this disease. It accounted for a staggering economic loss as well. The illness made people incapable of work, with the result that farms were not cultivated and other work projects were never completed. In 1955 the World Health Organization undertook the greatest public health venture of all time. It initiated an eradication program against malaria.

The disease is caused by a protozoan parasite that is transmitted by the anopheles mosquito. The mosquito spreads the disease by biting a person ill with malaria and thus picking up the infectious protozoans. It transmits these causative organisms by biting a well person. The campaign was started with DDT spraying to kill the mosquitoes, and with the use of antimalarial drugs for those already infected. The malaria eradication program has made significant progress, and 5 more countries and territories have been registered as malaria-free, bringing the total of malaria-free areas up to 18. The malaria eradication program consists of four phases:

1. Preparatory Phase: geographical reconnaissance and training of staff.
2. Attack Phase: house spraying or other attack methods are applied.
3. Consolidation Phase: attack measures are stopped and surveillance is carried out.
4. Maintenance Phase: vigilance operations aim at preventing the reestablishment of the disease.

[9] Peter Wyden, *The Overweight Society* (New York: Pocket Books Cardinal Edition, 1966), p. 44.

In 1970 it was estimated that of the 1,802 million people who originally lived in malarious areas, 1,340 million (or 74 per cent) were in areas where malaria had now been eradicated or where programs were in progress.

The cry against the use of DDT that has arisen from Western Europe and North America has restricted its use in these areas. Fears from malarious areas is that this restriction will inhibit malaria eradication programs, as in fact it has. For example, as a result of premature cessation of spraying in Ceylon, their malaria rate went from 110 cases in 1961 (after a 15-year campaign against malaria) to 2.5 million in 1968–1969. This DDT controversy has made the research concerning the development of a vaccine against malaria increasingly significant. Biological means of controlling mosquitoes are being explored in Nigeria, for example, where a minnow-sized fish that feeds on mosquito larvae is being studied; and in India, genetically altering the male mosquito renders it sterile. Effective alternatives must be developed so that the relentless attack against malaria may continue.

Tuberculosis. There are still 15 million cases of tuberculosis, and 3 million deaths a year are caused by it. There has been a rapid decline in the death rate for tuberculosis in the economically developed countries. The development and use of effective drugs have been responsible in great part for the decline. The disease remains, however, a significant worldwide public health problem. In some countries 70 per cent of the children are infected before the age of 14. This does not mean that these children have active tuberculosis. It indicates that they have been in contact with the disease, as revealed by tuberculin testing, and *could* become active cases. A committee on tuberculosis of the World Health Organization stated that tuberculosis could not be eliminated as a public health problem until less than 1 per cent of the children in a country became infected by age fourteen. No country of the world as yet can meet that criterion.

The BCG (bacillus Calmette-Guerin) vaccine is one of the major weapons in the effort to control tuberculosis. It is 80 per cent effective in preventing the disease in those who have been so vaccinated. In India, there are over 5 million cases of tuberculosis, and two-thirds of the population are carriers of the virulent tubercle bacillus. In a ten-year period, 50 million Indian children have been given BCG vaccine.

Another giant step forward was taken with the development of antituberculosis drugs, namely streptomycin, PAS (para-aminosalicylic acid), and isoniazid. These drugs are not only effective against the disease, but inexpensive as well, making their extensive use feasible. The drugs represent a major breakthrough in tuberculosis control.

With the BCG vaccine and the antituberculosis drugs, man now has the weapons to eliminate another disease. It is now a matter of producing them in sufficient quantities and getting them to the right places at the right times. Not an easy task! The BCG vaccine has seen very limited use in this country. Most American physicians feel that it is more appropriately used in countries where the tuberculosis incidence is higher. The vaccine masks the results of tuberculin tests designed to determine if a person has had contact with the tuberculosis germs. Anyone who has had the vaccine will automatically register a positive reaction on a tuberculin test. In this country it is felt that finding specific individuals who are serving as sources of infection through tuberculin testing is a more effective approach than mass BCG vaccinations. Some American physicians and public health authorities feel that the use of the BCG vaccine has value even in the United States. Some studies are being conducted in high-incidence areas (overly populated, low-income areas in cities) utilizing the vaccine. The results of these studies will shed some light on this controversy.

Leprosy (Hansen's Disease). The inhuman segregation of patients with leprosy is finally becoming a thing of the past. However, in some areas, getting lepers to register is still difficult because of the stigma long associated with the disease. In Africa, for example, only 50 per cent of the registered cases were under treatment, even though dapsone, one of the sulfone drugs taken orally, can cure the disease completely if it is detected early. It is estimated that there are approximately 10 million cases of leprosy in the world.

Leprosy, which is caused by a bacillus, has an incubation period of from one to several or many years. Its period of contagion is only that stage when the lesions on the skin are open and can discharge bacilli. This period of communicability can be shortened by the administration of drugs. In areas where it is common, leprosy is often contracted in childhood and may not appear until adulthood. Children appear to be more susceptible to the disease than adults. Educational efforts are being made to stress the greater risk of the disease when the individual is exposed early in life. As effective treatment for this condition is being recognized, the unreasoned fear that has been associated with it has been diminishing.

River Blindness is prevalent in tropical Africa as well as in the central portions of S. America. Tiny black flies (simulium damnosum) transmit the disease by carrying microscopic young forms of parasitic worms. These are transmitted to the human bitten by an infected fly. In the human, when the worms reach the adult stage, they produce nodules under the skin in which they develop hundreds of thousands of young. These microscopic worms then invade the tissues of the skin and eyes, with blindness a frequent outcome. The disease is often referred to as river blindness because of its high incidence in river valleys. The fly that transmits the disease is known to thrive best in quick-running water.

New drugs developed for the treatment and control of the disease leave much to be desired. Some drugs are effective only on the adult worm and others only on the embryo form of the worm. In some areas, spraying with insecticides (DDT) has been effective in exterminating the tiny black fly. More than 250 million people are still affected by river blindness (onchocerciasis) and attempts are being made to organize mass programs for its eradication.

Cholera is an intestinal disease that is caused by bacteria and spread via food and water contaminated by human waste. Sanitation and personal cleanliness almost eliminate the transmission of this disease from man to man. In fact, the likelihood of the disease spreading is so rare in areas where hygiene is good that the United States no longer demands a certificate of cholera vaccination from international travelers. The cholera patient suffers from vomiting, diarrhea, dehydration, and collapse. Death from severe dehydration can occur with frightening suddenness. The fatality rates range anywhere from 10 to 80 per cent, depending on the availibility of early treatment, which includes the replacement of body fluids and antibiotics. Control measures that are taken include the boiling of water for drinking and dishwashing. Cholera vaccine is administered despite its uncertain value. The control of flies is also important in reducing the spread of the infection.

In the mid-nineteenth century, cholera raged throughout the world, killing tens of thousands of people. In Europe, it precipitated the development of the first public health measures that included a clean water supply and proper disposal of sewage to prevent the spread of the disease. There was an outbreak of cholera in the West Bengal in 1961, in which 1,422 people died during a six-month siege. Cholera moved north and westward and appeared in the Mediterranean area in 1965, and in 1970 reports of cholera came from Africa, Turkey, and Russia. *World Health* reported that "one of the outstanding events of 1970 was the extension of the seventh pandemic[10] of cholera, which began in 1961, to countries far from the traditional endemic areas in Asia."[11] The year 1970 was the worst year of the pandemic, with at least 46 countries reporting the disease. The summer of 1973 saw a cholera epidemic in Italy where 22 people died of the disease. The last epidemic had occurred in that country in 1911.

Though health officials of the United States have been warned that the disease will continue westward and ultimately reach this country, they see it as no immediate threat because of adequate water supplies and sanitation.

Trachoma and infectious conjunctivitis represent a leading cause of blindness in the world, affecting some 500 million people. It is particularly prevalent in North Africa, Asia, and parts of deeper Africa and South America, particularly in dry, desert regions. In certain areas, practically the entire adult population is infected. The rate of infection among preschool-age children runs between 70 and 90 per cent in areas where poor hygiene, poverty, and crowded living conditions exist. A study conducted in India revealed a 78 per cent infection rate among rural school children. A pilot project on Taiwan uncovered a 48 per cent incidence among its children. Antibiotics are effective in clearing

[10] The end of the 6th pandemic came around 1923 when cholera retreated to its "homeland" in the deltas of the Ganges and Brahmaputra rivers.

[11] *World Health,* May 1971.

up the condition. Mass campaigns on a national level are being encouraged to bring this disease under control.

Snail Fever (Schistosomiasis or Bilharziasis) has plagued man for thousands of years. Egyptian medical men refer to remedies for the disease as far back as 3000 B.C. It is recognized as the greatest unconquered parasitic disease afflicting more than 200 million people. In terms of its damaging effects it ranks close to malaria. The disease is characterized by skin rash, headache, loss of appetite, nausea, fever, blood in the urine, and difficulty in breathing. In the chronic cases, there is liver damage, an enlarged spleen, a bloated abdomen, and an emaciated body. Treatment for the disease is far from satisfactory, since the drugs available are toxic and take several days or weeks to administer. The cause of the difficulty is a schistosome, a small worm whose life cycle involves both man and snail. To date, scientists have not found a weak link in the life cycle to effect a means of eradicating the schistosome. Scientists endeavoring to use chemical means to destroy the snail are discouraged by the high costs and loss of other forms of aquatic life resulting from this method. Biological control is also being investigated with the introduction of the snail-eating larvae of the marsh fly. These larvae seek and destroy only the snail. Irrigation projects have served as a means of further spreading the snails and the disease, so that the incidence is considered to be 50 per cent higher in areas where water improvement projects have taken place. Some authorities predict that the economic benefits of the Aswan Dam in Egypt will be canceled out by the further spread of this disease, since reinfection takes place easily with the first trip back to the rice field or other common sources of infection. Control of the disease, in addition to finding a suitable drug for its treatment, must include the elimination of the snail and careful control of irrigation systems as well as improved overall sanitation procedures.

Sleeping Sickness (trypanosomiasis) is a disease found in most of Africa south of the Sahara Desert. Several types of protozoa are responsible for sleeping sickness. The disease is transmitted by the tsetse fly, and animals as well as humans are susceptible to the illness. Some protozoa causing the disease are harmless to animals but dangerous to man. The animals in these cases act as reservoirs of infection. The tsetse fly, by first biting the animal and then man, transmits the disease. The opposite is sometimes found to be true where some protozoa causing the disease are harmless to man but fatal to the animals. In these cases, the people are deprived of animals that are needed as a source of protein or to help cultivate the land for the growth of crops. Either directly or indirectly the disease is a source of hardship to man.

Insecticides are now used in many areas to eradicate the tsetse fly. Drugs are also used to treat people who have contracted the illness. In the past, sleeping sickness was invariably fatal, but it can now be cured if treated in the early stages. Programs of prevention and treatment of the disease need to be continued and further extended.

REVIEW QUESTIONS

1. Why are public health organizations necessary to maintain acceptable levels of community health?
2. What are the major functions of the local health department?
3. Why do voluntary health organizations have greater flexibility in their mode of operation? What has been the nature of their contribution?
4. How is the role of the hospital changing from that of serving solely as a treatment center?
5. What has been the contribution of the United States Hospital and Medical Facilities Survey and Construction Act (Hill-Burton)?
6. What are the medical care functions of the nursing home?
7. How are some of the early abuses occurring in nursing homes being overcome?
8. What is the role of the state health department?
9. What contributions can the school make in the health area?
10. How are the free clinics and some neighborhood health centers changing the nature of health care delivery?
11. Why is interest in world health becoming a necessity?
12. What factors in addition to poverty contribute to the incidence of kwashiorkor in the world?
13. To what extent is snail fever (schistosomiasis) a threat in the underdeveloped regions of the world? Why are drugs that are effective in curing this disorder not a complete solution to the problem?
14. To what extent has the World Health Organization's program for the eradication of malaria progressed since its inception in 1955?
15. Why have American physicians had some reservation with regard to the use of the BCG vaccine for tuberculosis in the United States?
16. Since there is now effective treatment for leprosy, what problems must now be overcome in order to eradicate this disease?
17. Describe the structure of the World Health Organization.
18. Describe some of the far-flung activities of the World Health Organization. To what extent do the health problems differ for each of its regional offices?
19. What are the major functions of The United Nations Children Fund (UNICEF)? Why does this organization work very closely with the World Health Organization?

20 What are the purposes of the Food and Agriculture Organization (FAO)?

21 What was the contribution made by Dr. Thomas A. Dooley and MEDICO?

22 How did the ship SS *Hope* serve as more than a hospital ship? Why are its contributions to underdeveloped areas of the world long-lasting ones?

Appendix

Emergency First Aid

Artificial Respiration

An adult at rest breathes about 12–18 times a minute, taking in about a pint of air with each breath (slightly faster for children).

Breathing may stop as a result of gas or drug poisoning, electric shock, choking, drowning, suffocation, injuries to the head, neck, or chest, poliomyelitis, or convulsions.

Most persons can live only about 6 minutes after breathing stops. Artificial respiration must begin as soon as possible after natural breathing has been interrupted or when natural breathing is so irregular or shallow as to be ineffective.

Artificial respiration is a method of getting air into and out of a person's lungs until he can breathe for himself. It is a lifesaving measure.

Mouth-to-Mouth Method

One of the simplest and most effective ways to give artificial respiration is by the mouth-to-mouth (or mouth-to-nose) method. This method is effective for both children and adults and can be used even when there are injuries to the chest and arms.

Here is how to do it:

1. Place the person who has stopped breathing on his back.
2. Open his mouth and clear out any foreign matter such as food or dirt, with your fingers or a cloth wrapped around your fingers. If the person has false teeth, remove them.

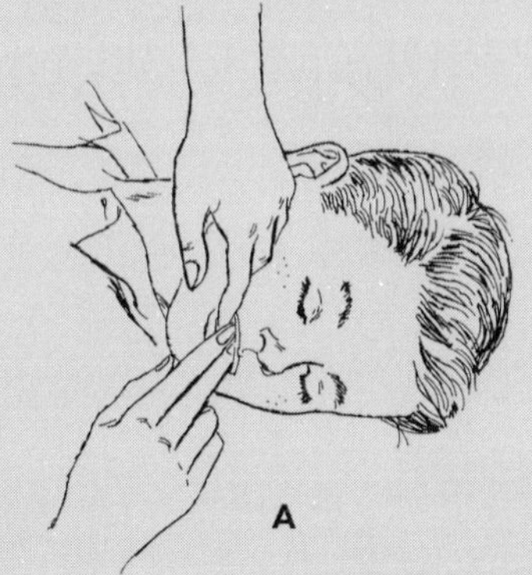

A. Before starting any type of artificial respiration be sure that the mouth and throat are completely clear of mucus and foreign objects. Use your fingers to clean the mouth. You may cover fingers with a piece of cloth to help remove mucus and slippery objects.

3. Tilt his head back so that his chin points upward and lift his lower jaw from beneath and behind so that it juts out. This moves the base of the tongue away from the back of the throat, so it does not block the air passage to the lungs. *Unless this air passage is open, no amount of effort will get air in.*

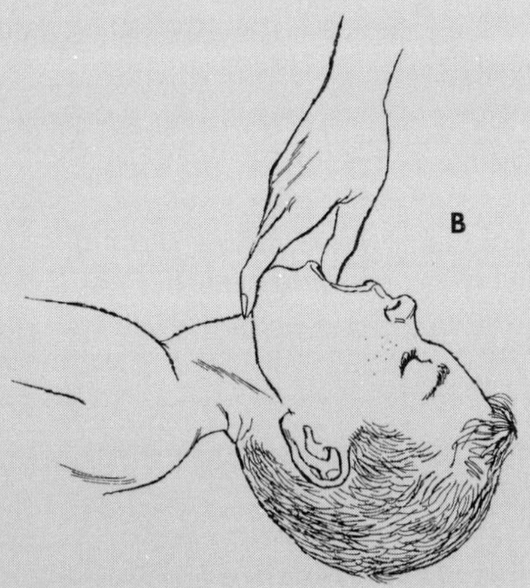

B. The head must be tipped back to allow a free air passage with the jaw held in a jutting out position. The more you can achieve the "sword swallower" position the better.

4. You can blow air into a person's lungs through either his mouth or nose. Open your mouth wide and place it tightly over the person's mouth. Pinch his nostrils shut to prevent air from escaping through the nose. *Or* close the victim's mouth and place your mouth over his nose. *With an infant or small child, place your mouth over both his nose and mouth, making an airproof seal.* Air can be blown through an unconscious person's teeth even though they may be clenched.

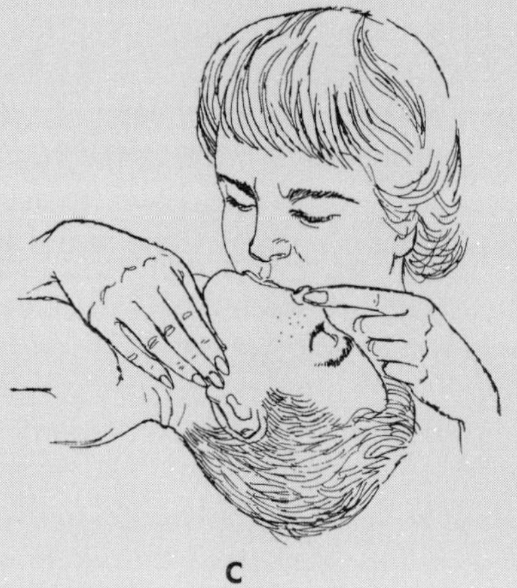

C

C. Remember—Don't blow too hard. Your mouth and the mouth of the person receiving treatment should be wide open with a complete seal between them. Inhale more than usual before exhaling into person's mouth. In this way he will get more oxygen. Pinching the nostrils prevents air from escaping through the nose. With your right hand be sure to hold the jaw in a jutting out position.

5. Blow into the mouth or nose, continuing to hold the unconscious person's lower jaw so that it juts out to keep the air passage open.

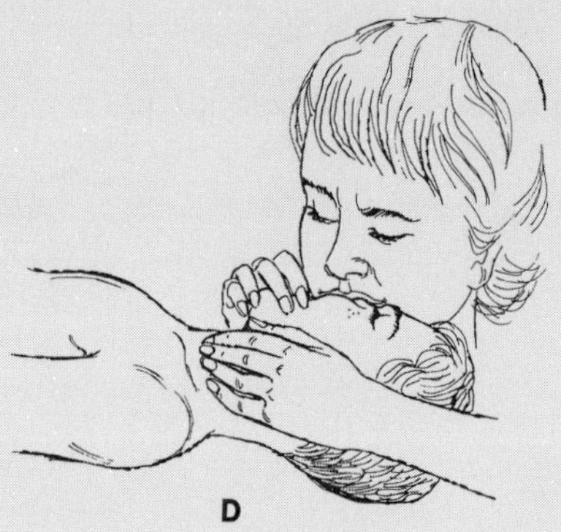

D

D. This is the mouth-to-nose type of respiration with lips being sealed by the two fingers of the right hand. This would be used when an obstruction is in the mouth that cannot be removed, or a severe mouth injury prevents proper contact.

6. Remove your mouth from the patient's mouth. Turn your head to the side and listen for the return outflow of air coming from the patient's lungs. If you hear it, you will know that an exchange of air has occurred.
7. You can then continue your breathing for the patient. Blow vigorously into his mouth or nose about 12 times each minute (or 1 breath every 5 seconds). Remove your mouth after each breath and listen for the exchange of air. In the case of an infant or child, blow less vigorously, using shallower breaths about 20 times a minute (or every 3 seconds).
8. If you are not getting an exchange of air, turn the person on his side and strike him several times between the shoulder blades, using considerable force. This will help dislodge any obstruction in the air

passages. Check the position of the head and jaw. Again make sure there is no foreign matter in his mouth. If you wish to avoid direct contact, you may hold a cloth (piece of gauze, handkerchief, or other material) over the victims' mouth or nose, and breathe through it. The cloth does not greatly affect the exchange of air. However, do not waste precious seconds looking for a cloth if one is not handy.

Normal breathing may sometimes start up again after 15 seconds of artificial respiration. But if it doesn't, you should continue the procedure, especially in cases of electric shock and carbon monoxide poisoning. Alternate with other persons, if possible, so as to maintain maximum efficiency.

The first signs of restored breathing may be a sigh. There may be irregular breathing at first. Artificial respiration should be continued until regular breathing occurs. If vomiting occurs at this time, turn the victim on his side so that vomitus can be cleared from his mouth.

Mouth-to-Neck Method

A laryngectomee or individual who has lost his larynx (voice box) requires some modification of the resuscitation technique. These individuals breathe through openings in their necks either completely or partially. The *total* laryngectomee does not breathe from his nose or mouth at all; all his air is drawn in from the neck opening (or stoma). In resuscitating this person, therefore, placing the mouth and lips tightly over the neck opening and blowing into the stoma should make the chest rise. If the chest fails to rise and the rescuer hears air escaping from the victim's nose or mouth, he can assume the victim is a *partial neck breather.* In this case the mouth

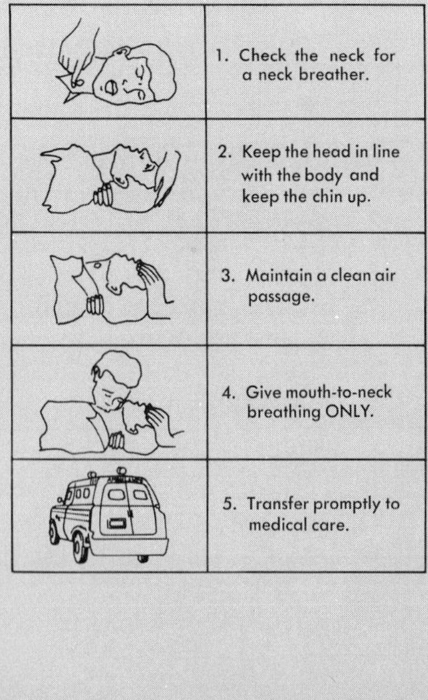

	1. Check the neck for a neck breather.
	2. Keep the head in line with the body and keep the chin up.
	3. Maintain a clean air passage.
	4. Give mouth-to-neck breathing ONLY.
	5. Transfer promptly to medical care.

Mouth-to-Neck Respiration

(reproduced by permission of the International Association of Laryngectomies, sponsored by: The American Cancer Society, Inc. Copyright issued to American Cancer Society, Inc.)

must be closed and the nose pinched during the mouth-to-neck resuscitation.

Chest-Pressure Arm-Lift Method (or Silvester Method)

The Silvester Method of artificial respiration is the only alternate manual method suggested in cases where the first aider is a laryngectomee or where facial wounds are so severe mouth-to-mouth cannot be used.

1. Place the non-breathing person on his back, clearing the mouth and maintaining an open air passage. This may be facilitated by placing something under the victim's shoulders enabling the head to drop backward.
2. Turn the victim's head to the side.
3. Kneel at the victim's head taking his wrists and crossing them over the lower chest.

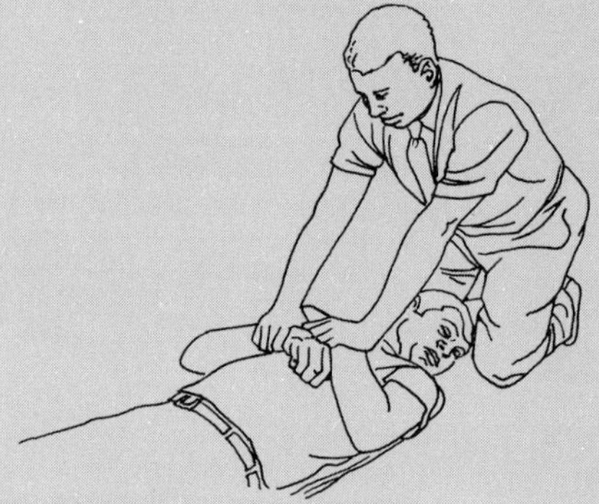

(Courtesy American National Red Cross)

4. Rock forward and apply steady even pressure downward on the chest.

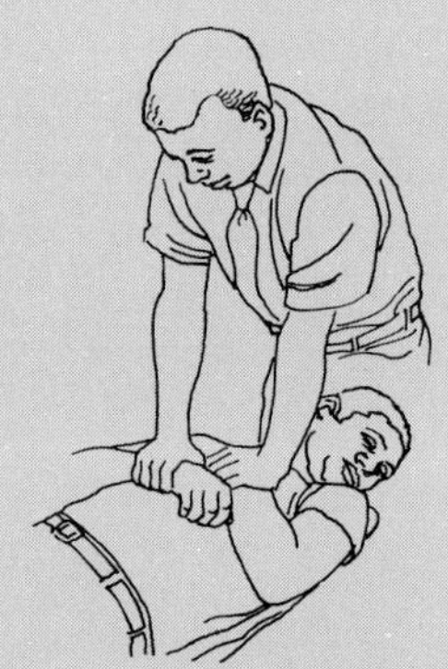

5. Immediately release this pressure by rocking back, pulling the victim's arms outward and upward over the victim's head and backward as far as possible.

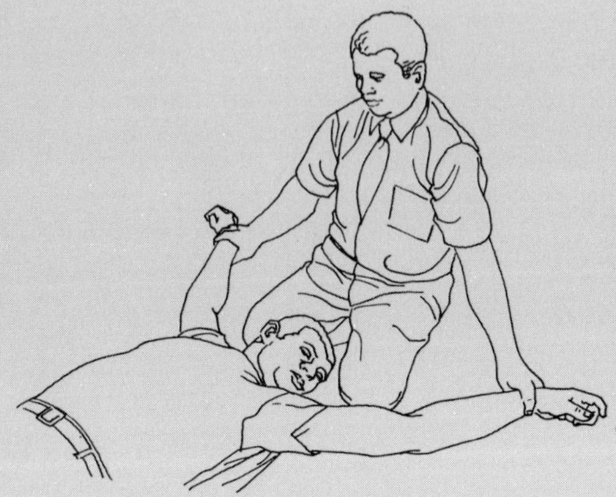

6. Repeat about 12 times per minute.

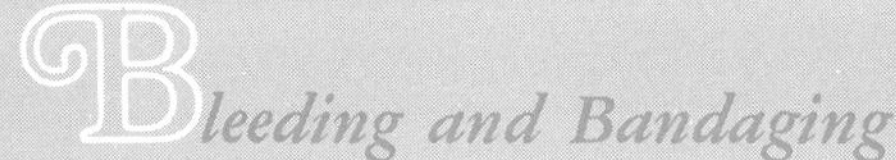

Bleeding and Bandaging

What to Do

1. Apply dressing or pad directly over wound.
2. Apply direct even pressure—use your bare hand if necessary when bleeding is serious, and dressing not immediately available.
3. Leave dressing in place.
4. Continue pressure by applying bandage.
5. Secure bandage in place—check to be sure bandage is not too tight and cutting off circulation.
6. Elevate limb above heart level except where there is a possible broken bone.
7. Treat for shock.
8. IF BLOOD SOAKS THROUGH DRESSING DO NOT remove but apply more dressings.

ATTENTION!!

Do not use a tourniquet unless it is impossible to stop excessive life-threatening bleeding by any other method.

Excessive Bleeding

Bleeding needs immediate attention. Even the loss of small amounts of blood will produce weakness and can cause the condition known as shock. The loss of as much as a pint of blood by a child or a quart of blood by an adult may have disastrous results.

The first step in controlling bleeding is to exert direct pressure over the wound area. You can do this best by placing the cleanest material available (a pad of sterile gauze is best) against the bleeding point, and applying firm pressure with your hand until a bandage can be applied.

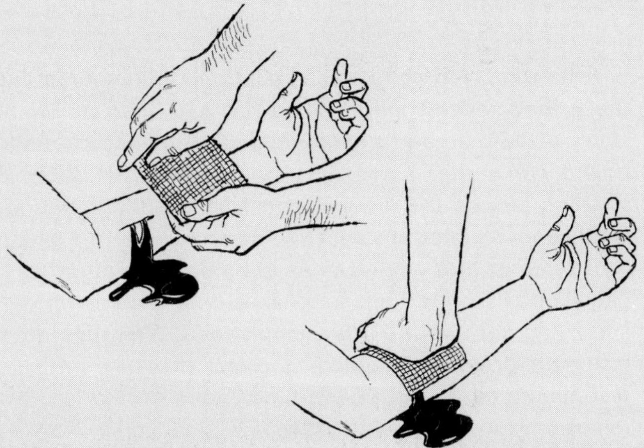

To stop bleeding apply dressing or pad directly over the wound and then apply pressure. Remember—immediate, direct pressure—even with the bare hand—is the important action to stop bleeding. Continue the pressure until the bleeding has stopped or slowed to the point that you will be able to apply a bandage. Don't be in a hurry to stop the pressure.

When bleeding is serious you may have to use your bare hand while waiting for someone else to get material for a dressing. This can place dangerous germs in the wound and cause infection, but it is obviously better to run the risk of infection than to let the person bleed to death. The pad should be large enough to overlap the edges of the wound and, if possible, the pressure should be applied in a manner that brings the edges of the wound together.

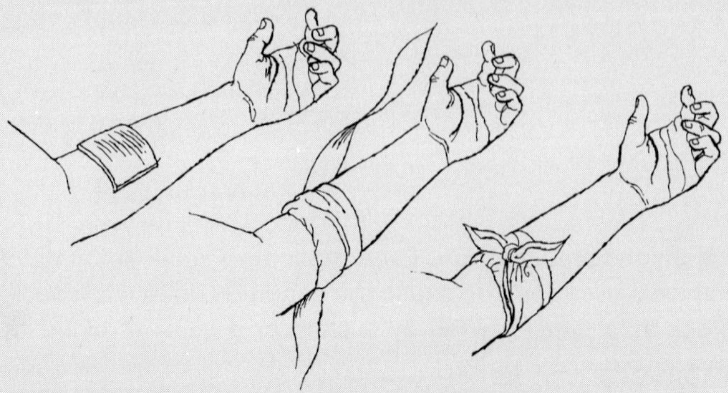

Apply the bandage firmly over the dressing to continue the pressure and thus continue to stop the bleeding.
CAUTION—Check the bandage after you have tied the knot to be sure it is not too tight and is not cutting off circulation.

After the bleeding has been controlled, do not remove the dressing from the wound, even though blood has saturated it. Simply apply additional layers of cloth to form a good-sized covering and bandage snugly and firmly.

A bandage that is too tight can cause further injury. Because of possible swelling around the wound, check the bandage periodically and loosen it if it seems to interfere with the circulation of the blood.

If a leg or arm wound does not stop bleeding after direct pressure and elevation of the limb has been executed, then direct pressure on the artery supplying the wound may be needed. Pressure on the brachial artery (pressure point) *in addition* to direct pressure and elevating the arm is recommended. If the severe bleeding is on the leg, then pressure on the femoral artery is recommended.

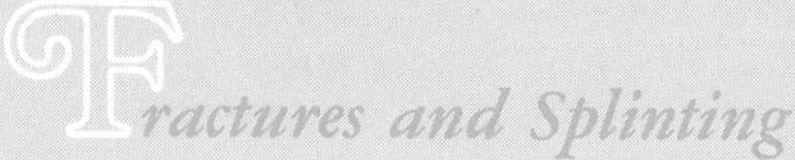

Fractures and Splinting

What to Do

1. Look for bleeding and control it.
2. Whenever in doubt, treat as a fracture.
3. Apply the splint at the site of the accident.
4. Never move the person before splinting unless his life would be further in danger.
5. Prevent shock, further injury]and infection.

6. Splint securely enough to prevent any voluntary or involuntary motion at the point of fracture.
7. Check splint ties frequently to be sure it does not interfere with circulation of blood.

In most cases of severe injury there is the possibility that the person may stop breathing. If this should occur stop all other lifesaving procedures and administer artificial respiration.

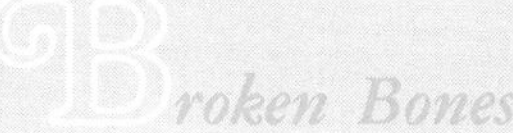

Broken Bones

Any break in a bone is called a fracture. If the ends of a broken bone do not come through the skin, the break is called a closed (or simple) fracture. If one or both ends of a broken bone come through the skin, the break is called an open (or compound) fracture. An open fracture is serious because germs can get in and cause infection.

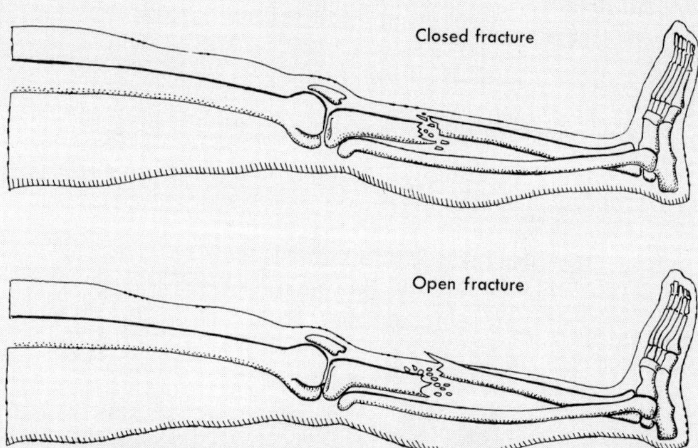

The top figure is a closed fracture but with improper handling it can very easily become a fracture such as you see in the bottom picture. All fractures or suspected fractures should be handled very carefully to avoid further injury.

In an open fracture, you will be able to see the wound where the bone breaks the skin. The bone itself may not be visible; it may slip back under the skin after breaking through.

In the case of a closed fracture, it is obviously more difficult to be sure that a break has occurred. One sign is pain at or near the break and tenderness and swelling around it. By running your finger gently along the bone, you may be able to feel an irregular piece of bone. A more obvious sign of a closed fracture may be the twisted or crooked unnatural position of an arm or leg or its appearance of being shorter than normal. The injured person may find it painful or impossible to move the limb.

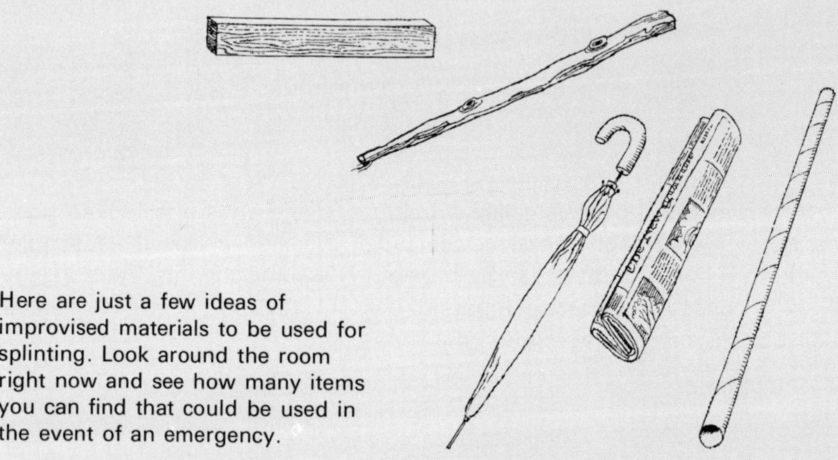

Here are just a few ideas of improvised materials to be used for splinting. Look around the room right now and see how many items you can find that could be used in the event of an emergency.

Whenever there is any reason to believe that there may be a broken bone, treat the injury as though it actually is a fracture. Otherwise, you may cause further injury.

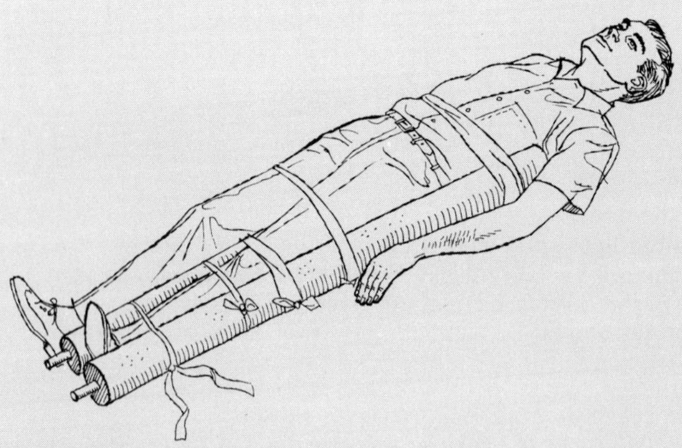

Apply splints so that they extend beyond the joints above and below the fracture.

If you are alone with an injured person who must be moved, and are unable to *carry* him, you may be able to *pull* him to safety. He should be pulled in the direction of the long axis of his body, not sideways. Danger of injuring him is less if a blanket (or similar object) can be placed under him, so that he can ride the blanket.

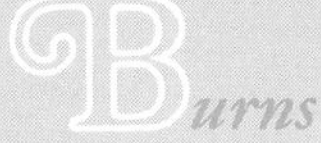

Burns

What to Do

1. Apply cold water applications or submerge part in cold water for first degree burns.
2. Treat for shock.
3. Relieve pain.
4. Prevent infection.
5. Cover burned area with dry sterile or clean cloth.
6. Encourage fluids to replace fluid loss from body.
7. Give water, salt, and soda solution: 1 teaspoonful salt and ½ teaspoonful soda to 1 quart water for third degree burns.

What Not to Do

1. DO NOT pull clothes over burned area.
2. DO NOT remove pieces of cloth that stick to burn.
3. DO NOT try to clean the burn.
4. DO NOT break blisters.
5. DO NOT use grease—ointment—petroleum jelly or any type of medication on severe burns.
6. DO NOT use iodine or antiseptics on burns.
7. DO NOT touch burn with anything except sterile or clean dressing.
8. DO NOT change dressings that were initially applied until absolutely necessary. They may be left in place 5–7 days.

The seriousness of a burn depends upon its extent (amount of body surface involved) and "degree" (depth of destruction of tissues). There are three recognized degrees:

A. In first degree burns, the skin is merely reddened as by a slight sunburn.
B. In second degree burns, blisters develop.
C. In third degree burns, there is deeper destruction, and the burned area may appear either charred or white.

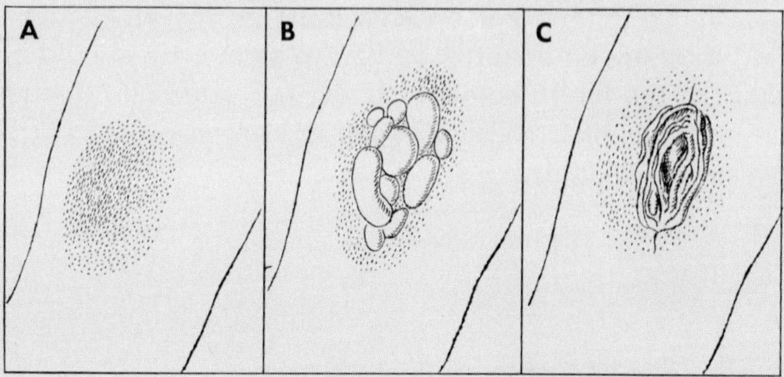

A. a first degree burn only reddens the skin and if it does not cover more than 25 percent of the body, usually is not serious. B. In second degree burns blisters develop and there is now the very real danger of infection. Extensive second degree burns will require giving additional fluids to the burned person. Do not apply grease or salve. Cover with sterile or clean dressing. C. Third degree burns even in a relatively small area are serious. The injury is deep and the underlying tissue has been destroyed. Keep this type of burn clean to avoid infection.

It is difficult or impossible to determine the degree of a burn at first. It often appears less deep than it actually is. The degree may differ in different parts of the affected area.

If a sterile dressing is not available, or is not big enough to cover a large burned area, use a clean towel or sheet. The dressing should be thick enough to keep air out of the burned area. Do not touch a burn or breathe directly on it. Do not attempt to open blisters or remove bits of dirt or debris from the burned surface. The blisters are not harmful and they protect the underlying tissues against entry of germs until the dressing is applied.

If adjoining surfaces of skin are burned, be sure they are separated by gauze—for example, between toes and fingers, between ears and head, between folds of the groin and genital region, and in the armpits. Otherwise they may stick together. The dressing on a serious burn should be left on as long as possible.

No ointments or salves should be used on burns. Never use iodine or any other antiseptic on burns. Dressings should be dry.

Transportation of the Injured

What to Do

1. Before transporting any sick or injured person:
   Bleeding should be stopped.
   Breathing should be established.

Fractures should be splinted.
Shock should be treated.
All other lifesaving methods completed.

2. Determine carefully the type and seriousness of the injuries and condition of the injured person.
3. Give complete emergency treatment *before moving* the injured.
4. Be gentle in moving the injured person; have enough help to assure safe moving.
5. Always carry a stretcher to an injured person, not the person to the stretcher.
6. Stretchers should be used for the more seriously injured persons and for transporting the injured over a long distance.
7. Be sure the person will not slip or fall from the stretcher while being carried. Belts or strong cloth bindings such as sheets may be used to secure the person to the stretcher.
8. Always use a two-man carry in preference to a one-man carry, if a hand carry is used. This helps to make the person being carried more

A. This saddle-back carry is simple and effective for moving an injured person a short distance, when his injuries are not serious. B. The four-hand seat carry shown is an excellent method for carrying conscious, not too seriously injured persons a short distance. C. This is an effective method of carrying an unconscious injured person a short distance provided it is not necessary to keep him flat.

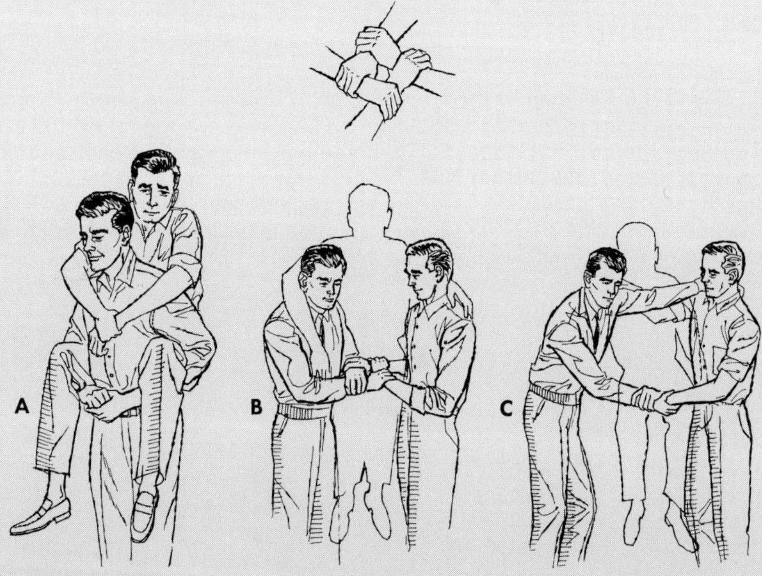

comfortable, enables him to be carried farther, and is less likely to aggravate fractures or other serious injuries.

9. The various hand carries should not be used unless the person needs only slight support for short distances; or in case of emergencies where delay will endanger life. Examples—fire or explosion.

Transporting Injured Persons

Do not be in a hurry to move an injured person. First aid authorities report that more harm is probably done through improper transportation of injured persons than through any other measure of emergency assistance. The danger of causing paralysis or death in moving persons with head, back, or neck injuries has already been noted. Thus, before considering moving an injured person, except under the most urgent conditions, such as exposure to fire, you should make a careful check for all possible injuries so that you will know the right method of transporting him.

There are many ways of moving an injured person, depending upon the nature and location of injuries. Some of the most useful are illustrated. It is important to lift and carry a person gently, moving him slowly and carefully without jerky movements.

If it becomes absolutely necessary to move a person to safety *before* a thorough check of injuries can be made, you should try to *protect all parts of his body from the tension of lifting.* A body should never be jacknifed (lifted by head and heels only). Try to give adequate support to each extremity, to the head and the back, and to keep the entire body in a straight line.

A. This is the first step in the correct method of using four people to load a seriously injured person on a stretcher. In this first step the fourth man does not touch the injured person. B. The three persons now lift slowly and all together and roll the injured person gently toward them on injured side. C. The fourth man now places the stretcher into position and then assists in lowering the person into the stretcher. Even, slow motion assures greatest safety and comfort of the injured person.

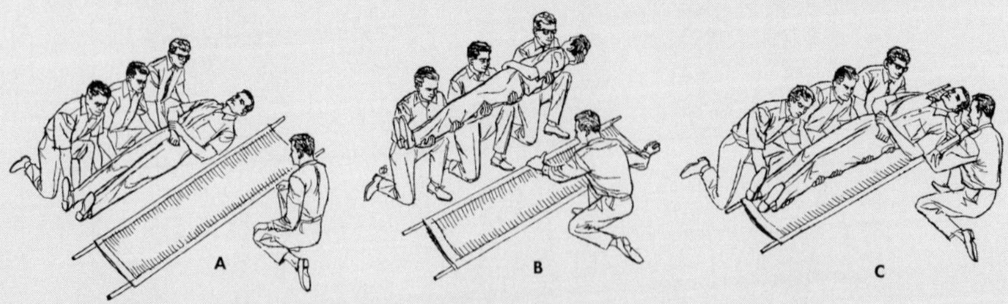

Shock

What to Do

1. Keep the person lying down.
2. Keep head lower than legs and hips if no chest or head injury.
3. Have head and shoulders slightly raised with chest or head injury or difficulty in breathing.
4. Keep the person from chilling.
5. Offer fluids by mouth if person is conscious and medical help is not available for an hour or more. Use solution of 1 teaspoonful salt and $\frac{1}{2}$ teaspoonful baking soda to a quart of water. Give $\frac{1}{2}$ glassful every 15 minutes.

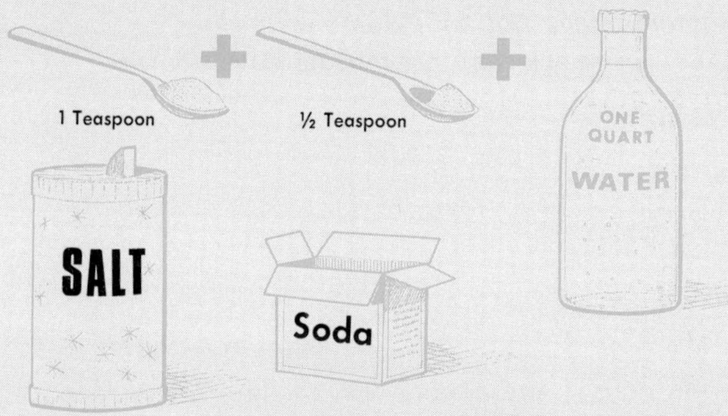

6. Never attempt to give fluids to an unconscious person.
7. Alcohol should not be used as a stimulant.

"Shock" as used in this section refers to a condition that frequently comes with serious injury such as severe wounds, burns, bleeding, and broken bones. It is due to a shortage of blood in various parts of the body. This causes the heart to beat faster in order to pump more blood, resulting in a rapid pulse. Lack of enough circulation through the brain causes unconsciousness.

Obviously a large amount of bleeding increases the danger of shock. In severe burns the oozing of blood fluids from the burned area increases the danger. *Shock may cause death if not treated promptly even though the injury which causes it may not itself be enough to cause death.*

Shock is easy to recognize. The skin gets pale and clammy, with small drops of sweat particularly around the lips and forehead. The person may complain of nausea and dizziness. His pulse may be fast and weak and his breathing shallow and irregular. His eyes may be dull with enlarged pupils, or he may be unconscious. A person may not be aware of the seriousness of his injury, then suddely collapse.

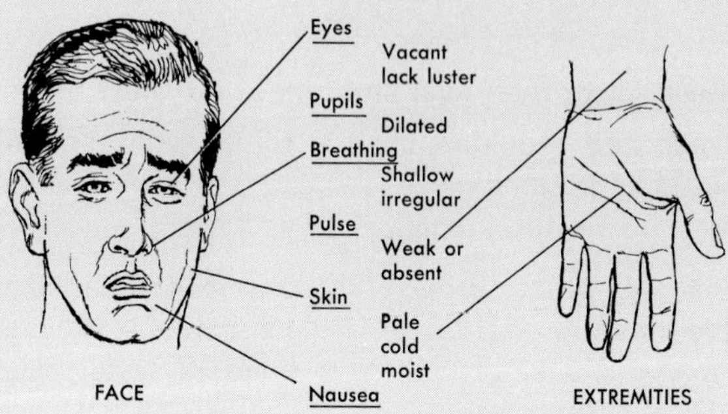

All seriously injured persons should be treated for shock even though all of these symptoms have not appeared and the person seems normal and alert. Treatment for shock may prevent its development.

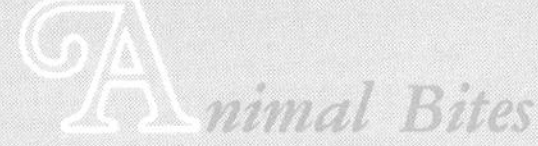

Animal Bites

What to Do

1. Wash the wound thoroughly with soap and water.
2. Catch the animal and confine for 14 days (if practical).

Animal bites (those made by dogs and cats are most common) always involve the danger of infection since there are many germs on an animal's teeth and in its mouth, but in addition such bites may carry the greater risk of rabies, sometimes called hydrophobia. The virus or germ of this disease is present in the saliva of rabid animals. Rabies can attack humans as well as animals. Rabies is usually a fatal disease once it has developed; however, the incubation period is such that if the animal can be confined and watched for a period of 14 days and it is determined that the animal was rabid, the Pasteur treatment may be given to the person who has been bitten. This treatment consists of a series of injections usually given one a day for 14 days. The incubation period is rarely less than 15 days. If it is suspected that the person may have been bitten by a rabid animal, this person should commence rabies immunization after being seen by a physician.

It is unlikely that adequate laboratory facilities will be available to determine whether or not the animal was rabid; however, if the animal has been confined and has not died in 14 days the chances are excellent that it was not rabid. If it is rabid, it will, after several days, show what are called "furious" symptoms. Shortly thereafter the animal becomes paralyzed and dies.

Scratches caused by animals with other than their teeth should be washed thoroughly with soap and water and then treated as any other injury.

Blisters

What to Do

1. Wash blister area clean.
2. Sterilize a needle.
3. Open blister from edge.
4. Gently squeeze out fluid and cover with dressing.
5. Keep it clean.

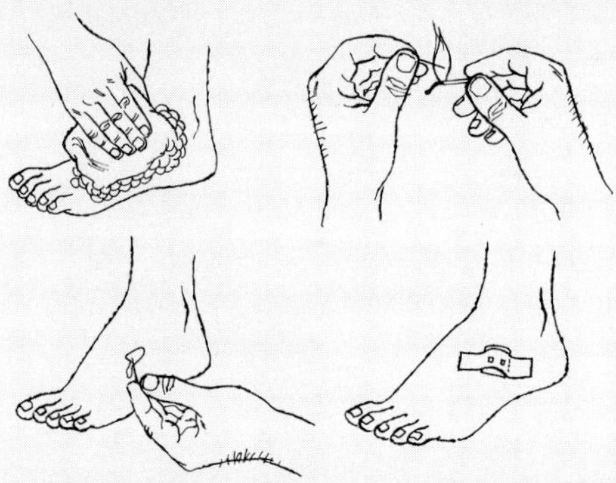

Blisters not caused by burns may result on the skin when it has been subjected to repeated pressures and excessive rubbing. They are not uncommon on the feet from poorly fitting stockings or shoes, or on the hands from using unfamiliar equipment or doing unaccustomed work. They should be cared for to prevent serious infection from developing.

Do not attempt to remove the dead skin which formed the blister. Let it stay on as long as possible to provide protection to the tender underlying tissue and assist in the prevention of infection.

Convulsions

What to Do

1. Keep the person from hurting himself.
2. Give mouth-to-mouth or mouth-to-nose resuscitation if breathing stops.

What Not to Do

DO NOT attempt to restrain the person having the attack, except to prevent his injuring himself. No matter what the cause of the convulsion, little can be done to shorten the attack. *The most important thing is to prevent the person from hurting himself.*

If he has fallen to the floor, move objects that he might strike. Put a pillow or some rolled clothing under his head. If his teeth are clenched don't try to pry them loose. A blanket wrapped loosely around his legs will tend to control their thrashing about. If due to epilepsy, the convulsion will soon end. When it does, the person will be sleepy and should be allowed to sleep as long as he wishes. He may be very irritable and have no memory of the convulsion.

In a child or infant, convulsions may occur with high fever. It is recommended that medical help be sought immediately if repeated convulsions occur.

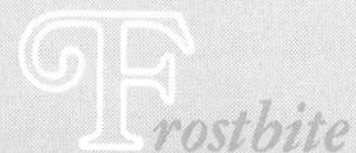

What to Do

1. Rapidly thaw frostbitten part of body.
   a. Place affected part next to warm part of your body or warm part of somebody else's body, or
   b. Place frostbitten part of body in lukewarm water (102° to 105° F.).
   c. Cover affected area with scarves, clothing, blankets, or other material.
2. Give hot coffee or hot tea.
3. Handle affected part with great care and gentleness.

What Not to Do

1. DO NOT rub the affected part.
2. DO NOT use *hot water.*
3. DO NOT use hot water bottle or heat lamps.
4. DO NOT disturb blisters if they develop.
5. DO NOT *rub with ice or snow.*

Exposure to dry cold causes the local injury known as frostbite. Parts of the body most likely to be frostbitten are the cheeks, nose, chin, ears, forehead, wrists, hands, and feet. Most cases of frostbite are caused by exposure to air below freezing temperatures.

The symptoms of frostbite vary depending on the severity of the injury. The frostbitten part is usually not painful, but is numb and stiff. The skin is first white or grayish white in color and then it becomes bright pink. If the exposure to cold continues the skin becomes white again.

When the frostbitten area is warmed it immediately becomes red and swollen and large blisters may develop. Severe frostbite causes the condition known as gangrene in which soft body tissue and sometimes even a bone are permanently destroyed. In the course of healing, a gangrenous tissue is slipped off and leaves healthy tissue underneath, but if deep tissue has been destroyed, the injured part may require amputation.

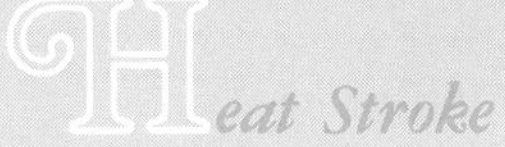

Heat Stroke. This is a serious condition. In contrast to heat exhaustion and heat cramps, a patient with heat stroke usually has a high fever (105 or higher), and no evident perspiration. His skin is hot and dry.

Symptoms include headache, dizziness, irritability, and seeing objects through a red or purplish haze. The patient may suddenly become unconscious, the pulse is full and strong, breathing is noisy like snoring, and there may be convulsions.

What to Do

1. Undress the person and put him to bed in the coolest available area.
2. Sponge body freely with water or alcohol to reduce his temperature to 102°F.
3. Cold packs may be applied or the victim may be placed in a tub of cold water. Do not chill the victim once the temperature is lowered to 102°F. Dry him off and keep him cool with fans or air conditioning.
4. *Do not* give stimulants such as coffee or tea.

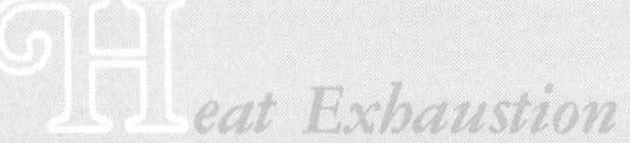

Heat Exhaustion

Heat Exhaustion.—This condition may be mild or severe. In mild cases, the patient usually feels tired and may experience headache and nausea. In severe cases, perspiration is profuse, weakness extreme, and the skin is pale and clammy. *The temperature is usually normal or subnormal.* Vomiting may occur. Unconsciousness is rare, but often the patient will be unable to stand. Painful cramps in leg, or arm muscles may begin suddenly and continue for as long as 24 hours.

What to Do

1. Put the victim to bed or lay him down in a cool place.
2. Give him cool salted water to drink (1 teaspoonful of salt per glass) over a period of one hour.
3. Apply cool wet cloths and fan the victim.

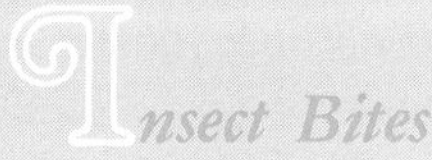

Insect Bites

What to Do

Bees, Wasps, Hornets

1. Remove the stinger.
2. Apply paste of baking soda or soothing lotion like calamine.
3. Apply ice to the site of the sting.

Scorpions

1. Apply constricting band above the sting on the side toward the heart. *Caution:* Band should be loose enough to allow finger to slide under it.
2. Apply ice pack if available; otherwise, cold wet cloths.
3. Keep affected arm or leg *lower* than rest of body for about 2 hours.

Spiders (Black Widows and Brown Recluse)

1. Keep person quiet.
2. Elevate hips and legs in shock position.
3. Apply hot packs if abdominal cramps develop.

Ticks

1. Cover the tick with heavy oil. If the tick does not withdraw immediately, allow the oil to remain a half hour.
2. Then carefully remove the tick with tweezers being sure all parts are removed.
3. Thoroughly scrub the area with soap and water.

Severe Reactions to Insect Stings

Occasionally there will be a severe reaction to an insect bite from a victim with a history of allergic reactions. Persons with this kind of history should be taken to the nearest hospital immediately. Nausea, vomiting, shock, difficulty in breathing, convulsions, or coma may manifest themselves.

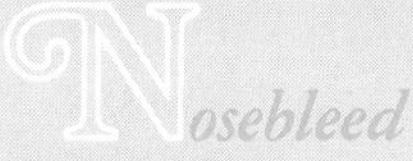

Nosebleed

What to Do

1. Place person in sitting position, leaning forward if possible.
2. Gently grasp the lower end of the nose between the thumb and index finger, firmly press the sides of the nose against the center for 5 minutes.
3. Release pressure gradually.
4. Apply cold cloths to back of neck or over nose.

Note: If bleeding persists, plug the bleeding nostrils with small strip of gauze rolled up loosely. Leave part of roll sticking out of nose so it can be easily removed later.

Nosebleeds occur both spontaneously and as a result of injury. There may be an underlying disease, such as high blood pressure, but in many cases there is no disease. Some people, particularly young people, develop nosebleed following strenuous activity, colds, or exposure to high altitude. The bleeding is usually more annoying than serious. Occasionally, where disease is involved there may be sufficient bleeding to be dangerous.

Anyone with a nosebleed should remain quiet. A sitting position, or a lying position with head and shoulders raised, is best. Walking about, talking, laughing, or blowing the nose may cause increased bleeding or start bleeding again after it has stopped.

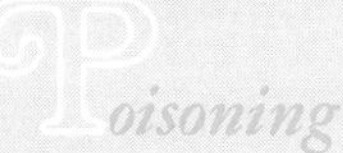

What to Do

1. First aid must be given immediately, minutes count. The general aim is to dilute and neutralize the poison. Give the victim a glass of water or milk (either or both).
2. In strong acid (e.g., toilet bowl cleaner), strong alkali (e.g., drain cleaner) or petroleum product (e.g., kerosene, gasoline, furniture polish) poisoning, dilute and neutralize, *but do not induce vomiting.*
3. Vomiting should be induced only if the person is conscious and you know the type of poison used is noncorrosive. Vomiting may be induced by touching the back of the throat with the fingers or handle of a spoon. The patient should be placed face down with his head lower than his hips to prevent the matter vomited from entering his lungs and causing further damage.
4. If you can find the package from which the poison came, its antidote may be given on the label. If available without delay, use the antidote as directed or bring the container with you to the hospital.
5. If the poison was a sedative, keep him awake by talking to him and encourage him to walk about. Give him several cups of black coffee every 2 hours.
6. Respiration must be maintained if breathing has stopped.

Special Procedures for Special Poisons

Acids. Dilute quickly with a glass of water and then give milk of magnesia, or if it is not available, baking soda solution, to neutralize the acid. Several glassfuls may be given *but do not give enough to cause vomiting.* Then give milk, olive oil, or egg white to protect the digestive tract lining.

Alkalies. Give a glass of water quickly, then vinegar or lemon juice in the diluting fluid to neutralize the alkali. Follow with milk, olive oil, or egg white. *Do not cause vomiting.* The only reason for giving plain water first is that it is quickly available.

Kerosene Poisoning. Give a half cup of mineral oil, if available, to protect the digestive tract lining, and use strong coffee or tea as a stimulant. *Do not cause vomiting.* Keep the patient warm and combat shock. Be prepared to use artificial respiration if the patient stops breathing.

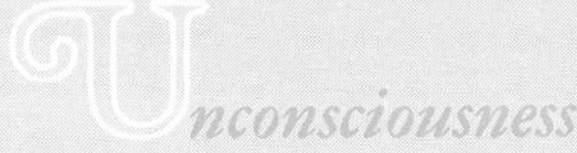

Unconsciousness

What to Do

(When Person Is Flushed—Red Faced—With Strong Slow Pulse)

1. Lay person down with head *slightly raised* above level of rest of body.
2. Apply cold wet cloth to head.
3. If breathing stops start artificial respiration.

(When Person Is Pale—Cold—Clammy to Touch—With Weak Pulse)

1. Lay person down with head *slightly lower* than rest of body.
2. Keep him warm.
3. If available hold aromatic spirit of ammonia under nose (except where head injury is suspected).
4. If breathing stops start artificial respiration.

(When Person Has Bluish-Face, Weak Pulse, Irregular Breathing)

1. Lay person down.
2. Keep him warm.
3. Start artificial respiration immediately if breathing stops.

What Not to Do

1. DO NOT give stimulant.
2. DO NOT give food or drink.
3. DO NOT move (except to remove from danger).

Unconsciousness may occur in such conditions as fainting, apoplexy (sometimes called a stroke), shock, and diabetes. (See treatment of shock, and discussion of diabetes.)

Simple fainting occurs when not enough blood reaches the brain. This may be due to hunger, fatigue, emotional distress, or severe injury.

Warnings of faintness are blurring of the vision, weakness, paleness, and giddiness. If you should have these symptoms, lie down immediately if possible. If not, sit or kneel and bend forward at the waist, putting your head down to get it lower than your heart.

Apoplexy (or stroke) should be suspected whenever an elderly person faints. Apoplexy is caused by interference with the blood supply to the brain. It may occur when a blood vessel in the brain bursts or becomes blocked.

Sometimes a person with apoplexy will collapse but not completely lose consciousness. His face may become red and congested. One side of his body or parts of one side may become paralyzed. His speech may be affected, blurred, and stumbly. He may have difficulty swallowing.

Index